Pharmacy Education

What Matters in Learning and Teaching

Edited by

Lynne M. Sylvia, PharmD

Senior Clinical Pharmacy Specialist
Department of Pharmacy
Tufts Medical Center
Boston, Massachusetts

Adjunct Clinical Professor
School of Pharmacy
Northeastern University
Boston, Massachusetts

Judith T. Barr, ScD, MEd

Associate Professor
Director, National Education and Research
Center for Outcomes Assessment
School of Pharmacy
Northeastern University
Boston, Massachusetts

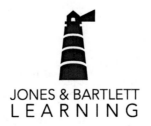

JONES & BARTLETT
LEARNING

World Headquarters
Jones & Bartlett Learning
40 Tall Pine Drive
Sudbury, MA 01776
978-443-5000
info@jblearning.com
www.jblearning.com

Jones & Bartlett Learning Canada
6339 Ormindale Way
Mississauga, Ontario L5V 1J2
Canada

Jones & Bartlett Learning International
Barb House, Barb Mews
London W6 7PA
United Kingdom

Jones & Bartlett Learning books and products are available through most bookstores and online booksellers. To contact Jones & Bartlett Learning directly, call 800-832-0034, fax 978-443-8000, or visit our website, www.jblearning.com.

Substantial discounts on bulk quantities of Jones & Bartlett Learning publications are available to corporations, professional associations, and other qualified organizations. For details and specific discount information, contact the special sales department at Jones & Bartlett Learning via the above contact information or send an email to specialsales@jblearning.com.

The authors, editor, and publisher have made every effort to provide accurate information. However, they are not responsible for errors, omissions, or for any outcomes related to the use of the contents of this book and take no responsibility for the use of the products and procedures described. Treatments and side effects described in this book may not be applicable to all people; likewise, some people may require a dose or experience a side effect that is not described herein. Drugs and medical devices are discussed that may have limited availability controlled by the Food and Drug Administration (FDA) for use only in a research study or clinical trial. Research, clinical practice, and government regulations often change the accepted standard in this field. When consideration is being given to use of any drug in the clinical setting, the health care provider or reader is responsible for determining FDA status of the drug, reading the package insert, and reviewing prescribing information for the most up-to-date recommendations on dose, precautions, and contraindications, and determining the appropriate usage for the product. This is especially important in the case of drugs that are new or seldom used.

Production Credits
Publisher: David Cella
Acquisitions Editor: Katey Birtcher
Associate Editor: Maro Gartside
Editorial Assistant: Teresa Reilly
Senior Production Editor: Renée Sekerak
Associate Production Editor: Jill Morton
Marketing Manager: Grace Richards
Manufacturing and Inventory Control Supervisor: Amy Bacus
Composition: Glyph International
Cover Design: Kristin E. Parker
Cover Image: Courtesy of Kristin E. Parker
Printing and Binding: Malloy Incorporated
Cover Printing: Malloy Incorporated

Library of Congress Cataloging-in-Publication Data
Pharmacy education : what matters in learning and teaching / edited by Lynne
M. Sylvia, Judith T. Barr.
    p. ; cm.
  Includes bibliographical references and index.
  ISBN-13: 978-0-7637-7397-7
  ISBN-10: 0-7637-7397-2
  1. Pharmacy—Study and teaching. I. Sylvia, Lynne M. II. Barr, Judith T.
  [DNLM: 1. Education, Pharmacy. 2. Learning. 3. Teaching—methods. QV
18 P5364 2011]
  RS101.P43 2011
  615'.1071—dc22

                                                2010013262

6048

Printed in the United States of America
14 13 12 11 10   10 9 8 7 6 5 4 3 2 1

Contents

Preface xi

About the Authors xv

Contributors xvii

SECTION I   EVIDENCE MATTERS 1

Chapter 1   **What Matters in Plotting Your Journey to
            Effective Teaching and Learning?** 3
            Lynne M. Sylvia, PharmD
            Introduction 3
            What Matters in Teaching and Learning? 4
            What Are the Characteristics
                of an Effective Teacher? 9
            Plotting Your Journey: Post-Chapter Exercise 19
            References 22

Chapter 2   **What Matters in a Student-Centered
            Approach?** 25
            Laura L. Harris, PhD, ATC, LAT
            Jill Clutter, PhD, CHES
            Introduction 25
            What Are the Types or Domains of Learning? 27
            How Do We Learn? 33
            What Are Learning Styles? 38
            How Does One's Generation Influence
                Learning? 44
            Integrated Model 46
            Closing Thoughts 50
            Scenarios 50
            Additional Considerations and Resources 51
            References 52
            Appendix 2–1 Pharmacists' Inventory
                of Learning Styles 54

Chapter 3   **What Matters in a Systems Approach to
Learning and Teaching?** 57
Judith T. Barr, ScD, MEd
Introduction 57
What Is a System, Systems Thinking, and
a Systems Approach? 58
What Matters in the Systems Approach
to Education? 60
What Matters in Applying the Systems
Approach to Pharmacy Education? The Four
Pharmacy Education Scenarios 61
Summary 80
References 80
Additional Resources 82

Chapter 4   **What Matters in Assessment?** 85
Katherine A. Kelley, PhD
Introduction 85
What Are the Terms and Concepts Associated
with Assessment? 87
What Techniques and Tools Are
Used in Assessment? 91
How Do I Use Assessment Information to
Improve My Teaching, My Courses, and
the Curriculum? 98
References 101

SECTION II   **WHAT MATTERS IN LEARNING AND
TEACHING SETTINGS?** 103

Chapter 5   **What Matters in Large Classroom Teaching?** . . . 105
Judith T. Barr, ScD, MEd
Introduction 105
What Matters in the Traditional Passive
Lecture? What Are Some Suggestions
for Beginning to Move into
Active Learning? 106
The Transformation from Teaching
to Learning 111
What Matters in Increasing Active Learning
Experiences: Getting Ready for Inclusion
of Active Learning Activities in
Your Large Class 116

Active Learning in Action in Large Classes:
   Pedagogies of Engagement 118
Lessons from Undergraduate Physics
   Education Reform Efforts 126
Be Prepared for Student Push Back 127
One Last Consideration 128
References 129
Additional Resources 132

**Chapter 6   What Matters in Applying Technology to
            Teaching, Learning, and Assessment?** **133**
Evan T. Robinson, RPh, PhD
Introduction 133
What Is the Role of Educational
   Technology? 135
What Are the Considerations to Implementing
   Technology Initiatives? 137
Why Consider Applying Technologic
   Innovations? 141
Summary 150
References 150

**Chapter 7   What Matters in Facilitation of
            a Small Group or Seminar?** **153**
Zubin Austin, PhD, MBA, MIS, BSPharm
Introduction 153
What Is Small-Group Teaching
   and Learning? 154
What Is My Job? The Role of Facilitator in
   Small-Group Teaching and Learning 155
How Do I Get Things Started with Small-Group
   Teaching and Learning? 158
What Is Their Job? The Role of Learners in
   Small-Group Teaching and Learning 159
How Do We Work Together as Facilitators and
   Learners in Small-Group Collaboration? 163
What Matters in Assessment of
   Small-Group Learning? 166
How Do We Put It All Together?
   Pearls for Educators 167
Summary 172
References 173

Chapter 8   **What Matters in Laboratory Learning
and Teaching?** 175
Jennifer Kirwin, PharmD, BCPS
Jenny A. Van Amburgh, BSPharm, PharmD, CDE
Introduction: Why a Chapter About
Laboratory Teaching? 175
Why Include a Laboratory Course? 176
What Matters About Learning in
the Laboratory? 177
What Matters in the Design of
a Laboratory Course? The Foundational
Principles of Laboratory Experiences 178
As the Laboratory Coordinator, What
Operational Issues Need to Be Considered? 185
Who Will Maintain and Service Laboratory
Supplies and Equipment? 186
What Matters with Applications
to Pharmaceutical Science Laboratories? 189
What Matters About Continuous Quality
Improvements and Feedback? 191
What Will Matter in the Future? 192
Summary 192
Acknowledgment 193
References 193
Appendix 8–1 Your Course Mapping Process 196

Chapter 9   **What Matters in Experiential Education?** 197
Lynne M. Sylvia, PharmD
Introduction 197
What Is Experiential Education? 198
What Matters in Learning in Experiential
Education? 199
What Matters in the Design of Experiential
Education? 203
What Matters in the Role of the Preceptor? 209
What Matters in Teaching Strategies
That Promote Learning in Experiential
Education? 212
What Matters in Assessment? 217
What Matters in Providing Feedback? 220
Summary 222
References 222
Appendix 9–1 Mapping Exercise 224

SECTION III   **WHAT MATTERS IN DEALING**
                     WITH STUDENTS? **225**

Chapter 10   **What Matters in Developing Professionals**
                     and Professionalism? **227**
                     Dana P. Hammer, RPh, MS, PhD
                     Introduction 227
                     Why Professionalism Matters 228
                     What Is Professionalism? 229
                     How Does Professionalism Relate to Teaching,
                     Learning, and Assessment? 231
                     What Works with Regard to Developing
                     Professionalism in Students? 233
                     What Works with Regard to Assessing
                     Professionalism? 242
                     What Should You Do When Unprofessional
                     Behavior Occurs? 244
                     Summary 246
                     References 246

Chapter 11   **What Matters in Advising and Mentoring**
                     Students? **251**
                     Lisa A. Lawson, PharmD
                     Eric G. Boyce, PharmD
                     Introduction 251
                     What Is the Difference Between Advising
                     and Mentoring? 251
                     Student Advisement: General Philosophy
                     and Goals 252
                     What Are the Roles and Responsibilities
                     of a Faculty Advisor? 254
                     What Types of Student Advising Might
                     I Provide? 255
                     What Are the Legal Aspects of Advising? 260
                     What Are the Benefits of Advising? 261
                     What Are the Pitfalls of Advising? 261
                     How Do I Assess and Document
                     My Advising Activities? 262
                     What Resources Are Available to
                     Learn More About Advising? 262
                     Student Mentoring: General Philosophy
                     and Goals 263
                     What Are the Roles and Responsibilities
                     of a Mentor? 264

What Are the Attributes of a
   Successful Mentor? 265
How Do I Get Started as a Mentor? 266
What Are the Essential Components
   of a Student Mentoring Program? 266
What Types of Mentoring Might I Provide? 266
What Are the Benefits of Mentoring? 268
What Are the Pitfalls of Mentoring? 268
How Do I Assess and Document My Mentoring
   Activities? 268
Summary 269
References 269

SECTION IV   WHAT MATTERS IN FACULTY ADVANCEMENT? 271

Chapter 12   What Matters in Faculty Development? 273
Eric G. Boyce, PharmD
Introduction 273
What Is Faculty Development? 274
What Is the General Philosophy and Approach
   to Faculty Development? 274
Who Is Responsible for Faculty
   Development? 275
What Are the Components of a Faculty
   Development Program? 276
What Opportunities Are Available for
   Development in Specific Areas? 281
Faculty Development in Service
   and Administration 285
How Should I Document My
   Development? 286
How Is Development Assessed and
   Evaluated? 287
Summary 287
References 289

Chapter 13   What Matters in Faculty Service? 291
John R. Reynolds, PharmD
Introduction 291
What Is Service? 292
How Are People Organized to Accomplish
   Service? 296
What Are the Motivations to Serve? 297

How Should You Respond to a
Call for Service? 299
How Can You Balance Service Commitments
with Other Commitments? 301
General Recommendations and Guidelines
on How to Approach Service 302
Summary 305
References 305

Chapter 14   **What Matters in the Scholarship
of Teaching and Learning?** 307
Donna M. Qualters, PhD
Judith T. Barr, ScD, MEd
Introduction 307
What Is the Scholarship of Teaching
and Learning (SoTL)? 308
What Is the Difference Between Scholarly
Teaching and SoTL? 308
Why Is SoTL Important Today? 310
How Can I Do SoTL? 310
What Are Other Ethical Considerations
in SoTL? 322
Summary 323
References 323
Additional Resources 324

Index **325**

Preface

Where did it all start . . . this teaching and learning thing? When Socrates taught from his porch? When the discoverer of fire taught the technique to another caveman? When God instructed Adam and Eve not to eat the apple?

Well, whenever it started, in writing this book we recognize that we are standing on the shoulders of giants. Our premise is that the ultimate goal of a teacher is not teaching, but rather the facilitation of student learning. Socrates encouraged students to find their own truth and knowledge through questioning and debate (a form of active learning). John Dewey said that "Learning is doing,"[1] and Chickering and Gamson included student engagement in their 1987 "Seven Principles of Good Practice in Undergraduate Education."[2] These pioneers have encouraged us to center our teaching on the learner and on our subject, rather than on ourselves as teachers. However, most contemporary faculty agree that the seismic shift from an emphasis on teaching to a focus on student learning can be traced to the essay "From Teaching to Learning—a New Paradigm for Undergraduate Education" by Robert Barr (no relation to one of the present authors) and John Tagg. We quote from this classic 1995 article in *Change* magazine: "In its briefest form, the paradigm that has governed our colleges is this: A college is an institution that exists *to provide instruction*. Subtly but profoundly we are shifting to a new paradigm: A college is an institution that exists *to produce learning*."[3]

Now, 15 years later, within our institutions we have teaching and learning centers, divisions of education technology, and other resources to help faculty adopt the learning-centered philosophy. Neuroscientists are showing with functional magnetic resonance imaging studies that active learning is deeper learning. Accreditation bodies in education call for active learning in classrooms, and commercial electronic companies provide clickers to engage students in course-embedded electronic responses to assess learning in real time. The movement toward learner-centered teaching and student engagement is supported by evidence of higher rates of retention and application of knowledge. The answer is clear, but the question is whether we are prepared to meet this call for a shift from transmission of knowledge to the facilitation of learning. This book was written with this intent in mind: to help you, both new and experienced faculty, plan and execute educational activities within a learner-centered environment, particularly in schools of pharmacy.

In this book we will guide you in a journey to learner-centered teaching with the understanding that each of you have different experiences and backgrounds in pharmacy education. The workbook style of this text, with integration of reflective exercises and self-diagnostic questions, will allow you to customize the presented material to your current situation as a prospective, new, or experienced faculty member. Our muse in this journey is Parker Palmer, and our compass is his inspirational text *The Courage to Teach*,[4] which recently celebrated its 10th year in print.

Palmer reminds us that the road to effective teaching and student learning starts with an exploration of our inner landscape. As such, your journey will begin with a discussion of the teacher within. In Chapter 1, you will be challenged to examine your current teaching philosophy and role as a teacher. What do you currently believe constitutes good teaching and the promotion of learning, and how does your person, or the way you identify with the world, influence the way you teach? In subsequent chapters in the first section of this text (Chapters 1 through 4), a foundation will be laid for the application of learner-centered teaching. Chapter 2 will offer an understanding of the learner, the most important member of our teaching and learning community. This chapter addresses how a student's preferred learning style and generational characteristics influence learning and how knowledge, skills, behaviors, and reflective thinking are developed and nurtured using a learner-centered approach to education. Chapter 3 delves into the systems approach and all of the inputs and processes that need to be considered when planning a lecture, coordinating a course, or participating in the revision of a pharmacy curriculum. Using systems thinking, you will be able to identify how the content that you teach interrelates and connects with the course in which you are teaching, the curriculum in total, and the longitudinal development of your students. In the last chapter of this section, the focus is on assessment. With a clear understanding of the learner, your role as teacher, and the systems approach, how will you measure whether you have met the goal of student learning? Chapter 4 will provide an assessment toolbox that can be used in the various settings of pharmacy teaching and learning.

Section II of this text is devoted to the environment of teaching and learning. In this section, you will explore the large classroom, the clinical site, the laboratory, and the small classroom as environments of teaching and learning. What are the inherent challenges to both teaching and student learning in these environments? Which teaching strategies have been shown to be most effective in *facilitating* learning, and which assessment techniques are best suited to *measure* learning in these settings? How can technological advances, ranging in complexity from PowerPoint slides to virtual reality, enhance your teaching and promote student learning? Each of these questions will be posed to deepen your self-discovery of what matters in teaching, learning, and assessment.

Section III focuses on your role as a faculty member, advisor, and mentor in the professional maturation of the pharmacy student. In his essay "On Professionalism," Michael Lacombe, MD, advises us to "Teach professionalism. Gently. Make the student proud of themselves, have them respect each other, and teach them to respect the patient."[5] Chapter 10 provides recommendations on how to enact these words and nurture student professionalism in and out of the classroom. Beyond your role as a faculty member and model of professional behavior, you also influence the professional growth of your students through your roles as an academic advisor and mentor. How can you optimize these roles? Using a case-based approach, Chapter 11 outlines the responsibilities and potential pitfalls of each position and addresses the legal issues that are specific to advising and mentoring.

The last section of this text focuses on you, the faculty member, and your professional development. This section begins with a global view of the faculty development process. Chapter 12 outlines the opportunities for your development in teaching, service, and scholarship and how to maximize them, from the initial stages of your academic career through the tenure and promotion process and beyond. Of the three primary components of faculty contribution, service has been referred to as being victim to the middle-child syndrome, suffering in attention and appreciation.[6] Chapter 13 focuses on your role in service, how to develop a service plan, and how to balance service contributions to the university, the college or school of pharmacy, your profession, and your clinical practice, if applicable. Finally, in Chapter 14, the topic of discussion is the scholarship of teaching and learning. In this chapter you are asked to challenge your understanding of scholarship as it relates to your teaching and your students' learning. You will be guided in the development of an individualized plan for the study of your teaching and learning strategies with the ultimate goal of sharing your findings with the greater community of scholars.

As you follow our lead through this journey in *Pharmacy Education: What Matters in Learning and Teaching*, we encourage you to embrace the workbook style of the text. Opportunities have been provided in each chapter for goal setting, self-diagnosis and rediagnosis of learning needs, and reflection. The value of reflection cannot be overstated. It allows for "future behaviors to be guided by a systematic and critical analysis of past actions and their consequences."[7] So before you adopt any of the practices or strategies recommended in this text, it is important for you to reflect on your past and current practices in teaching, learning, and assessment. Where are you in this journey to effective teaching and facilitation of learning? What strategies and practices will fit your person, and what can you learn from your past experiences in teaching and learning? After you have implemented some changes in teaching and learning strategies, reflect on the following questions: What worked? What didn't work? And if you could do it again, what would you change?

Our goal in *Pharmacy Education: What Matters in Learning and Teaching* is to empower you along this journey to examine your teaching with the goal of facilitating and promoting student learning. As such, we are guided by Parker Palmer's words from *The Courage to Teach*: "I have no question that students who learn, not professors who perform, is what teaching is all about. Students who learn are the finest fruit of teachers who teach."[4]

Bon voyage!

References

1. Dewey J. *The School and Society.* New York, NY: Phoenix Books; 1956.
2. Chickering AW, Gamson ZF. *Applying the Seven Principles for Good Practice in Undergraduate Education.* San Francisco, CA: Jossey-Bass; 1991. A summary of these principles appeared as an article, "Seven Principles for Good Practice in Undergraduate Education," in the *American Association for Higher Education Bulletin* (1987;39:3–7). http://honolulu.hawaii.edu/intranet/committees/FacDevCom/guidebk/teachtip/7princip.htm. Accessed December 28, 2009.
3. Barr RB, Tagg J. From teaching to learning—a new paradigm for undergraduate education. *Change.* November–December 1995:13–25. http://ilte.ius.edu/pdf/BarrTagg.pdf. Accessed December 28, 2009.
4. Palmer PJ. *The Courage to Teach: Exploring the Inner Landscape of a Teacher's Life.* San Francisco, CA: John Wiley and Sons; 1998.
5. Lacombe ML. On professionalism. *Am J Med.* 1993;94:329.
6. Brazeau GA. Revisiting faculty service role—is "faculty service" a victim of the middle-child syndrome? *Amer J Pharm Ed.* 2003:67(3):article 85.
7. Driessen E, van Tartwijk J, Dornan T. Teaching rounds: the self-critical doctor: helping students become more reflective. *BMJ.* 2008;336:827–830.

About the Authors

Lynne M. Sylvia, PharmD, is a senior clinical pharmacy specialist in the Department of Pharmacy at Tufts Medical Center, Boston, Massachusetts. She also holds the position of adjunct clinical professor at Northeastern University, School of Pharmacy, also in Boston. Lynne coordinates a 12-week advanced pharmacy practice experience at the medical center for pharmacy students in their fourth professional year, she serves as a pharmacy residency preceptor, and she contributes to direct patient care in the areas of drug allergy, cardiology, and drug-induced diseases. She has been a pharmacy practitioner–educator for the past 30 years; for more than 20 years, she was a full-time pharmacy faculty member in both tenure- and nontenure-track positions. For the past eight years, she has facilitated the Residents Teaching Seminar, an annual seminar series offered to all pharmacy residents in Massachusetts. She is a member of the editorial boards of *Pharmacotherapy* and the *Annals of Pharmacotherapy*. Lynne earned her bachelor of science in pharmacy from the Massachusetts College of Pharmacy and Health Sciences in 1980 and her doctor of pharmacy from Duquesne University School of Pharmacy in 1983. She completed a residency in clinical pharmacy at the Rhode Island Hospital and a residency in hospital pharmacy at Mercy Hospital of Pittsburgh.

Judith T. Barr, ScD, MEd, is an associate professor and director of the National Education and Research Center for Outcomes Assessment in Healthcare at the School of Pharmacy, Northeastern University, Boston. She received her bachelor of science degree from Simmons College, her masters in education from University of Massachusetts–Boston, and her doctorate in health policy and evaluation from the Harvard School of Public Health. Judy has extensive experience in healthcare professional education. Within the School of Pharmacy she has taught large classes such as pharmacoeconomics, healthcare systems, and research methodology as well as designed and taught healthcare professional education courses for graduate and undergraduate students in the health professions. She has also precepted advanced practice pharmacy students in campus-based education experiences and chaired the curriculum and assessment committees. All of her courses extensively involve in-class active learning activities and group project assignments. In addition to educational research and scholarship, she conducts patient-centered outcomes research. She has written more than 75 journal articles, monographs, chapters, and other publications.

Contributors

Zubin Austin, PhD, MBA, MIS, BSPharm

Associate Dean, Academic Associate Professor

OCP Professor in Pharmacy Practice Research

Leslie Dan Faculty of Pharmacy

University of Toronto, Canada

Eric G. Boyce, PharmD

Associate Dean for Academic Affairs

Professor of Pharmacy Practice

Thomas J. Long School of Pharmacy and Health Sciences

University of the Pacific

Stockton, California

Jill Clutter, PhD, CHES

Assistant Professor

School of Allied Medical Professions

The Ohio State University

Columbus, Ohio

Dana P. Hammer, RPh, MS, PhD

Director

Bracken Pharmaceutical Care Learning Center

Teaching Certificate in Pharmacy Education

University of Washington School of Pharmacy

Seattle, Washington

Laura L. Harris, PhD, ATC, LAT

Director of Athletic Training Clinical Education

School of Allied Medical Professions

The Ohio State University

Columbus, Ohio

Katherine A. Kelley, PhD

Assistant Dean for Assessment

Clinical Assistant Professor

College of Pharmacy

The Ohio State University

Columbus, Ohio

Jennifer Kirwin, PharmD, BCPS

Associate Clinical Professor

School of Pharmacy

Bouvé College of Health Sciences

Northeastern University

Boston, Massachusetts

Lisa A. Lawson, PharmD

Philadelphia College of Pharmacy

Dean, Barbara H. Korberly Professor in Women's Leadership and Health

University of the Sciences in Philadelphia

Philadelphia, Pennsylvania

Donna M. Qualters, PhD

Director and Associate Professor

Center for Teaching Excellence

Suffolk University

Boston, Massachusetts

John R. Reynolds, PharmD

Dean and Professor

School of Pharmacy

Bouvé College of Health Sciences

Northeastern University

Boston, Massachusetts

Evan T. Robinson, RPh, PhD

Professor and Dean

School of Pharmacy

Western New England College

Springfield, Massachusetts

Jenny A. Van Amburgh, BSPharm, PharmD, CDE

Associate Clinical Professor

School of Pharmacy

Bouvé College of Health Sciences

Northeastern University

Boston, Massachusetts

Evidence Matters

CHAPTER 1

What Matters in Plotting Your Journey to Effective Teaching and Learning?

Lynne M. Sylvia, PharmD

Introduction

You have chosen the path of a teacher. Most likely, you made this decision because you had some positive experiences with teaching as a tutor, teaching assistant, graduate student, or pharmacy resident. You have most likely observed good teachers, those who empower students to self-learn by facilitating lifelong learning skills and a passion for self-discovery. There is also a good chance that one of your teachers made a lasting impression on you, either good or bad, and this impression has influenced your decision to teach. Now that you have chosen the path of a teacher, where do you begin? First, accept that you are embarking on a journey that will include many pleasurable excursions, some rough tracks, and few worthy shortcuts. The metaphor of a journey is often used in teaching, and aptly so. Becoming a good teacher requires purposeful travel. Nothing is gained from adopting another teacher's bag of teaching tricks in an attempt to race to the finish line. Instead, you are more likely to achieve your goal of good teaching by mapping out a journey that includes time for you to self-reflect, to read and think about teaching and learning, to take risks with your teaching, and to actively participate in professional development activities and peer review.

To start your journey to effective teaching, this chapter will attempt to answer some fundamental questions about teaching and learning:

- What is the relationship between teaching and learning?
- What constitutes good teaching?
- How do you find your own passion for teaching and stimulate a passion for learning in your students?

What Matters in Teaching and Learning?

Teaching has historically been described as *what teachers do* and learning as *what students do*; however, teaching and learning do not exist as separate and distinct activities. As explained in this section, there is a unique relationship or interdependence between teaching and learning, and this relationship is influenced by many intellectual, attitudinal, and environmental factors. Most important, learning should be recognized as the primary goal or outcome of your teaching. The facilitation and promotion of learning, rather than the transmission or telling of knowledge, should be at the forefront of all of your actions as a teacher. No assumption should be made that your teaching will lead to student learning. Your ability to facilitate learning will depend on your level of knowledge of the student as a learner, your ability to translate sound educational theory into practice, and your depth of knowledge of your subject matter. In addition, the ability to facilitate learning will require a keen awareness of how you influence both the learning environment and your student's interest and motivation to learn.

Before you set out to travel, it is usually best to know your destination. Using our metaphor that teaching is a journey, we will start by defining learning. As teachers, our final destination is the facilitation of learning, and we achieve this goal through effective teaching.

What Is Learning?

We all know what learning feels like and what it often looks like, but it is far more difficult to define. Some describe it as an *aha moment*, that instant when all things become clear and understandable. Others use phrases such as *something clicked* or *the light has been turned on* to describe a feeling of enlightenment or clarity. Based on these examples, should learning be defined as a process or an outcome? According to *Webster's* dictionary, *learning* is "knowledge or skill acquired through instruction or experience."[1] Using this definition, learning is quantitative, a product or outcome in terms of knowledge or skills that result from a process. But does *knowing a lot* best define learning? Can something as lifeless and sterile as having a lot of knowledge capture the wonder of an aha moment? According to Ramsden, learning "should be seen as a qualitative change in a person's way of seeing, experiencing, understanding, conceptualizing something in the real world—rather than as a quantitative change in the amount of knowledge someone possesses."[2(p271)] Rogers describes learning as "the insatiable curiosity that drives the adolescent boy to absorb everything he can see or hear or read about gasoline engines in order to improve the efficiency and speed of his 'cruiser.'"[3(pp18,19)] The words *self-discovery*, *change*, and *invention* are frequently used by psychologists to describe the transformational aspects of learning. Overall, learning can be defined as a multidimensional, complex, internal process that results in a change or modification in behavior. The depth or nature of the change in behavior will differ depending on the individual and the learning experience. Using the latter definition, learning is both a process and an outcome, and there is a personalized or individualized aspect to it. Rather than a possession, such as a vast amount of knowledge, learning will be viewed as something that you do to better relate to the world around you.

If you appreciate that learning is an internal process, then you must also appreciate that the learner or student must accept some of the responsibility for learning. It has been said that students themselves decide whether to learn or not.[4(p27)] The willingness of a student to accept responsibility for learning is influenced by a number of factors. In Chapter 2, the authors discuss how people learn, and they review the various theories and models of how people process and integrate information. Chapter 2 also focuses on how you can identify your student's learning style and preference for receiving and processing information. *Learning styles* are defined as "characteristic cognitive, affective and psychological behaviors that serve as relatively stable indicators of how learners perceive, interact with and respond to the learning environment."[5] Basically, if you are aware of your student's preferred learning style, you will be more aware of the set of behaviors and expectations that the student will bring to the learning environment. In addition to style of learning, other factors that influence a student's willingness to learn are level of motivation (e.g., need for extrinsic motivators to learn), attitude about teaching and learning, approach to learning (surface, deep, or strategic), response to different learning environments, orientation to studying, and the ability to set goals and self-regulate.[6] All of these factors need to be considered before you can serve as a true partner in your student's learning.

What Is the Relationship Between Teaching and Learning?

Reflective Exercise

The relationship between teaching and learning has been described as linear, cyclical, and bidirectional (as illustrated below and in **Figure 1–1**). Which illustration best represents your vision of the relationship between teaching and learning? Why?

$$\text{Subject} \rightarrow \text{Teaching} \rightarrow \text{Learning} \rightarrow \text{Outcome}^{7}$$

$$\text{Teaching} \leftrightarrow \text{Learning}$$

> We [teachers] can only provide the opportunity, the environment, the encouragement . . . but the learning belongs ultimately with the learner.
>
> D. Schon *Educating the Reflective Practitioner;* 1987

If you subscribe to the theory that learning is largely an outcome measured quantitatively in terms of knowledge or skill, then you will most likely view teaching as the process by which knowledge is imparted, transmitted, or transferred to the student. In this regard, teaching would be synonymous with filling a cup. The subject matter will reside in you, the teacher, and it would be poured or transferred from you (the one who knows) to the student (the empty vessel). Based on this description of teaching, a linear relationship exists between teaching and learning:

$$\text{Subject} \rightarrow \text{Teaching} \rightarrow \text{Learning} \rightarrow \text{Outcome (Grade)}^{7}$$

In this relationship, learning is the dependent variable and teaching is the independent variable. Thus, learning will be largely dependent on the teacher's mastery of the subject matter and his or her ability to effectively

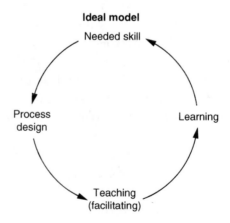

Figure 1–1 Cycle of Teaching and Learning

Source: Courtesy of Nasseh B. Changing definition of teaching and learning. http://www.bsu.edu/classes/nasseh/bn100/change.html. Published 1996.

convey the subject matter. Is learning totally dependent on teaching and the teacher? As discussed in the previous section, the learner is largely responsible for his or her ability to learn. If intrinsically motivated, a learner will learn independent of the teacher. The teaching model conveyed by this linear relationship has been referred to as *teacher-centered teaching* because it focuses on the teacher, the subject matter or content of instruction, and the delivery of content. In this model, the teacher primarily serves as an instructor, content expert, or information giver, and he or she is the sole evaluator as to whether learning has occurred. The content and assignments are predefined by the teacher, and the student primarily assumes a passive role in the learning process. Teacher-centered teaching is based on the concept of objectivism, a quantitative learning process, whereas *learner-centered teaching* focuses on a qualitative learning process. Figure 1–1 depicting a cyclical relationship between teaching and learning, can be used to describe learner-centered teaching.

In Figure 1–1, described by Nasseh,[7] the teaching–learning relationship begins with the identification of a skill that is needed, relevant, and applicable in the real world. Determination of the needed skill is based on input from a variety of sources, including the learner and the teacher. Thus, this cycle of teaching and learning begins with a partnership between the teacher and learner. The second step in the cycle is the design of the teaching–learning process. Note the emphasis in this model on learning as a process rather than solely as an outcome. In this second step, attempts are made by the teacher to identify what students currently know or understand about the subject matter before any additional content is introduced. This step is based on the concept of constructivism, a theory that knowledge is not shared or transmitted but is constructed within each individual. Constructivists believe that learners develop their own mental schema or *scaffolding* from which they construct new knowledge. Basically, previously formulated ideas and knowledge stored in the learner's mental scaffolding are used as raw material for the construction of new knowledge. Constructivism requires a shift in the role of the student from a passive recipient to an active participant in the teaching–learning process. Learners need to be physically and actively engaged in a variety of activities that allow them to question, experiment, and reflect on the course content. To facilitate learning, the teacher's role must also change. Teachers who are committed to learner-centered teaching primarily serve as coaches, guides, and facilitators of student learning, as opposed to instructors.

In Chapter 5, active learning strategies used in learner-centered teaching will be presented. To appreciate the relationship between teaching and learning as described by this model, consider the words of Maryellen Weimer, author of *Learner-Centered Teaching*: "When instruction is learner-centered, the action focuses on what students (not teachers) are doing.

To facilitate learning that changes how students think and understand, teachers must begin by discovering students' existing conceptions and then design instruction that changes those conceptions."[4(pxvi)] In a learner-centered teaching model, the relationship between teaching and learning is represented as a cycle to depict the opportunity for change in the relationship. In this cycle, teaching influences learning; however, what is learned from teaching influences the design of future learning and teaching processes.

A third representation of the relationship between teaching and learning is depicted as follows:

Teaching ↔ Learning

> If he [the teacher] is indeed wise, he does not bid you enter the house of wisdom, but rather leads you to the threshold of your own mind.
>
> Kahlil Gibran

This illustration, in all of its simplicity, supports an interdependence or bidirectional relationship between teaching and learning. In this relationship, teaching influences learning and learning influences teaching. This interdependence can be explained by the Latin proverb, "By learning you will teach, by teaching you will learn."[8] This relationship between teaching and learning appears to be fluid, open to change, and never static. The teacher in this relationship appreciates that he or she is also a learner. What is learned from one's teaching and one's students is fed back into the teaching–learning cycle. This relationship suggests that learning leads to more effective teaching. It also suggests that teaching and learning are equal, connected partners. Based on the extent of the connectedness between teaching and learning in this relationship, teaching would never be viewed as an entity separate from learning.

In summary, teaching and learning are not one and the same. Optimally, they exist in an interdependent, dynamic relationship. Regardless of which educational theory or teaching model you subscribe to, learning must be recognized as the ultimate goal of your teaching.

In this section of Chapter 1, learning was examined as a process and an outcome, both quantitatively and qualitatively. The student was identified as being primarily responsible for his or her own learning. Thus far, the role of the teacher in the teaching–learning process has not been defined. According to Barr and Tagg, "teachers are instructional designers who put together challenging and complex learning experiences and then create environments that empower students to accomplish the goals."[9] Palmer, author of *The Courage to Teach*, describes a teacher as one who *leads out*.[10(p32)] How do you, as the teacher, lead your students out such that they maximize their potential for learning? The next section of this chapter will begin the discussion of the teacher by describing the characteristics of an effective teacher. Chapters 5 through 9 will extend the discussion of effective teaching by exploring how your choice of course content, teaching strategies, learning environment, and assessment technique can influence the student's ability to learn.

> Fact or misconception? Teaching = Learning

What Are the Characteristics of an Effective Teacher?

Reflective Exercise

Sit back and try to recall a teacher from grade school, high school, or college who made a lasting impression on you. This person could have been an athletic coach, religious educator, or any other individual serving in the role of teacher. What was it about this teacher that made him or her effective as a facilitator of learning? List the characteristics of that good teacher.

_____

_____

_____

_____

Everyone has their own story about a teacher who made a difference in their life. Those who are most fortunate can recall more than one teacher who had a lasting, positive influence on them. Looking back, what did that teacher do that made you excited about learning? Also, what was it about their person—who he or she was as an individual—that motivated you to learn?

For the past nine years, I have posed these two questions to a group of 20 to 40 pharmacy residents at the start of our annual seminar series on teaching and learning.[11] Each year, the residents have provided a similar set of characteristics of an effective teacher. The characteristics are as follows:

- Enthusiastic about the subject matter
- Open-minded
- Encouraging
- Knowledgeable about the topic
- Caring
- Confident
- A good listener
- Patient
- Has a good sense of humor
- Treats me as an individual
- Balances between holding my hand and letting me go on my own
- Is an effective communicator
- Takes the time to get to know his or her students
- Is available
- Holds the student accountable
- Is challenging

- Is humble enough to realize that learning can go two ways: from teacher to student and from student to teacher
- Is fair
- Passionate about teaching, the subject matter, and students

Are these the key characteristics of an effective teacher? If so, are any of them more important than others in terms of facilitating learning? A number of surveys and research projects aimed at identifying the characteristics of effective teachers and good teaching have been published. Study methods have varied, yet each study provides some level of evidence as to what constitutes effective teaching. After presenting the evidence from a number of longitudinal, peer-reviewed studies in higher education, you will be asked to reflect on the common themes that emerged from the evidence.

The Evidence

> Education is the kindling of a flame, not the filling of a vessel.
>
> Socrates

In 1987, Chickering and Gamson first described the seven principles for good practice in undergraduate education.[12] Published in the *AAHE Bulletin* (American Association for Higher Education), the seven principles were intended as a guideline for use by faculty, administrators, and students to improve undergraduate teaching and learning. Chickering and Gamson's work, supported by the Lilly Endowment, has led to the development of the Seven Principles Faculty Inventory and Institutional Inventory used by many undergraduate colleges to assess the quality of teaching and learning.[13] Based on 50 years of research on the way teachers teach and students learn, the seven principles focus on the *how* of teaching, not the *what* (the subject matter). The premise of Chickering and Gamson's work is that "undergraduate education should prepare students to understand and deal intelligently with modern life."[12] To do so, adherence with the following principles is advised:

- Encourage contact between students and faculty
- Develop reciprocity and cooperation among students
- Encourage active learning
- Give prompt feedback
- Emphasize time on task
- Communicate high expectations
- Respect diverse talents and ways of learning

Chickering and Gamson stated that each principle, when employed, has a powerful influence on the teacher's ability to facilitate learning. When all are employed, the effects on learning multiply by creating a synergy among diversity, expectations, cooperation, interaction, activity, and responsibility.

Bain, the author of *What the Best College Teachers Do*, observed and interviewed 60 to 70 faculty members from more than two dozen academic institutions to answer the question, What do outstanding teachers do and think that may help us in the quest to tie teaching to learning?[14] Bain defined an *outstanding teacher* as one who had "achieved remarkable success in helping students learn in ways that made a sustained, substantial and positive influence on how those students think, act and feel."[14(p5)] Bain and his colleagues interviewed hundreds of students and solicited nominations from professors throughout the country to identify potential candidates for inclusion in the study. The nature of the evidence supporting the notion that a professor "regularly fostered exceptional learning" varied with the individual candidate and his or her discipline. For example, success in helping students learn could have been determined from student testimony, through direct observation of the teacher by a study group, from examples of student work, or from a combination of these items. After observing and interviewing the study subjects, Bain summarized what outstanding teachers do and think by providing answers to six broad study questions[14(pp15–20)]:

> Teach only when cornered, otherwise let the people learn.
>
> Keith King

1. What do the best teachers know and understand?
2. How do they prepare to teach?
3. What do they expect of their students?
4. What do they do when they teach?
5. How do they treat students?
6. How do they check their progress and evaluate their efforts?

The messages about teaching and learning delivered in *What the Best College Teachers Do* cannot be distilled into a compact 100-word summary. Each of the six questions posed by Bain is addressed in a separate chapter of the text. To fully appreciate the scope and value of this work, the book should be read in its entirety. Outstanding teachers, as Bain describes, know that knowledge is constructed (not received), that teaching by questioning is crucial, and that caring is crucial. They know their subject matter very well, and they create learning environments in which the learners are confronted with important problems related to real-world issues. One of the central messages conveyed by Bain is that good teaching can be learned. As he states, "Part of being a good teacher (not all) is knowing that you always have something new to learn—not so much about teaching techniques but about these particular students at this particular time and their particular sets of aspirations, confusions, misconceptions, and ignorance. To learn from the best teachers we must recognize that we can learn—and that we will still have failures."[14(p174)]

In 2008, Walker presented the results of a longitudinal, qualitative study conducted over a 15-year period that was designed to answer the question, What are the characteristics of an effective teacher?[15] The study subjects were more than 1,000 undergraduate and graduate students in education. The study population was diverse, with representation from private and public colleges, as well as males and females of various ages and nationalities. Students in the study were asked to write an essay on their most memorable teachers, defined as those who had the greatest impact on their lives, those who were most effective in teaching their subject matter, and those who had the greatest impact on their decision to enter teaching. *Effective* was defined in terms of level of success in helping the students to learn. After reviewing 15 years' worth of essays, Walker summarized what he described as the 12 identifiable personal and professional characteristics of effective teachers. The characteristics that emerged from the study are as follows, in no particular order:

- Came to class prepared
- Maintained positive attitudes about teaching and students
- Held high expectations for all students
- Showed creativity in teaching
- Treated and graded students fairly
- Displayed a personal and approachable touch with students
- Cultivated a sense of belonging in the classroom
- Dealt with student problems compassionately
- Had a sense of humor
- Were forgiving and did not hold grudges
- Respected students
- Admitted mistakes

In addition to the aforementioned studies, there are countless other sources of information on what makes a good teacher. Each year, the Carnegie Foundation invites teachers to compete in the U.S. Professors of the Year program by submitting an essay on what constitutes good teaching. In 1996, 20 of the essays were compiled in a book titled *Inspiring Teaching: Carnegie Professors of the Year Speak*.[16] In one of these essays, Peter Beidler, a professor of English from Lehigh University, described 10 qualities that are vital for success as a teacher.[17] The essential qualities include a positive attitude, the ability to listen to your students, taking risks, instilling confidence in your students through the facilitation of learning, and having the desire to be a good teacher. In her essay, Sally Phillips, a professor of nursing at the University of Colorado Health Sciences Center, described four specific characteristics (the four Cs) that teachers must possess to facilitate learning: competence, creativity, collaboration, and caring.[17] According to Phillips, by practicing the four Cs, the teacher can effectively transition from being an instructor to being a guide in the student's personal discovery of knowledge.[17]

Common Themes: What Constitutes Effective Teaching?

A number of common themes or messages about what constitutes good teaching emerged from the evidence. Overall, most of the components of good teaching are intangible. As noted by Walker, the personal, subjective traits of a teacher (e.g., enthusiasm, positive attitude) were routinely emphasized by his study sample over any objective trait of the teacher (e.g., the specific degree earned by the teacher, what schools the teacher attended, or whether or not the teacher had received a teaching award).[15] What appears to matter most to students and learners is not necessarily what teachers do, but who they are and how they convey their person to their students. In the following six statements, an attempt is made to summarize the common themes that emerged from the evidence.

> The curriculum is so much necessary raw material, but warmth is the vital element for the growing plant and for the soul of the student.
>
> Carl Jung

Good Teachers Know Their Students

> *To know how to suggest is the great art of teaching. To attain it, we must learn to read the student's soul as we might read a piece of music.*[18]
>
> Amiel HF

> *What we teach will never take unless it connects with the inward, living core of our students' lives, with our students' inward teachers.*[10(p32)]
>
> Palmer PJ

How well do you know your students? What do you know about their perceptions of your subject matter? Do you know what your students value and care about in and out of the classroom? The words *connectedness* and *partnership* saturate the literature on effective teaching. When the teacher and the learner are partners in the learning process—and there is a connectedness among the student, teacher, and subject—the opportunity for learning is maximized. Establishing this connection requires that you share your person with your students and that you take the time to learn about their person. Knowing students does not just mean knowing their names, although this is not a bad place to start. Connectedness *begins* by building rapport with your students by learning their names, their short- and long-term goals, and by sharing personal experiences. However, to establish a connection that promotes learning and an enthusiasm for the subject matter, you will need to know much more about your students. Chapter 2 will focus on getting to know your students and how their preferred styles of learning and the generation in which they were born influences the teaching–learning process. Knowing your students will require that you care enough to invest time in and out of class to listen to them and to seek out their individual and collective stories, ideas, and perceptions.

Good Teachers Focus on Learning, Not on Teaching Strategy or Teaching Technique

Technique is described by Palmer as something that the teacher uses until the real teacher arrives.[10(p6)] Bain states that "the second biggest obstacle to becoming a good teacher is the simplistic notion that good teaching is just a matter of technique."[14(p174)] These educators are not suggesting

> Learning is not a spectator sport. Students must talk about what they are learning, write about it, relate it to past experiences, apply it to daily lives. They must make what they learn part of themselves.
>
> A.W. Chickering

that teaching technique is not important. In fact, good teaching requires that you be organized, creative, take risks by trying new assessment strategies and teaching techniques, and remain open to new technology. Instead, the message that these authors are conveying is that technique is overemphasized. Before adopting the latest teaching technique, ask yourself whether the teaching strategy has been shown to increase learning. Will use of this technique enhance your ability to connect with your students such that the potential for learning will increase? Does this technique fit your person, and will it extend your reach to your students? Remember that teaching techniques are tools that will help you connect your subject and yourself with your students, but no technique is the universal solution to effective teaching.

Good teachers also share what they have learned with their students, thereby encouraging their students to learn. Good teachers recognize that they are experienced at learning. They begin class by sharing what they learned that day in their practice site or what they are discovering through their research. They serve as role models for learning, offering their students the opportunity to witness the excitement and enthusiasm that is associated with learning.

Good Teachers Engage Students in the Learning Process

> Good teachers, like good midwives, empower. Good teachers find ways to activate students, for they know that learning requires active engagement between the subject and object matter. Learning requires discovery and invention. Good teachers know when to hang back and be silent, when to watch and wonder at what is taking place all around them. They can push and they can pull when necessary—just like midwives—but they know they are not always called upon to perform. Sometimes the performance is and must be elsewhere.[19(p50)]

> All genuine learning is active, not passive. It is a process of discovery in which the student is the main agent, not the teacher.
>
> M.J. Adler *The Paideia Proposal: An Education Manifesto*; 1982

Good teachers recognize that their place in the classroom, the laboratory, or the practice site is not at center stage. They place the student's ability to learn the subject matter and to relate the subject to the world around them as central to all they do. Good teachers achieve this goal by balancing the power in the classroom or practice site.[4(p28)] They loosen the reins of control by placing responsibility for learning on their students. In the practice site, the student is empowered to learn by being held responsible for designing a patient's care plan or for assessing a patient's level of adherence with a complex drug regimen. In the classroom, students are given the opportunity to talk about what they are learning, write about what they are learning, and question what they are learning. Balancing the power between teacher and learner requires that the teacher relinquish some control and assume a variety of roles, from instructor to coach to guide to facilitator. Observation and listening become second nature to the good teacher. The learning environment that they create is open and communal and is one in which their students are actively engaged in the teaching–learning–assessment process.

Student engagement is currently a benchmark by which the quality of a college or university is measured. The National Survey of Student Engagement (NSSE) is an annual survey completed by first-year and senior students at 470 four-year colleges and universities.[20] Student engagement is measured based on how colleges contribute to learning in five areas: level of academic challenge, active and collaborative learning, student–faculty interaction, enriching educational experiences, and supportive campus environment. By promoting student engagement as a characteristic of an effective learning environment, the NSSE has challenged colleges and universities since 2001 to examine the extent to which students are actively involved in their learning. As such, good teaching in higher education has become synonymous with student engagement.

Good Teachers Have Self-Knowledge

When I don't know myself, I cannot know who my students are. When I do not know myself, I cannot know my subject—not at the deepest levels of embodied, personal meaning.[10(p2)]

Palmer PJ

Teachers who are able to understand and manage their own emotions are better able to understand and manage those of their pupils.[21]

Goleman D

The self is a crucial element in the way teachers construe and construct the nature of their work.[22(p7)]

Day C

To what purpose and to what end do you teach? Who is the self who teaches? In *The Courage to Teach*, Palmer asks us to answer these two questions to gain the self-knowledge that we need as teachers.[10(p4)] The premise of his text is that good teaching comes from the identity and integrity of the teacher. We are asked to explore our inner landscape to learn more about how our selfhood—the way we view ourselves in the world—influences the way we connect or fail to connect with our students. Palmer is direct in his questioning, asking us to reflect on how our person comes across to students and how what we feel about teaching and learning is translated to our students through our words and actions. We are reminded that who we are as individuals often speaks louder to our students than does our subject. Palmer is not alone in his message that our identity heavily influences our ability to connect our students to our subject. In *What the Best College Teachers Do*, Bain dispels the notion that personality plays a role in successful teaching. Outstanding teachers

> By first knowing ourselves as thinkers and learners, we can gain the self-knowledge that we can build and capitalize on in our teaching.
>
> Ron Ritchhart

that Bain encountered were both "bashful and bold, restrained and histrionic."[14(p137)] What they had in common was that they were authentic, true to themselves, and they "saw themselves as students of life, fellow travelers in search of some small glimpse of the truth."[14(p143)] Day describes such authenticity in terms of having "strong emotional and intellectual identities."[22] The message is clear; good teachers know who they are as individuals and how their perceptions of themselves and their beliefs about teaching, learning, and their subject can and will influence their students' abilities to learn.

Good Teachers Are Passionate Teachers

Passion is not a luxury, a frill or a quality possessed by just a few teachers. It is essential to all good teaching.[22(p11)]

Day C

Read anything about good teaching and you will find the word *passion*. Good teachers are said to have passion for their subject, for their students, and are passionate about what they do overall. But what is passion and what does a passionate teacher look like? Fried, the author of *The Passionate Teacher*, describes passion as "not just a personality trait that some people have and others lack, but rather something discoverable, teachable and reproducible."[23(p6)] Fried writes of the teachers he has observed in hundreds of classrooms. He reminds us that passion is not the goal of teaching, but it is a bridge that allows us to connect with our students. Most encouraging to the reader of Fried's text is that passionate teaching is attainable and it can take many different forms. "Sometimes that passion burns with a quiet, refined intensity; sometimes it bellows forth with thunder and eloquence. But in whatever form or style a teacher's passion emerges, students know they are in the presence of someone whose devotion for learning is exceptional."[23(p17)] What passionate teachers have in common is that they dig deep into the heart of their topic, share what excites them about their own learning in their field of study, and engage students in a journey of mutual discovery.

So, how does one develop the passion that Fried describes, that which is essential for good teaching? It is achieved by looking within yourself and by taking a holistic approach to your development as a teacher. Day, the author of *A Passion for Teaching*, has illustrated the core elements of passionate teaching (see **Figure 1–2**).[22] Many of the seemingly elusive, qualitative characteristics of an effective teacher described by others are captured in Day's work. Note the essential elements of passionate teaching in the center of the figure—being hopeful about what, how, and who you teach; having and revealing a commitment to your subject and your students; remaining curious and sharing your curiosity with others; knowing and revealing your sense of self or identify; and displaying the five major virtues: honesty, courage, caring, fairness, and practical wisdom. In the

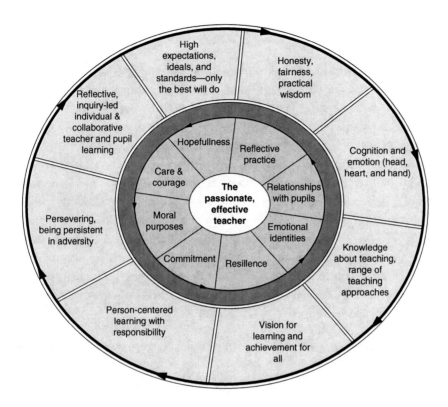

Figure 1–2 The Passionate, Effective Teacher

Source: Courtesy of Day C. *A Passion for Teaching.* London, England: RoutledgeFalmer; 2004:21.

outer circle of the figure, Day translates these core elements of passion into a holistic agenda for the continuing development of the teacher. This agenda calls for a merger of the emotional and intellectual identities (the mind and the heart) of the teacher with ideology and practicality.

The passion that Fried and Day describe as a component of good teaching has strong implications for those who educate pharmacists. The core elements of passionate teaching—caring, courage, resilience, hopefulness, integrity—are important for teachers to model in a professional, humanistic educational program such as pharmacy. Humanism, a way of being that is deeply rooted in the five virtues, is taught through the study of humanities, experiential education, service learning, and reflection. It is also learned through example, particularly through that set by preceptors, mentors, and teachers. As discussed in Chapter 10, professionalism and its intimate partner, humanism, are largely learned through observation, modeling, opportunity, and empowerment. Teaching that involves the whole person, not just the intellect—also known as passionate teaching—allows us to reach our students through humanism and to model the behaviors that are essential for development as a pharmacist.

Good Teachers Are Reflective and Open to External Review

To reflect is to think about your teaching practice and to critique what you did. What did you attempt with your teaching, and was it effective? How did you measure its effectiveness or lack thereof? What were your observations of your class today? If the class discussion was lively and engaging, what were the circumstances that may have led to this outcome? A reflection can relate to a past or current action, and it can also allow for future planning (i.e., how should I approach that issue next time?). Reflection should not be limited in scope but address the what, the how, and the why of teaching. Brookfield, in his text *Becoming a Critically Reflective Teacher*, states that critical reflection is important to ground teachers emotionally, to enable teachers to provide a rationale for their actions, and to enliven the classroom by making it challenging and stimulating.[24] Brubacher and colleagues described three primary reasons why we should be reflective practitioners:

- Reflective practice helps to free teachers from impulsive, routine behavior.
- Reflective practice allows teachers to act in a deliberate, intentional manner.
- Reflective practice distinguishes teachers as educated human beings because it is one of the hallmarks of intelligent action.[25]

Reflective practice typically begins as a solitary process of revisiting one's teaching, but it should evolve into a collective practice. Good teachers make their thinking public and subject their work to external review. They share their assumptions about teaching and learning with their colleagues, and they are open to critical appraisal by their peers.

Reflective Exercise

Of the six good teacher statements discussed in this section, which do you most identify with? Which statement addresses an aspect of teaching that you should further explore?

_____

_____

_____

_____

Plotting Your Journey: Post-Chapter Exercise

This chapter started the journey to effective teaching by defining the end point, the facilitation of learning. The term *learning* was defined, and *good teaching* in higher education was characterized based on the evidence. This chapter also asked you to closely examine the relationship between teaching and learning and to reflect on the qualities of good teaching. Following your review of the concepts presented in this chapter, you are now in a good position to articulate your beliefs about teaching. What are your current beliefs about the teaching of pharmacy or about teaching in general? These beliefs will set the framework for your teaching philosophy statement, a standard component of any teacher's portfolio. A statement of teaching philosophy is typically a one- to two-page document that offers a glimpse of the teacher within to the outside world. The statement should answer a number of questions about the teacher, such as what, how, and why the teacher teaches. Whether you are new to teaching or midcareer, there is value to putting down on paper what you currently believe about teaching. Please consider drafting a teaching philosophy statement now, before you move on to other chapters in this text. In subsequent chapters, you will be asked to revisit this statement and to reexamine your beliefs.

To help you write your statement, consider answering the following questions. The first four were posed by Palmer in *The Courage to Teach*[10(pp4,5)]:

- What subject do you teach? (What is your discipline—a core science, clinical problem solving, hospital pharmacy practice, specialty practice?)

  _____

  _____

- What techniques do you currently use and find to be effective in facilitating learning?

  _____

  _____

- For what purpose do you teach?

  _____

  _____

- How does your selfhood influence the way you connect with your students?

  _____

  _____

- If someone were to ask your students about your teaching, what would they say?

  _____

  _____

For those who are midcareer, consider these additional questions:

- What was your position on teaching when you started teaching? How has it changed, and what made it change?

  _____

  _____

- What are your current beliefs about teaching and learning?

  _____

  _____

- What have you tried in your teaching and found to be effective? Not effective?

  _____

  _____

- What have you learned about yourself through your teaching?

  _____

  _____

Brainstorming: My Teaching Philosophy Statement

References

1. *Webster's New Collegiate Dictionary*. Springfield, MA: G&C Merriam Company; 1979.
2. Ramsden P. Studying learning: improving teaching. In Ramsden P, ed. *Improving Learning: New Perspectives*. London, England: Kogan; 1988:271.
3. Rogers CR. Freedom to learn for the 80s. Columbus, OH: Charles Merrill; 1983:18–19.
4. Weimer ME. *Learner-Centered Teaching: Five Key Changes to Practice*. San Francisco, CA: John Wiley and Sons; 2002.
5. Keefe JW. Learning style: an overview. In: Keefe JW, ed. *Student Learning Styles: Diagnosing and Prescribing Programs*. Reston, VA: National Association of Secondary School Principals; 1979.
6. Silverman SL, Casazza ME. *Learning and Development. Making Connections to Enhance Teaching*. San Francisco, CA: Jossey-Bass; 2000:17.
7. Nasseh B. Changing definition of teaching and learning. http://www.bsu.edu/classes/nasseh/bn100/change.html. Published 1996. Accessed April 14, 2009.
8. ThinkExist. Latin proverb quotes. http://thinkexist.com/quotation/by_learning_you_will_teach-by_teaching_you_will/334478.html. Accessed November 25, 2009.
9. Barr RB, Tagg J. From teaching to learning—a new paradigm for undergraduate education. *Change*. November–December 1995:13–25.
10. Palmer PJ. *The Courage to Teach: Exploring the Inner Landscape of a Teacher's Life*. San Francisco, CA: John Wiley and Sons; 1998.
11. Sylvia LM. Mentoring prospective pharmacy practice residents: a monthly seminar series on teaching for pharmacy residents. *Am J Pharm Educ*. 2004;68(2):38.
12. Chickering AW, Gamson ZF. Seven principles for good practice in undergraduate education. *AAHE Bull*. 1987;39:3–7.
13. Paulsen SJ; Johnson Foundation. *Faculty Inventory: Seven Principles for Good Practice in Undergraduate Education*. Racine, WI: Johnson Foundation; 1989.
14. Bain K. *What the Best College Teachers Do*. Cambridge, MA: Harvard University Press; 2004.
15. Walker RJ. Twelve characteristics of an effective teacher: a longitudinal qualitative quasi-research study of in-service and pre-service teachers' opinions. *Educational Horizons*. Fall 2008:61–68. http://www.pilambda.org/horizons/v87-1/walker.pdf. Accessed January 14, 2009.
16. Roth JK, ed. *Inspiring Teaching: Carnegie Professors of the Year Speak*. San Francisco, CA: Jossey-Bass; 1996.
17. Rodgers AT, Cross DS, Tanenbaum BG, Tilson ER. Reflections on what makes a good teacher: Carnegie Foundation Professor of the Year winners. *Radiol Technol*. 1997;69(2):167. http://jan.ucc.nau.edu/~slm/AdjCI/Teaching/Teacher.html. Accessed March 25, 2009.
18. Amiel HF. *Amiel's Journal*. Ward H, trans. London, England: Macmillan and Company; 1895.
19. Ayers W. Thinking about teachers and the curriculum. *Harv Educ Rev*. 1986;56(1):49–51.
20. National Survey of Student Engagement. The 2001 national report. http://nsse.iub.edu/2001_annual_report/index.html. Accessed March 25, 2009.
21. Goleman D. *Working with Emotional Intelligence*. New York, NY: Bantam Books; 1998.

22. Day C. *A Passion for Teaching*. London, England: RoutledgeFalmer; 2004.
23. Fried RL. *The Passionate Teacher: A Practical Guide*. Boston, MA: Beacon Press; 1995.
24. Brookfield SD. *Becoming a Critically Reflective Teacher*. San Francisco, CA: Jossey-Bass; 1995.
25. Brubacher JW, Case CW, Reagan TG. *Becoming a Reflective Educator: How to Build a Culture of Inquiry in the Schools*. Thousand Oaks, CA: Corwin Press; 1994.

CHAPTER 2

What Matters in a Student-Centered Approach?

Laura L. Harris, PhD, ATC, LAT
Jill Clutter, PhD, CHES

Introduction

In Chapter 1, you were introduced to the relationship between teaching and learning. You learned that a good educator focuses on student learning first and foremost. To meet this end, you must appreciate how individuals learn and mature throughout their careers, both as students and as professionals. This chapter will help you understand and apply existing cognitive educational theories and learning style inventories to your classrooms, laboratories, and clinical settings to create a student- or learner-centered environment.

In rather simplistic terms, one might think of the difference between educator-centered and student- or learner-centered education as being a shift from *how to teach* toward *how to foster learning*. Student- or learner-centered instruction has been defined simply as "an instructional approach in which the students influence the content, activities, materials, and pace of learning."[1] As such, this educational approach necessitates some changes in your role as educator and in the balance of power in the classroom.[2] Although you will need to create conditions conducive to learner-centered education, students will also need to take a more active role in their own learning, accepting responsibility for their own growth and educational maturity. Consequently, with the student- or learner-centered approach, it is imperative that we, as educators, understand cognitive development, as well as learning style preferences, inherent in college students to better facilitate student growth and maturity.

> The telephone book is full of facts, but it doesn't contain a single idea.
>
> Mortimer Adler

Although higher levels of cognitive development are desired, it is important to recognize up front that a low level of development in a student does not imply a lack of intelligence. The same is true for learning styles. Intellectual ability is something that an educator cannot change; in education, intelligence is not the focus. Instead, the focus in education should be to challenge students to develop more advanced levels of cognitive development and an ability to use all learning styles as outlined in the following sections. Nonetheless, failure to achieve higher levels of development and balanced learning styles does not assign a student to a lower level of intelligence. As an educator, you are encouraged to think of developmental levels and learning styles as being independent of intelligence. As an example, young children entering kindergarten may be highly intelligent as assessed by an intelligence test; however, their developmental levels and learning styles will be immature at age 5 years. This is reflected in children's lack of compromise, resistance to change, limited vocabulary, and inability to solve complex problems. The goal of education is to challenge these students throughout the next 13 to 17 years such that they develop learning strategies that will encourage compromise, flexibility, improved communication, and enhanced problem-solving skills. As an educator, your ability to foster and facilitate such learning is grounded in an understanding of cognitive development.

Throughout this chapter, several theories will be presented as the foundation for creating a student- or learner-centered environment. For the novice educator, the thought of having to learn and use each of these theories is viewed as not only a complicated task, but also a daunting endeavor. It is not our purpose to overwhelm you, but rather to give you a foundation upon which to ground your teaching in purpose. We will begin with a description of the domains of learning (cognitive, psychomotor, and affective). Bloom's Taxonomy will be introduced as a tool for creating increasingly difficult learning and assessment strategies. Next we will present two of the more commonly referenced cognitive theories, Perry's Schemes of Intellectual and Ethical Development as well as Kitchner and King's Reflective Judgment Model. We will also investigate learning styles (Felder's Dimensions of Learning Style and Austin's Pharmacists' Inventory of Learning Styles) and generational influences on learning. In the end, our journey through educational theories will conclude with a combined model referencing all previously presented theories and models (Perry's Schemes, Kitchner and King's Model, Felder and Austin's Learning Styles, and generational influences). This integrated model should simplify the material and facilitate your initial attempts at creating a student- or learner-centered environment. Our promise is that the more you use and base your teachings in these theories and models, the more unconsciously you will root your teaching in a student- or learner-centered purpose.

To continue your exploration of effective teaching, this chapter will provide you with the tools to answer the following questions:

- How do people learn in the cognitive, psychomotor, and affective domains?
- How can an educator successfully implement Bloom's Taxonomy to develop a teaching strategy that fosters learning?
- What are some teaching techniques that you can use to challenge students in cognitive, affective, and psychomotor domains?
- What are the available theoretical frameworks and inventories that educators can use to challenge students' maturity and coping strategies throughout their young adulthood?
- What are the available theoretical models and tools that educators can use to familiarize themselves with individual learning styles?
- How do generational differences impact teaching and learning?
- How will you apply the various frameworks and inventories presented in this chapter to your teaching?

Consider the following scenario: You are a newly employed clinical faculty member with a practice in adult internal medicine. As you enter the first week of your academic position, you feel ready for the challenges that await you. Your residency experience provided you with the opportunity to gain solid clinical practice skills, and you are confident that you can teach students how to care for patients with hypertension, diabetes, and other common disease states. During the first week of your employment, you attend your first department of pharmacy practice and school of pharmacy faculty meetings. During these meetings, you are introduced to terms such as *pedagogy, andragogy, domains of learning*, and *assessment strategies*. As you exit these meetings, you realize that you have a lot to learn. But where do you begin? How will you facilitate learning in others if you have so much to learn about learning?

What Are the Types or Domains of Learning?

In Chapter 1, learning was described as both a process and an outcome. In this chapter, we will begin by expanding the discussion of learning as a process. Before you can facilitate your students' learning, you first need to understand how people learn and the different domains of learning. As a reminder, the constructivism theory supports that learning is an internal process in which individuals develop their own mental scaffolding from which they construct new knowledge. Based on this educational theory, learning is not achieved through transmission of knowledge from teacher to learner. Rather, as illustrated in **Figure 2–1**, it is acquired through a complex internalized process in which the learner uses previously learned

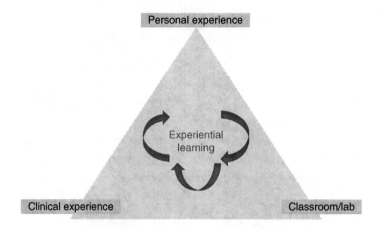

Figure 2–1 Influences on Learning

material, formulated ideas, and perceptions based on life experiences to build new knowledge. With this understanding, we can now discuss the different domains or types of learning.

In 1956, Bloom outlined three domains of learning: cognitive, psychomotor, and affective.[3] Each domain describes a category of learning. Although most individuals initially associate learning with the acquisition of facts or knowledge, not all learning is cognitive. Additional types of learning involve the development of psychomotor skills (e.g., operating a motor vehicle, dancing, playing an instrument) and values or attitudes (e.g., expressing empathy, caring, healthy skepticism). Bloom outlined the three domains of learning using classification systems referred to as taxonomies.[3] These taxonomies describe the different levels of progressive development within each domain of learning. **Table 2–1** outlines the stages of increasingly complex learning within each domain. Today, these taxonomies are used by many professional educators, including pharmacy faculty, to define learning outcomes and educational competencies required of an entry-level professional. Chapter 4 will provide more detail in using Bloom's Taxonomy to measure educational outcomes.

To comprehend each domain and apply them to your teaching and learning, let us assume that you will be responsible for teaching students how to obtain and interpret blood pressure readings in your experiential setting. During your pharmacy residency, you became quite proficient in this area of practice; however, how will you teach students using a student- or learner-centered approach such that they acquire this skill? What type(s) of learning does this activity entail? Before undertaking this educational activity, you need to consider the nature and extent of the student's past experiences with blood pressure determinations. What perceptions, understandings, and opinions does each student currently have based on his or

---

Table 2–1 The Three Domains of Learning

Stage of Difficulty	Cognitive*	Psychomotor†	Affective
1	Remember (*recall, recognize*)	Imitation (*modeling*)	Receiving (*listen, ask, reply*)
2	Understand (*interpret, explain*)	Manipulation (*instruct, practice*)	Responding (*participate*)
3	Apply (*execute, implement*)	Precision (*continual refinement*)	Valuing (*share beliefs*)
4	Analyze (*organize, attribute*)	Articulation (*coordination of skills*)	Organizing (*professional ethics*)
5	Create (*generate, plan*)	Naturalization (*unconscious use of skills*)	Internalizing values (*self-reliant, cooperative*)
6	Evaluate (*critique*)		

*The revised domain is presented. The original domain was defined as knowledge, comparison, application, analysis, synthesis, and evaluation.

†The psychomotor domain was never completed by Bloom. Several different versions of the psychomotor domain exist. The one presented here was developed by Simpson.[4]

---

her individualized experiences, and how will your educational activity allow for students to build on their learning? In addition, prior to exposing students to this activity, you need to consider the following three questions: What foundational or factual knowledge do your students need to have about blood pressure to obtain and interpret measurements accurately? What are the steps that a student must follow to obtain and assess blood pressure correctly? What information must a student be able to interpret to assess blood pressure accurately? Keep these questions in mind as we discuss each of Bloom's three domains.

The cognitive domain pertains to the acquisition of knowledge and intellectual skills.[3] The knowledge domain is comprised of six increasingly difficult stages of cognition: (1) *remembering or recalling* newly learned information, (2) *understanding and interpreting* new information, (3) *applying or implementing* new information into healthcare scenarios, (4) *analyzing or organizing* information in a usable format separate from memorization, (5) *creating or planning* health care based upon newly learned information, and (6) *evaluating or critiquing* newly learned information based upon evidence. (The latter two stages of Bloom's Taxonomy have been reversed by Simpson,[4] who argues that creating something original, built on previous stages of the domain, is the highest level of cognitive complexity.) This taxonomy or classification system reminds us that cognitive development is progressive and occurs in stages starting with basic recall or memorization and culminating in the ability to critique and evaluate newly learned information. The first question we referenced in the previous paragraph regarding foundational knowledge about blood pressure, and the third question addressing the interpretation of blood pressure measurements, fit into the cognitive domain. To meet the educational outcomes of correctly obtaining and interpreting blood pressure measurements, your students will need to display comprehension of basic factual information about blood pressure. Competency-based objectives reflecting cognitive development would include (1) to define a normal blood pressure, (2) to compare and contrast blood pressure measurements based on the stages of high blood pressure, and (3) to determine the goal blood pressures for patients with diabetes, heart disease, and end-stage renal disease. Now that you appreciate the cognitive domain of learning, the next step would be to design a student- or learner-centered teaching approach to ensure that your student can meet these learning objectives.

The psychomotor domain of learning involves the necessary motor skills that are required of a pharmacist.[3,4] It is composed of five increasingly difficult stages of learning: (1) *imitating or modeling* new skills, (2) *manipulating or practicing* newly learned skills, (3) gaining *precision or continually refining* newly acquired skills, (4) *coordinating* newly acquired skills with past skills, and (5) *unconsciously using* newly acquired skills. The second question that we previously posed, which addressed the steps necessary for assessing blood pressure accurately, fits into the psychomotor domain. Competency-based objectives specific to development in the psychomotor domain include the ability to accurately position the blood pressure cuff, position the stethoscope, and inflate the cuff. As you will learn in subsequent chapters, teaching within the psychomotor domain largely involves modeling and coaching on the part of the educator rather than lecturing or other forms of didactic instruction. In Chapters 8 and 9, teaching in a laboratory setting and the roles of modeling and coaching are described as they relate to experiential education.

The final domain, affective, also has five stages. Each stage describes a level of development and learning relative to attitudes, values, and beliefs.[3] The progressive stages within the affective domain are (1) *receiving, listening, and posing questions* about new information, (2) *responding and participating* in the use of newly learned information, (3) *valuing* information or beginning to build a personal belief or opinion, (4) *organizing* values and beliefs, and (5) *internalizing* personal values and beliefs. When analyzing the affective domain, it should be obvious that we failed to ask a question about affective learning. This is a common mistake for many educators. In many ways, the affective domain is the most important domain because it is this area where educators encourage their students to become reflective practitioners. This is where discussions and purposeful questions about healthcare beliefs and values aimed at a student's personal and professional development can be very important. It is also where the value of the clinical experience becomes the obvious complement to didactic and more traditional modes of education. Based on the blood pressure educational activity, a question specific to affective learning is, What student or patient behaviors, values, or attitudes may influence the acquisition of accurate blood pressure readings?

Reflective Exercise

In **Table 2–2**, the three domains of learning are applied to the educational activity of obtaining and interpreting blood pressure measurements. After reviewing this table, please attempt to apply this concept to the design of one of your educational activities. Are you developing a new lecture in medicinal chemistry, pharmacology, or therapeutics? Are you designing a new laboratory exercise or experiential activity? Which domains of learning will be addressed in your educational session? What learning objectives will you attempt to achieve in your session?

Reflective Exercise

Your educational activity:

_____

_____

_____

_____

Table 2–2 Applying the Domains of Learning: Blood Pressure Assessments

Cognitive Domain	Psychomotor Domain	Affective Domain
1. Define normal blood pressure.	1. Appropriately position the patient to obtain an accurate reading.	1. Appropriately introduce yourself to the patient.
2. Compare and contrast blood pressure measurements based upon the stages of high blood pressure.	2. Appropriately position the blood pressure cuff and stethoscope.	2. Identify whether the patient has concerns or apprehensions regarding the procedure.
3. Identify the goal blood pressure for a patient with no risk factors, with diabetes, with heart disease, or with end-stage renal disease.	3. Choose the appropriate cuff size for children, normal-sized adults, and patients with obesity.	3. Explain the process of blood pressure determination to the patient.
4. List factors, both drug and nondrug related, that can affect the measurement of blood pressure.	4. Inflate the cuff to appropriate levels of pressure.	4. Display empathy.
5. Determine the number of blood pressure readings necessary to assess blood pressure accurately.	5. Record the systolic and diastolic readings accurately.	

Cognitive Domain	Psychomotor Domain	Affective Domain

Using the Learning Taxonomies in a Student-Centered Approach

In pharmacy education, students must progressively develop within each of the three domains of learning to meet the educational outcomes of an entry-level PharmD program. Beginning with the lower level of the cognitive domain, *remembering* and *understanding* are usually the appropriate levels of complexity for initial educational encounters with students. During the early professional years, educational objectives aimed toward recalling, recognizing, interpreting, classifying, comparing, explaining, and summarizing blood pressure measurements are appropriate. However, as the experience of the student increases within a specific course and throughout the professional program, so should the difficulty of the learning objectives and tasks. Asking the student to apply, analyze, evaluate, and create are ways to challenge higher-order thinking skills within the cognitive domain. Examples of higher-level cognitive learning include evaluating a series of blood pressure measurements pre- and post-drug therapy or designing appropriate antihypertensive drug regimens for a patient with diabetes or heart disease who is receiving other medications for chronic conditions.

This same concept can be applied to increase the level of learning within both the psychomotor and affective domains. Basic psychomotor skills would start with the student simply modeling the steps to assess blood pressure and should advance by not only independently performing the steps, but also obtaining the correct measurements. Affectively, an educator would begin by asking students to identify their patients' healthcare beliefs about high blood pressure and advance to more abstract discussions or reflective writing assignments where students are asked to describe how patients should be informed of their blood pressure measurements. Another example would be to identify when and how to discuss hypertension with a patient or how to appropriately discuss weight loss or medication options.

Reflective Exercise

Revisit the previous exercise. What levels of learning (e.g., lower levels such as recalling or modeling, or higher levels such as creating or naturalizing) were conveyed in each of the domains? Do your learning objectives address a wide range of levels of learning? Most important, are the levels of learning appropriate? Were the students previously exposed to this educational area or activity, or are you initially exposing them to this content or skill area? Revise your educational plan accordingly.

How Do We Learn?

Now that you are aware of the domains or types of learning, it is important to know *how* students learn. Cognitive theories are an excellent tool to describe how learning occurs. These theories are focused on how individuals form cognitive structures to construct meaning in their worlds. In essence, cognitive theories describe *how* students think and the changes that will ultimately occur in their reasoning. For an educator, cognitive theories can provide a theoretical model upon which to challenge the cognitive and psychomotor domains and evaluate the advancing complexity of students' cognitive structures. Good educators continually walk the line between teaching to students' current cognitive developmental level and challenging students' growth to the next level of cognitive development.

> Higher cognitive development does not equate to higher intelligence.

Perry's Schemes of Intellectual and Ethical Development

Facilitating the development of sound clinical judgment and decision making in pharmacy students is a common challenge to all pharmacy educators. Students often seem locked in the black and white of pharmacy practice and have difficulty accepting the shades of gray. As educators, how can we identify the stage of learning in our students so we can facilitate this transition from black and white reasoning to acceptance of the shades of gray? Perry's Schemes of Intellectual and Ethical Development is a cognitive theory that helps explain the progressive development of cognitive reasoning.[5] This theory was developed based on information obtained through interviews with Harvard males beginning in 1955.[6] Although Perry's theory appears to be a stage model, it is best to think of the stages as categories that contain positions. The categories are static stages that mark the cognitive complexity of an individual, but the positions connote a more transient process that allows one to see the evolution of and movement toward increasing cognitive complexity.[5,7] There are nine positions conveniently grouped into four categories. **Table 2–3** outlines each category and corresponding position.[5]

The first category is *dualism,* which comprises positions one and two. Students who are in dualism believe that knowledge is absolute and that their worlds are dichotomous. At positions one and two, tasks that require thinking about more than one point of view are often confusing and frustrating. Concepts that are explained by *it depends* or *maybe* are difficult for these students to grasp. Dualistic students believe that authority figures (e.g., faculty and preceptors) hold all the answers. The second category, *multiplism,* refers to positions three and four. At these points, students can recognize that multiple perspectives exist on any given issue, thus *it depends* and *maybe* answers are tolerated but not completely comprehended. In multiplism, all opinions are equally valid, with the exception of that of authority figures, who are still believed to know the absolute truth. *Relativism* is the third category and consists of positions five and six, where students now realize that knowledge is contextual and relative. Analytical skills are developed, and judgments are possible. Complex concepts that are defined by gray areas are now not only tolerated but are comprehended. The fourth and final category is *commitment in relativism,* consisting of positions seven, eight, and nine. Students are now able to make commitments to values, ideas, and behaviors as they explore to find their own truths. At this stage, students possess the ability for affective learning as described in Bloom's Taxonomy. Commitments are made, but they are revised in light of new evidence and new choices. Students can

Table 2–3 Perry's Schemes of Intellectual and Ethical Development

Categories	Positions	Description
Dualism	1 + 2	Knowledge is absolute World is dichotomous
Multiplism	3 + 4	Recognizes multiple perspectives Authority holds truth
Relativism	5 + 6	Knowledge is contextual Analytical skills exist
Commitment	7 + 8 + 9	Commit to values, ideas, and behaviors through exploration Knowledge changes as evidence changes

Source: Adapted from Perry WG. *Forms of Intellectual and Ethical Development in the College Years: A Scheme.* Troy, MO: Holt, Rinehart & Winston; 1970.

accept that no one person ever has all the answers and that most knowledge will continue to be molded and changed as their experiences change.

Reflective Exercise

Think back on your own education. Identify an example to illustrate when you were functioning in *dualism*, *multiplism*, and *relativism*. Next relate Perry's Schemes to a first-year pharmacy student versus a more advanced student. What are the differences in their cognitive structures?

_____

_____

_____

_____

Using Perry's Theory in a Student-Centered Approach

As an educator, it is important to reflect and connect your teaching and learning strategies (e.g., Bloom's Taxonomy) to theories like Perry's to challenge students within the appropriate cognitive stages. For example, teaching traditional college-aged freshmen and sophomores often requires an educator to be comfortable with dualistic minds. Students early in their collegiate careers, especially those who are just beginning to learn the foundational knowledge of their chosen professions, are incapable of seeing complex or contextual discipline-specific knowledge. They must first understand facts and concepts in black and white terms. This provides the foundation for more complex knowledge to be introduced. A good educator will allow dualistic students the opportunity to gain confidence in their budding knowledge while periodically challenging the same students to see emerging complexities. Take, for example, an advanced pharmacy course designed to teach students how to select appropriate drug therapies for chronic diseases. Earlier in the curriculum, these students were taught the pharmacology and pharmacokinetic behaviors of antihypertensive medications and the pathophysiology of hypertension. Now you are building on their foundational knowledge by teaching them how to select appropriate antihypertensive medications for actual patients with a number of chronic conditions. When the students were introduced to the Joint National Committee on Prevention, Detection, Evaluation, and Treatment of High Blood Pressure (JNC 7) guidelines, you must be aware that they simply memorized the guidelines. Resultantly, they are not yet applying the guidelines to the care of specific patients. Using your knowledge of Perry's Schemes, you know that you would like to stretch them into more multiplistic thinking. By designing your instruction to address some of the more advanced levels of learning in Bloom's cognitive and psychomotor domains, you will be able to encourage students to move beyond dualism to multiplism. For example, because students memorized the JNC 7 guidelines, they will have a tendency to follow the guidelines blindly. You can stretch these students into multiplism by discussing the limitations to choosing hydrochlorothiazide as the preferred drug in all patients despite the fact that the guidelines list it as the drug of first choice for hypertension. This is an example of fostering a movement from dualistic to multiplistic thinking.

Kitchner and King's Reflective Judgment Model

Kitchner and King's Reflective Judgment Model can be used to identify the extent to which a person has the ability to view a problematic situation and "bring critical judgment to bear on the problem."[8] In the current climate, one might think of this as the discerning process of critically evaluating and using the evidence available for practice (i.e., evidence-based medicine). As students mature in this process, they become more adept at using the literature to inform and justify their practice. There is a reciprocal relationship between this developmental sequence and learning.

Each of the seven stages of the Reflective Judgment Model (see **Table 2–4**) includes assumptions about knowing and the "role of evidence, authority, and interpretation in the formation of solutions to the problem."[8] The first few stages of the model are mainly indicative of children and young adolescents and are considered to be *prereflective*. Stage one represents a single category belief system in very simplistic terms. Basically, seeing is believing. In stage two, while certainty in one answer is the predominant belief, there is a more dualistic shift in emerging knowledge. This is similar to Perry's Scheme where there can be more than one answer, but only one of the two answers can be correct (i.e., right answer and wrong answer).[8] Stage three

---

Table 2–4 Kitchner and King's Reflective Judgment Model

Categories	Stages	Description
Prereflective	1 + 2 + 3	Knowledge is concrete Knowledge is gained by direct observation or through authorities
Quasi-reflective	4 + 5	Knowledge is uncertain Knowledge is subjective
Reflective	6 + 7	Knowledge is constructed Analytical and evaluative skills exist

Source: Adapted from Kitchner KS, King PM. The reflective judgment model: transforming assumptions about knowing. In Arnold KD, King IC, eds. *College Student Development and Academic Life*. New York, NY: Garland Publishing Inc; 1997:141–159.

builds on the dualistic notion but refines the categories to *known* and *not known at this time*. There exists the faith that all questions and problems are now or will be answerable at some time in the future. This stage may be indicative of many early undergraduate students or professional students who are being introduced to new concepts.

The next two stages, considered to be *quasi-reflective*, venture beyond the more concrete epistemology (way of knowing) into increasingly elaborate schema. Students at stage four recognize that knowledge may be uncertain and authorities may be lacking. There might not be one right answer, and the process might be as important as the answer. This ability is usually found in upperclassmen in college. As an educator, the use of case studies that highlight ill-structured problems (i.e., real-world circumstances) is useful at this stage. At stage five, students, most typically graduate students, recognize that knowledge is contextual, but they may have trouble discerning different interpretations of the evidence connected with a given problem. In other words, they will do a thorough literature review but are still unable to distill the evidence into a judgment on the issue.

True *reflective* thinking does not occur until the sixth and seventh stages. The ability to come to individual decisions is indicative of stage six, where a student can discern that "some perspectives, arguments, or points of view may be evaluated as better than others."[8] Such abilities are generally found in advanced graduate and professional students. In stage seven, which typically becomes more developed in the years beyond the age of the traditional college student (e.g., 30s), people develop the ability to justify solutions to problems based upon critical evaluation of the evidence and synthesis of that evidence.

Using Kitchner and King's Theory in a Student-Centered Approach

As with Perry's theory, the cognitive stage is often dependent upon the age of the student. For example, freshmen and sophomores are more often experiencing the lower stages, and juniors and seniors are preoccupied with the mid to upper stages. Professional students, such as those in doctor of pharmacy programs, are mostly dealing with issues in the advanced stages due to their age (e.g., 22 to 30 years). Stage six is an example. At this point pharmacy students are contemplating their practice as a professional. What kind of pharmacist will I be? Who do I consider to be mentors? What theories do I value most in pharmacy practice? As students begin to move into the later stages of cognitive development (i.e., relativism and commitment to relativism), educators and mentors have an opportunity to begin to challenge students in a more affective realm. As skills or techniques are taught, students should be challenged to think and reflect on how these skills and techniques fit into their personal practice philosophies.

Let us revisit the idea of teaching blood pressure assessments and choice of antihypertensive medications. As with dualistic students, students who are prereflective will want to follow the JNC 7 guidelines and select hydrochlorothiazide without applying critical thought. However, quasi-reflective students are able to analyze case studies and will begin to look at mediating variables, such as patient comorbidities and drug interactions. Keep in mind that these students still require careful questioning and direction in correctly selecting the best medication for more complicated patients. Not until students are in a reflective stage do they possess the ability to evaluate each patient individually and develop the best treatment option while considering the JNC 7 guidelines, the patient's history, and available evidence.

Affective learning is also evident in quasi-reflective and reflective stages when moral and ethical dilemmas are posed. Consider the example of the controversial morning-after pill. Is this a medication that the student believes in advocating or supporting? How will the student handle a situation where such medication is dispensed by his or her employer, even when it is against his or her personal beliefs? These are primary questions that are key to developing the affective domain in students exhibiting more advanced developmental stages. Without an understanding and appreciation of educational theory, most educators are skilled only at educating and challenging cognitive and psychomotor aspects of students. Educational theory affords educators the opportunity to challenge students beyond the cognitive and psychomotor domains.

Reflective Exercise

Apply Kitchner and King's theory to yourself. In what stage are you currently? In what stage are most of your students?

_____

_____

_____

_____

What Are Learning Styles?

A learning style is defined as an individual's preferred method of interacting or processing information. Each person possesses his or her own preference for learning (e.g., visual or verbal learner). An easy way to conceptualize individual and differing learning styles is to think about corrective eye wear as an analogy for learning style. Consider a student who is farsighted. This student's vision is limited to seeing far away objects without correction. Likewise, a nearsighted student's vision is limited as well, but it is limited in a different way. The nearsighted student can only see nearby objects without correction. With the appropriate corrective lenses, both students will be capable of seeing more clearly. However, if these two students were to swap their corrective lenses, they would lose all clarity in their fields of vision. This is because each person sees best when he or she is wearing his or her personal prescription for eye wear. No two individuals' prescriptions (e.g., 20/15, 20/30) are the same, just like no two individuals' learning styles are the same. As an educator, recognizing learning styles allows us to see how our students see. If you want to gain insight into differing learning styles, wear someone else's corrective lenses for an hour and evaluate the quality of your vision.

Learning styles vary among both educators and students. No two individuals ever approach learning and processing information in the exact same way; therefore, the idea that an educator can create one style of teaching to reach all students is as irrational as thinking everyone has the same prescription for corrective lenses. Instead, educators must vary their styles in hopes that all students can see at several different points of an educational exercise. There are numerous tools available to assist educators in identifying their students' learning styles. The Myers-Briggs Type Indicator and Kolb Learning Style Inventory are two of the most common. Felder's survey, Austin's inventory, and Fleming's VARK are examples of others. This chapter will only address Felder and Austin's models. This does not imply that they are the best; they are just a few of the most available and commonly cited models in pharmacy education. As you read Felder and Austin's models, keep the following questions in mind: Do you know the preferred learning styles of your students? Are they visual, verbal, or sequential learners? How are you designing instruction to address these varied learning styles?

Felder's Dimensions of Learning Style

Felder believes that learning styles can be defined by five dichotomous, continuous dimensions.[9] The five dimensions are (1) Sensory–Intuitive, (2) Visual–Verbal, (3) Inductive–Deductive, (4) Active–Reflective, and (5) Sequential–Global. **Table 2–5** provides a brief description of each dimension. The first dimension, Sensory–Intuitive, describes what information is perceived. Sensory learners prefer factual information that can be sensed through sight, smell, sound, or touch; whereas intuitive learners favor conceptual and abstract information that can be created and imagined. In this regard, the sensory learner would more readily learn to use a stethoscope by directly seeing the patient or hearing the patient's heart sounds, whereas an intuitive learner could relate the use of a stethoscope to previously learned material or a referenced case study. The Visual–Verbal dimension

---

Table 2-5 Felder's Learning Style Dimensions

	Dimension	
Sensory	What type of information is preferentially perceived?	Intuitive
Visual	Through which sensory mode is information most effectively perceived?	Verbal
Inductive	How is information preferentially organized?	Deductive
Active	How is information preferentially processed?	Reflective
Sequential	With which process is understanding reached?	Global

Source: Adapted from Felder RM. Reaching the second tier—learning and teaching styles in college science education. *J Coll Sci Teach*. April–March 1993:286–290.

---

describes learners' preferences toward learning through visualization or verbalization. For example, visual learners have difficulty retaining information that is spoken, and they learn more readily when pictures, graphs, or visual aids are provided. On the other hand, verbal learners are likely to forget information that is simply illustrated through a diagram and not explained. The third dimension, Inductive–Deductive, explains a student's preference for organizing information. Students who prefer induction, learn by seeing cases (e.g., results or examples) first and then delving into the theories and principles. On the other hand, deductive students must first learn general principles (e.g., steps or procedures). By nature, deductive learners often prefer organization and structure leading to a step-by-step approach, whereas inductive learners can be stifled by too much structure. The Active–Reflective dimension is most easily understood by conceptualizing the difference between doers and thinkers. Active learners strive to process information by being actively involved and interacting with others or the environment, and reflective learners are far more introspective, wishing to process in solitude. The last dimension, Sequential–Global, describes how information is understood. Sequential learners process information in organized segments; global learners take holistic leaps. The disadvantage to sequential learning is that solutions can be derived without a full comprehension of the situation. The order to the learning can sometimes produce a correct answer without exactly knowing how or why. A disadvantage of global learning is the amount of time it takes to learn. These learners have to understand the big picture before they can solve a problem.

Felder has documented that most lectures are heavily biased toward the intuitive, verbal, deductive, reflective, and sequential learning dimensions.[9] On the other hand, laboratories tend to be more designed for sensory, visual, and active learners. With a combination of a lecture and a hands-on laboratory, two dimensions are still unaccounted for in teaching. One recommendation for addressing the unaccounted dimensions, Inductive and Global, is to encourage problem-based scenarios. An example would be to present pharmacy students with a case study of a patient who had been successfully taking the recalled medication Vioxx. In this case study, there would be several other medications that would be possible for the patient; however, the objective of the exercise would not be to find the best medication but rather to go through the process of thinking through a unique problem. For example, (1) students must recognize that Vioxx was recalled, (2) students must recognize why the patient was on Vioxx, and (3) students must select another appropriate medication. An exercise that encourages a process of thinking in reverse and universally would address both inductive and global practices.

Reflective Exercise

Log on to http://www.engr.ncsu.edu/learningstyles/ilsweb.html and take Solomon and Felder's Index of Learning Styles Questionnaire.[10] What is your learning style? How might your learning style affect your teaching? Evaluate a course, lecture, or lab that you have taught. Did you accommodate multiple learning styles? If not, how might you restructure your course or lecture to accommodate multiple learning styles?

_____

_____

_____

_____

Austin's PILS for Pharmacy Practice and Education

Austin's Pharmacists' Inventory of Learning Styles (PILS) is an instrument that was designed to identify the specific learning styles of pharmacists.[11] Extensive focus group work by Austin resulted in six dimensions to describe the learning styles of pharmacists. However, statistical analysis revealed that only two of the six dimensions were significant descriptors for pharmacists. Thus, PILS is based upon two dimensions or axes. **Figure 2–2** illustrates the two axes (unstructured and structured; doing and reflecting).

The Unstructured–Structured (U–S) dimension composes the vertical axis. Unstructured environments are environments where outcomes and processes are not clearly defined or assessed; instead, performance expectations are defined individually.[11] On the other end, structured environments are those where outcomes and processes are clearly defined and assessed.[11] The horizontal axis is formed by the Doing–Reflecting (D–R) dimension. Doing involves experimentation and trial and error; reflecting involves mental rehearsal and observation rather than active experimenting.

To acquire knowledge one must study; but to acquire wisdom, one must observe.
Marilyn vos Savant

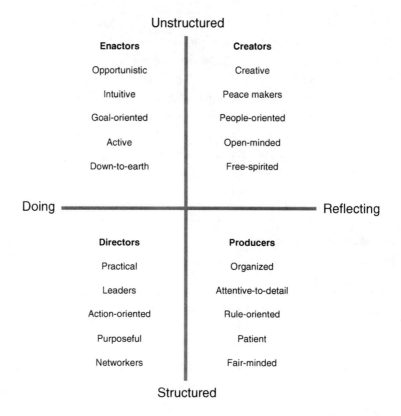

Figure 2–2 Typology for Pharmacists' Inventory of Learning Styles

Source: Courtesy of Austin Z. Development and validation of the Pharmacists' Inventory of Learning Styles (PILS). *Am J Pharm Educ.* 2004;68(2):1–10.

The advantage of the PILS is twofold. One, it was designed to explain the learning styles of pharmacists. Two, Austin offers the PILS free of charge and encourages its use amongst pharmacy educators.[11] A copy of the PILS is included in Appendix 2–1 at the end of this chapter.

Reflective Exercise

Complete the PILS (see Appendix 2–1). Do the results seem similar to the results from Felder's Dimensions of Learning Style questionnaire? Which instrument do you prefer to use in assessing your students' learning styles? How are you going to learn to teach in your weaker learning styles?

_____

_____

_____

_____

Using Learning Styles in a Student-Centered Approach

The true gift of Felder and Austin's learning styles assessment tools is in the justification for how educators should teach. When a student's learning style is a mismatch with the educator's teaching style, boredom and disengagement can result. The solution is for the educator to vary his or her teaching style to address a variety of learning styles within the classroom or clinical environment. This not only optimizes the willingness of students to learn, but it also encourages students to learn how to learn in different learning styles.[11]

Each learning experience should be constructed from the framework of multiple learning styles in hopes that all students are reached. Think about this in terms of teaching a group of students who do not speak the same language. For example, hypothesize what it would be like to teach 100 students in a classroom where 25 spoke Spanish, 25 spoke English, 25 spoke Japanese, and 25 spoke Russian. If you taught solely in English, 75 percent of the students would not learn as effectively. Varying your teaching style to accommodate the different learning styles allows you to instruct students in their native language. This is the most obvious benefit of teaching based upon learning styles.

Valuing the concept of teaching across different learning styles is the first step toward effective teaching. The second step is knowing what educational strategies align best with the different learning styles. **Table 2–6** and **Table 2–7** provide a summary of the preferred teaching and learning strategies according to the two different axes of PILS.

Table 2–6 Vertical Axis (U–S) Teaching and Learning Strategies

Unstructured

- Personalized feedback from educator or preceptor
- Educator or preceptor sharing affective stories from his or her experience
- Scenarios that force the student to apply skills to real situations
- Peer feedback on performance
- *Learns least from theory-based readings*

Structured

- Case studies
- Concept maps
- Brainstorming to create solutions to problems
- Theory-based readings
- Self-directed and autonomous activities (i.e., papers)
- *Learns least from group work*

Table 2–7 Horizontal Axis (D–R) Teaching and Learning Strategies

Doing	Reflecting
• Small-group discussions	• Expert advice
• Projects	• Discussions following readings
• Peer feedback on performance	• Journaling or logging
• Homework problems	• Lecturing
• Scenarios that force student to apply skills to real situations	• *Learns least from projects*
• *Learns least from lectures*	

How Does One's Generation Influence Learning?

Never before have there been the multifaceted influences of diversity affecting all aspects of our society, including education. This diversity causes multiple differences in worldview based upon each person's individual outlook, often referred to as the lens through which we view the world. In this respect, an additional aspect worth considering is that of generational influences on learning. Although there are some variations, most generations are defined in approximately 20-year intervals. The individuals born during these generational spans have been affected by the pervasive occurrences, technologies (or lack thereof), music, celebrities, and defining moments of that period.[12-14] Recognizing the characteristics inherent in a given generation assists in understanding some of the basic premises that color a generation's worldview (see **Table 2–8**). Although defining generations is not meant to stereotype individuals, it does provide broad strokes for consideration in both educational and professional interactions.

Do any of the descriptors in Table 2–8 resonate with you? Perhaps they are descriptive of you, a family member, or a coworker. Do keep in mind that these are very broad descriptions, but you can see how everyone's lens may be slightly colored by his or her generational standing, and that may provide a better understanding in both professional and educational venues.

More than any other generation, the Millennials have and will continue to greatly impact higher education in the United States. In an exploratory study, Sandfort and Haworth[15] found that this generation thinks a college degree is a way to guarantee a middle-class lifestyle. Ninety percent of the Millennials interviewed expected to attend college, and 70 percent expected to have professional jobs.[15] These students go one step further by correlating going to college with having a happy life. The National Center for Education Statistics reports that in 2002, there were 9.9 million students aged 18 to 24 years in higher education, and it is projected that by 2014, 11.5 million students in higher education will be aged 18 to 24 years.[16] All of these students will be considered Millennial students.

Table 2–8 Generational Comparisons

Generation/Age Span Defining Moments	General Characteristics	Educational/Work Implications
Veterans/traditionalists (Born 1922–1943) • Great Depression • World War II	• Built much of the nation's infrastructure • Believe in duty before pleasure • Financially conservative • Patriotic • Value home and family	• Strong work ethic • Loyal employees • Detail-oriented • Favor classroom or conference • Respect authority
Baby boomers (Born 1944–1960) • Vietnam War • Women's lib • Civil rights movement	• Grew up in times of economic expansion • Service-oriented • Tend to be competitive • Self-gratifying	• Success-oriented • Dedicated • Hardworking • Willing to put in long hours • Favor classroom or workshop
Generation X (Born 1960–1980) • Nixon resignation • Jim Bakker scandal • Beginning of digital era	• Many are products of nontraditional families • Latchkey children • Self-reliant • Challenge the status quo • Dislike being labeled	• Blurred work and life boundaries • Distrustful of authority • Independent workers • Interested in training • Online
Generation Y/Millennials (Born 1980–2000) • Columbine • 9/11 • The Internet	• More racially diverse • Indulged by parents • Lead busy, overplanned lives • Civic-minded • Well-mannered and polite	• Technologically savvy • Multitaskers • High tolerance • Collaborative • Achievement-oriented • Digital learning

Source: Adapted from Zemke R, Raines C, Filipczak B. *Generations at Work: Managing the Clash of Veterans, Boomers, Xers, and Nexters in Your Workplace.* New York, NY: AMACOM; 2000. Lovely S, Buffman AG. *Generations at School: Building an Age-Friendly Learning Community.* Thousand Oaks, CA: Corwin Press; 2007.

Comparisons of Millennials to previous generations are useful in that higher education exhibits an intergenerational mixture of faculty, staff, and students. A comparison study[17] of Generation X and Millennial medical students at one medical school (n = 809) revealed strong personality differences between the two generations. Millennial students were more open and more willing to change than the Generation X students. Jonas-Dwyer and Pospisil examined how the characteristics of Millennial students affect the academic environment.[18] Specifically, these students desire educational experiences that are active and relevant, flexible, include regular feedback, and include opportunity for social and interactive learning, all of which can be challenging to accomplish using traditional educational methods. Millennials are looking to faculty as leaders and role models, and they want the faculty to take the lead in the classroom. Yet Millennials demand respect for themselves and their ideas. The authors' research reveals that Millennials have always experienced challenges and pressures; thus, they want more challenges with projects and assignments in higher education. Clearly, the characteristics and preferences of the Millennial students challenge any currently static educational methodology.

Using Generational Differences in a Student-Centered Approach

Although some students have indicated resistance to the student- or learner-centered approach in the past, it may be that the current generation of college students (Millennials) is well-suited for this. Wilson illustrates how Chickering and Gamson's seven principles for good practice in undergraduate education are applicable even to the current Millennial generation of students.[19,20] These principles are (1) encourage contact between students and faculty, (2) develop reciprocity and cooperation among students, (3) encourage active learning, (4) give prompt feedback, (5) emphasize time on task, (6) communicate high expectations, and (7) respect diverse talents and ways of knowing.

Group work and teamwork activities are essential to energizing Millennial students in the classroom.[21] The educational literature also suggests that students learn more effectively in groups than on their own.[22] However, the research suggests that due to various challenges in curriculum development, designated courses on teamwork skills are rare.[23] One approach to this type of preparation would be to introduce Millennial students to team-based learning projects.

Reflective Exercise

Given the characteristics of Millennials, how would you restructure a traditional lecture to maximize their learning? For example, what do Millennials value? How do they learn?

_____

_____

_____

_____

Integrated Model

At the beginning of this chapter, the novice educator asked the question, Where do I begin in my quest to learn more about learning? We have attempted to outline key cognitive theories, compare and contrast learning styles, and discuss the generational influences on learning. Our promise is that the more you use and base your teachings in these theories and models, the more you will develop purpose in your teaching. To end and summarize the chapter, we will attempt to integrate and combine the theories, learning styles, and generational influences to assist you in your attempt to create a learner-centered teaching environment. Before doing so, please consider each of the concepts presented in this chapter as they relate to your individual growth as a teacher. Using the taxonomies as your foundation, conduct a personal inventory of your levels of learning in the cognitive, psychomotor, and affective domains. The key questions to ask are as follows:

> Growth demands a temporary surrender of security.
> Gail Sheehy

- What is my level of cognitive development with regard to student learning? Am I at the level of recall of theories and comprehension of theoretical information? Am I ready to apply these principles and theories to my teaching?
- What is my level of psychomotor development with regard to student learning? Am I modeling the use of technology in the classroom and laboratory? Have I mastered specific clinical skills so I am ready to teach these skills? What additional areas of psychomotor development should I work on?
- What is my level of affective development with regard to student learning? Am I currently posing new questions about my role as an educator? Am I listening to mentors and my students? Am I putting myself in situations where I can observe the classroom from the role of a learner?

Figure 2–3 provides an illustration of our integrated model. This model is designed to be used as a step process in teaching, which is represented by the increasing size of the arrows. Think of this model as additive, building from introductory knowledge to advanced knowledge throughout a curriculum. It is not practical to think that one educator or one class can

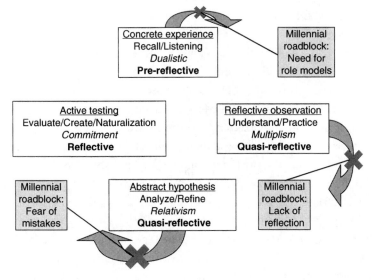

Figure 2–3 Integrated Theory and Educational Model

experience each step within this model. Instead, it is the role of the educator to facilitate movement along the model throughout a curriculum.

Within the model we have used Austin's PILS as our foundation. Within each text box (i.e., step), Austin's vertical axis (Unstructured = Concrete experience; Structured = Abstract hypothesis) and horizontal axis (Doing = Active testing; Reflecting = Reflective observation) are represented as the underlined text. Bloom's Taxonomy is shown in normal text, Perry's Schemes of Intellectual and Ethical Development is represented in italics, and Kitchner and King's Reflective Judgment Model is represented in bold. We have introduced the generational challenges provided by Millennials as black Xs. Please keep in mind that these are *potential* challenges, not absolutes. Your goal as the educator is to try to avoid these generational roadblocks by designing educational activities that address different levels of cognitive development in addition to various learning styles.

The first step is to teach introductory material in a manner that establishes concrete learning experiences. Bloom might describe this as recalling facts in his cognitive domain or listening to stories within his affective domain. Similarly, this step can be described as a dualistic phase where facts are viewed by the student in black and white terms; at this stage there is an outright lack of contextual understanding. This is purely a prereflective period in teaching, and ultimately learning, because students are not ready to digest the information. Instead, they are just beginning to get familiar with the amount of material before them. Just as we learned from the *Three Little Pigs*, a strong foundation must exist before we can withstand challenges (i.e., huffing and puffing). Our generational roadblock that can potentially block learning from progressing to the next stage is the Millennials' need to have a role model. Throughout their lives Millennials' parents have been the authority figures with all the answers. To be an effective educator at this stage, you must gain the trust of your students by being invested in them as human beings and by being a role model. This is where some individual attention can be helpful. Millennials will respond positively to boundaries and high expectations as long as those boundaries and expectations are believed to be personally aimed, not globally applied to all students. Millennials invest in those who invest in them, and a lack of investment from an educator can result in Millennials developing mistrust in the educator's opinions and teachings. This will interfere with a student's progression into the next step.

This poses a particular problem given the typically large size of many pharmacy classes. Try these suggestions for reaching a more personal level of investment with Millennial students. Learning each student's name is an important first step. Millennials need to feel special and appreciated. Another suggestion is to spend time to provide personalized comments when grading written assignments, such as essays. Even using chat room discussions in WebCT or Blackboard will lend a more personalized feel to a large class.

The second step in teaching is to encourage reflection from your students. Now is the time to ask them to connect their observations with what they have learned previously in the concrete step. This can occur simultaneously with introductory information. Bloom might liken this to understanding information within his cognitive domain or practicing within his psychomotor domain. Because students are now beginning to understand shades of gray in their knowledge, it is appropriate to discuss and challenge students to think in multiplism (i.e., contextual situations or scenarios). Kitchner and King would describe this as a quasi-reflective period where students are beginning to think about the information they have learned.[8] At this point, students are still not ready to digest the information, but they are ready to begin chewing on it. The biggest potential roadblock at this phase is the lack of reflection that is a germane characteristic of Millennials. Remember that this is a generation that has grown up with proficiency tests in high school; they believe there is one answer and that they only have to know material for a test and not apply it at a later time. Our advice is to avoid playing into their expectations for study guides at this stage. Provide them with stories and examples of why information must be known and not memorized. Rhetorically, ask students if they get to use a study guide when they are performing CPR on an unconscious patient. Without reflection, students will be paralyzed in their ability to hypothesize the next step.

The creation of structured hypotheses is the third step. This must occur in the mid- to upper-level courses within a curriculum. This is a continuation of reflection (i.e., quasi-reflective) because students are now ready to analyze information in the cognitive domain or refine skills within the psychomotor domain, thus implying a continual and constant reflection in an effort to develop a relativist means of thinking. Relativistic thinking refers to students' ability to see information as purely contextual and to understand multiple points of view. As students continually reflect on information, they are beginning the process of developing hypotheses that can be challenged via active testing. Perhaps the biggest potential roadblock to teaching Millennials is their fear of mistakes, which prohibits the testing of formed hypotheses. The proverbial Helicopter Parent has hovered above and protected the Millennial. Most Millennials have limited experience with mistakes; their parents have guarded them or fixed mistakes for them. As an educator, you must believe that the fear of mistakes is not a characteristic of arrogance or narcissism, but rather a symptom of Millennials' fear of disappointing their role models. Encourage mistakes in classroom activities and simulations! This is where real learning takes place, and it is the key to completing the learning cycle.

The last stage is doing and testing. This is a step in teaching that requires a solid foundation of knowledge from your students. Constant challenge and rationale should be encouraged as students evaluate in the cognitive domain and naturalize in the psychomotor domain. We liken this process to a carpenter who must select the appropriate tools to place in his or her toolbox. This is a period when students should be testing, critiquing, and analyzing different theories and skills to place in their toolboxes, where the toolbox represents their skill set as a pharmacist. This is truly the most reflective period because students are engaged in constant thought. This is the type of healthcare professional we should all hope to have care for us one day, a professional who thinks about the best analgesic to prescribe given our medical histories and comorbidities—a personalized plan that is contextual yet open to be modified in light of new evidence.

Closing Thoughts

Let us end with a personal example. One year we had the pleasure of having a senior-level student voluntarily serve as a teaching assistant in a freshman-level course for three consecutive quarters. This senior student was a very observant and intuitive individual, probably a creator in terms of PILS. After three quarters of assisting with the same course, he approached us one day with a very simplistic observation. He told us that he had figured us out. We were intrigued—and a little concerned—about what he had figured out. He continued his observation with the following statement: "You have a reason for everything that you do in a classroom; nothing is assigned or presented without you knowing exactly *why* you are doing it and *what* you want to achieve." We had never consciously thought of this, but after some reflection his assessment seemed fairly accurate. Not to insinuate that we are perfect in our delivery and methods, but that is exactly what we should strive to create. As educators, we should know exactly where our students are cognitively, we should also have an idea of their learning styles, and that should guide our purpose in class. Leave it to a student to provide one of the greatest epiphanies we have ever had as educators!

> Have a vision. Be demanding.
> Colin Powell

Scenarios

The following scenarios are provided as additional opportunities for reflection and application of the material addressed in this chapter. Based on what you have learned in this chapter, how would you address each of these teaching scenarios?

Scenario 1: The Concrete Thinker

Bob is the top student in a nationally renowned pharmacy education program. Bob is obviously highly intelligent, but he seems unable to grasp contextual concepts. He wants yes or no answers and is struggling with theoretical applications. How do you help Bob see the contextual nature of pharmacy practice? How can you challenge Bob to become more *relative* in his learning?

_____

_____

_____

_____

Scenario 2: The Reflective Learner

Amy is a third-year Millennial pharmacy student. During her first two years in pharmacy school, her academic progress was above average, but clinically she appeared to be underperforming. Whenever questions were posed during clinical exercises, Amy would stare at her preceptor and could not generate an answer. Most preceptors thought Amy was disinterested and lethargic. Upon taking the PILS, it was discovered that Amy is primarily reflective. How do you mentor Amy to use her natural reflective tendencies to facilitate a more productive clinical educational outcome? How do you challenge Amy to develop other learning styles that will be useful in actual practice as a future pharmacist?

_____

_____

_____

_____

Scenario 3: The Great Pontificator

Dr. George is a tenured professor who has been using a teacher-centered approach for years. He has traditionally received average teaching evaluations, but recently his evaluations have become increasingly more critical. Students remark that Dr. George's lectures do not encourage independent thought or application of material. What suggestions would you make for Dr. George that will engage his students in a more student- or learner-centered approach?

_____

_____

_____

_____

Additional Considerations and Resources

A number of additional resources applicable to the content of this chapter are recommended for your review. These resources compliment the material provided in this chapter.

Psychosocial Developmental Theory: Chickering and Reisser's Seven Vectors

Chickering's seven vectors represent a passage from the relatively linear developmental models to a more complex-stage psychosocial model aimed at outlining what preoccupies students as they move into adulthood. Chickering's original seven vectors, revised in 1993 with Reisser, are described as "major highways for journeying toward individuation."[6] Although the original version was based primarily on white, heterosexual males, the revised version is more comprehensive in recognizing additional research detailing the different struggles affecting women, minorities, and gay and lesbian students.[6] For more information on this model, refer to the following book:

Chickering AW, Reisser L. *Education and Identity*. 2nd ed. San Francisco, CA: Jossey-Bass; 1993:1–42.

Learning Styles: Kolb's Experiential Theory

Kolb's Learning Style Inventory is the foundational theory for PILS. Kolb believes that the most adept students are well-balanced learners and can complete the experiential learning cycle with relative ease.[24] To learn more about Kolb's experiential learning model, see Chapter 9. From the experiential learning model, Kolb developed specific learning styles. The four specific learning styles are (1) divergers, (2) assimilators, (3) convergers, and (4) accomodators.[24] To learn more about Kolb's learning styles, refer to the following book:

Kolb DA. *Experiential Learning: Experience as the Source of Learning and Development*. Upper Saddle River, NJ: Prentice Hall; 1984:2–40.

References

1. Collins JW, O'Brien NP. *Greenwood Dictionary of Education*. Westport, CT: Greenwood; 2003.
2. Weimer ME. *Learner-Centered Teaching: Five Key Changes to Practice*. San Francisco, CA: John Wiley & Sons; 2002.
3. Bloom BS. *Taxonomy of Educational Objectives, Handbook I: The Cognitive Domain*. New York, NY: David McKay Co Inc; 1956.
4. Simpson EJ. *The Classification of Educational Objectives in the Psychomotor Domain*. Washington, DC: Gryphon House; 1972.
5. Perry WG. *Forms of Intellectual and Ethical Development in the College Years: A Scheme*. Troy, MO: Holt, Rinehart & Winston; 1970.
6. Chickering AW, Reisser L. *Education and Identity*. 2nd ed. San Francisco, CA: Jossey-Bass; 1993:1–42.
7. Pascarella ET, Terenzini PT. *How College Affects Students: Findings and Insights from Twenty Years of Research*. San Francisco, CA: Jossey-Bass; 1991.
8. Kitchner KS, King PM. The reflective judgment model: transforming assumptions about knowing. In Arnold KD, King IC, eds. *College Student Development and Academic Life*. New York, NY: Garland Publishing Inc; 1997:141–159.

9. Felder RM. Reaching the second tier—learning and teaching styles in college science education. *J Coll Sci Teach*. April–March 1993:286–290.

10. Solomon BA, Felder RM. Index of learning styles questionnaire. http://www.engr.ncsu.edu/learningstyles/ilsweb.html. Accessed February 27, 2009.

11. Austin Z. Development and validation of the Pharmacists' Inventory of Learning Styles (PILS). *Am J Pharm Educ*. 2004;68(2):1–10.

12. Howe N, Strauss W. *Millennials Rising: The Next Great Generation*. New York, NY: Vintage Books; 2000.

13. Zemke R, Raines C, Filipczak B. *Generations at Work: Managing the Clash of Veterans, Boomers, Xers, and Nexters in Your Workplace*. New York, NY: AMACOM; 2000.

14. Lovely S, Buffman AG. *Generations at School: Building an Age-Friendly Learning Community*. Thousand Oaks, CA: Corwin Press; 2007.

15. Sandfort MH, Haworth JG. Whassup? A glimpse into the attitudes and beliefs of the millennial generation. *J Coll Character*. 2006;(2):2–27.

16. National Center for Education Statistics. Enrollment in degree-granting institutions. September 2005 [cited March 22, 2010] [online]. http://nces.ed.gov/pubs2006/2006030_3a.pdf.

17. Borges NJ, Manuel RS, Elam CL, Jones BJ. Comparing Millennial and Generation X medical students at one medical school. *Acad Med*. 2006;81(6): 571–576.

18. Jonas-Dwyer D, Pospisil R. The Millennial effect: implications for academic development. In: Proceedings from the 2004 Conference of Higher Education Research and Development Society of Australia; Sarawak, Australia July 2004 [cited March 22, 2010] [online]. http://www.herdsa.org.au/conference2004/ Contributions/Rpapers/P050-jt.pdf.

19. Wilson ME. Teaching, learning, and Millennial students. In: Coomes MD, DeBard R, eds. *Serving the Millennial Generation*. San Francisco, CA: Jossey-Bass; 2004:59–72.

20. Chickering AW, Gamson ZF. Seven principles for good practice in undergraduate education. *AAHE Bulletin*. 1987;39(7):3–7.

21. Mangold, K. Educating a new generation: teaching baby boomer faculty about Millennial students. *Nurse Educ*. January–February 2007:21–23.

22. Pfaff E, Huddleston P. Does it matter if I hate teamwork? What impacts student attitudes toward teamwork. *J Mark Educ*. 2003;25(1):37–45.

23. Rodger S, Mickan S, Marinac J, Woodyatt G. Enhancing teamwork among allied health students: evaluation of an interprofessional workshop. *J Allied Health*. 2005;34(4):230–235.

24. Kolb DA. *Experiential Learning: Experience as the Source of Learning and Development*. Upper Saddle River, NJ: Prentice Hall; 1984:2–40.

Appendix 2–1
Pharmacists' Inventory of Learning Styles

Source: Courtesy of Austin Z. Development and validation of the Pharmacists' Inventory of Learning Styles (PILS). *Am J Pharm Educ.* 2004; 68(2): 1–10.

Think about a few recent situations where you had to learn something new to solve a problem. This could be any kind of situation—while you were taking a course at school, learning to use new software, or figuring out how to assemble a barbecue.

Now circle the letter in the column that best characterizes what works best for you in situations like the ones you have thought about.

When I Am Trying to Learn Something New . . .	Usually	Sometimes	Rarely	Hardly
1. I like to watch others before trying it for myself.	B	D	C	A
2. I like to consult a manual, textbook, or instruction guide first.	B	C	D	A
3. I like to work by myself rather than with other people.	A	C	B	D
4. I like to take notes or write things down as I am going along.	B	C	D	A
5. I am critical of myself if things do not work out as I had hoped.	B	C	D	A
6. I usually compare myself to other people just so I know I am keeping up.	B	D	C	A
7. I like to examine things closely instead of jumping right in.	B	D	C	A
8. I rise to the occasion if I am under pressure.	C	A	B	D
9. I like to have plenty of time to think about something new before trying it.	D	B	C	A
10. I pay a lot of attention to the details.	B	C	A	D
11. I concentrate on improving the things I did wrong in the past.	C	A	D	B
12. I focus on reinforcing the things I got right in the past.	B	D	A	C
13. I like to please the person teaching me.	D	B	A	C
14. I trust my hunches.	D	C	A	B

When I Am Trying to Learn Something New . . .	Usually	Sometimes	Rarely	Hardly
15. In a group, I am usually the first to finish whatever we are doing.	A	C	D	B
16. I like to take charge of a situation.	C	A	B	D
17. I am well organized.	B	A	C	D

Now, add the number of times you circled each letter:

A =   B =   C =   D =

Your *dominant* learning style is the letter you circled most frequently:

Your *secondary* learning style is the next most frequently circled letter:

A = Enactor

You enjoy dealing directly with people and have little time or patience for indirect or soft-sell jobs. You enjoy looking for and exploiting opportunities as they arrive and have an entrepreneurial spirit. You learn best in a hands-on, unencumbered manner, not a traditional lecture-style format. Though you do not take any particular pleasure in leading others, you do so because you sense you are best-suited for the job. You are confident, have strong opinions, and value efficiency. You are concerned about time and like to see a job get done. Sometimes, however, your concern with efficiency means the quality of your work may suffer and you may not pay as much attention to others' feelings and desires as you ought to.

B = Producer

You generally prefer to work by yourself, at your own pace, and in your own time, or with a very small group of like-minded people. You tend to avoid situations where you are the center of attention or constantly being watched—you prefer to be the one observing (and learning) from others. You have an ability to learn from your own—and other peoples'—mistakes. You place a high priority on getting things done properly, according to the rules, but at times you can be your own worst critic. You value organization and attentiveness to detail.

C = Director

You are focused, practical, and to the point. You usually find yourself in a leadership role and enjoy this challenge. You have little time or patience for those who dither or are indecisive or who spend too much time on impractical, theoretical matters. You are good at coming to quick, decisive conclusions, but you recognize that at times your speed may result in less than perfect results. You would rather get a good job done on time than do an excellent job delivered late. You like being in a high-performance, high-energy, fast-paced environment.

D = Creator

You enjoy out-of-the-box environments where time and resources are not particularly constrained. You have a flair for keeping others entertained and engaged, and you sincerely believe this is the way to motivate others and get the best out of everyone. You are most concerned—sometimes too concerned—about how others perceive you, and you place a high priority on harmony. You find little difficulty dealing with complex, ambiguous, theoretical situations (provided there is not a lot of pressure to perform), but sometimes you have a hard time dealing with the practical, day-to-day issues.

CHAPTER 3

What Matters in a Systems Approach to Learning and Teaching?

Judith T. Barr, ScD, MEd

Introduction

As you begin a new educational assignment—whether it is a new class, a new course, or a new assignment to lead a curricular revision—you are entering a complex system with many interrelated and interdependent elements. Internal to your university, these elements may originate from the students themselves; the courses they are taking prior to, concurrent with, or after your course; the physical properties of the room in which you will teach; or other curricular requirements of the college or university. External to the institution, accreditation bodies, professional and scientific organizations, national health professional curricular recommendations, clinical practice guidelines, and government regulations are among the many factors that can influence the content of classes, courses, and the curriculum.

As you gain experience and success in your academic career, you will likely be given more responsibility. At first, you may be assigned a few lectures, then it may be a course, then the development of a clinical or scientific content theme across the curriculum, and perhaps a capstone assignment of coordinating a review of your institution's doctor of pharmacy curriculum. In this chapter, you will be guided on this journey of increasing complexity. Using a systems approach, you will explore the interconnected factors to consider as you move through four increasingly complex scenarios: planning a lecture, organizing a course, coordinating the longitudinal development of a clinical area across the curriculum, and conducting a curricular review. As you progress in your faculty career, you will also gain expertise in your understanding of the elements and their interrelationships of this complex enterprise we call pharmacy education.

This chapter will help you answer the following questions:

- What is the systems approach to education? What are its characteristics?
- What are elements of the input, process, and outcome components in each scenario? What are their interrelationships?
- How and why do the elements of these three components vary with the scenario?
- What internal and external influencers affect each scenario?
- What is meant by the nested nature of the curriculum, a system within a system, and a longitudinal content theme?

In many ways, we applied features of the systems approach when designing and organizing this book. The goal of this book is for you to gain a deeper knowledge of, and comfort with, learning and teaching in pharmacy education. To enable you to do that, we identified important components of pharmacy education, organized the content into chapters, and then within each chapter we provided you with reflective exercises to assist you in applying the specific chapter content to your situation. Throughout the book we will show you how the content of various chapters are interrelated and interconnected. Now it is time for you to apply the systems approach to different aspects of pharmacy education.

What Is a System, Systems Thinking, and a Systems Approach?

Let us start with four quotations and accompanying brief explanations to illustrate the characteristics of a system, systems thinking, and a systems approach. This will provide the background that you will need as you consider the pharmacy education scenarios that follow.

> System: a complex of elements standing in interaction.[1]
> L. von Bertalanffy

A *system* can be defined as a complex of elements standing in interaction. We must think in terms of systems of elements in mutual interaction.[1]

What is a system? In the 1940s, von Bertalanffy, a German biologist, began to study biologic systems by identifying their "complex of elements" (component parts) and then examining the connections and interactions among these elements. If this approach could work in biology, he thought, why couldn't it work in other fields? And it did. His concept of thinking of a system and its interacting components rapidly diffused into other disciplines. In 1968, his book *General Systems Theory* was published.[2] By late 2009, the United States Library of Congress listed 783 books with "systems approach" in their titles. The subjects range widely from business to sociology to engineering to financial control to ecology to environmental challenges to climate change—and to education.

> A *system* is a network of interdependent components that work together to try to accomplish the aim of the system. A system must have an aim. Without an aim, there is no system.[3]

To von Bertalanffy's elements (Deming calls then *components*) and interactions, Deming added the need to have the aim or goal of a system identified. He primarily studied economic, business, and quality control systems, but his addition of the concept of *aim, goal,* or *output* was an important expansion of the general systems theory.

> *Systems thinking* is a discipline for seeing wholes. It is a framework for seeing interrelationships rather than things, for seeing patterns of change rather than static snapshots. It is a set of general principles—distilled over the course of the twentieth century, spanning fields as diverse as the physical and social sciences, engineering, and management. . . . During the last thirty years, these tools have been applied to understand a wide range of corporate, urban, regional, economic, political, ecological, and even psychological systems. And systems thinking is a sensibility—for the subtle interconnectedness that gives living systems their unique character.[4]

Senge added the concept of *wholes.*[4] Working primarily with management, organizational change, and competitiveness. Senge expanded the systems theory by including the whole of the system or organization. He argued that rather than focusing on individuals within a management system, an organization needs to understand the *whole* of its complex and dynamic system and work to align the units within an organization to the overall aims of the organization.

The next quotation is from the world of education. In its book *A Systems Approach to Teaching and Learning Procedures: A Guide for Educators,* the United Nations Educational, Scientific and Cultural Organization (UNESCO) encourages an international audience of those "professionally involved in education" to apply a systems approach to identify strengths and weaknesses and to make improvements.[5]

> The *systems approach* is a method: it is not a science or even a particular interpretation of education or social facts. Its purpose is to enable all those working within complex situations, whatever their role, to analyze this complexity, describe it, recognize dysfunctions when they occur, and allow for the various levels of social or institutional realities.[5]

> The systems approach is a method.[5]
> UNESCO

In this chapter, we will use the systems approach method to begin to understand the complexity of pharmacy education. We do this so that we can better plan and execute our learning and teaching experiences. As we begin our journey across four levels of pharmacy education, remember that systems thinking and the systems approach have three important characteristics:

1. The system and its aims or goals are identified. For purposes of this book, pharmacy education is our overall system, and the preparation of pharmacists who are ready for current and future pharmacy practice is our overall goal.

2. The system is composed of many elements, components, or subsystems that are influenced by many internal and external forces or influencers. All elements of the system are interconnected and interrelated, and changes in one element can have a ripple effect that alters other components. Ultimately, this could cause us to redefine our goal.

3. To understand the overall system and its elements, all elements of the system must be identified and the system viewed *holistically*. In systems thinking, we must think holistically and identify all of those subsystems and influencers (e.g., classes, courses, students, faculty, environmental and regulatory factors) that shape, influence, and affect the achievement of the goals of the overall system. For example, what happens in one course may influence future classes in the curriculum and ultimately practice experiences.

Reflective Exercise

The respiratory system, a backyard garden, a baseball team, a university, and a city can all be considered systems. What are the aims of each? Considering the whole of each system, what are the elements of each, and how do they interconnect and interact? What other systems can you identify?

_____

_____

_____

_____

What Matters in the Systems Approach to Education?

For an education system, what matters? Cromwell and Scileppi called for a systems approach to provide "a better understanding of the complexity of schools and the education process."[6] Kaufman, also writing from a general education perspective, identified some of the components of an educational system as "teaching and instruction, management and administration, facilities and support, community, and learners."[7]

But is there evidence supporting the use of a systems approach in education, or is it all theory? For those interested in further background in the area, a series of Web-based exchanges in late 2009 provides a rich review of available evidence. Nora Bynum, project director of the Network of Conservation Educators and Practitioners, issued the following challenge to the e-community in an POD post: "While we support the need to approach teaching from an integrated, systems-based perspective that emphasizes interconnections and attenuating or reinforcing feedback interactions . . . we have had trouble locating published literature that talks about successes (or failures) trying to teach using systems-based approaches" (Nora Bynum, PhD, POD Listserve, October 19, 2009). She listed seven references (primarily from the intersection of ecology and economics education) and asked others to contribute to the evidence.

Richard Hake, emeritus professor of physics at Indiana University, responded with a bibliography of articles and postings documenting the effect of a systems approach in ecology and economics as well as university programs in physics,[8] ecosystems,[9] and other fields (Richard Hake, PhD, NET-GOLD listserv, October 27, 2009). Hake's 2002 article, "Lessons from the Physics Education Reform Effort,"[8] not only provided particularly valuable evidence of, and insight into, the effectiveness of the systems approach in physics education reform, but it also contained his subjective identification of 14 lessons learned from the experience. Several quotations from his lessons learned will appear among the marginal notes in the following sections. Last, at the end of 2009, Hake expanded his online bibliography to over 200 annotated citations on systems thinking across many fields, including applications in education.[10]

Published studies of the use of a systems approach in pharmacy education are sparse. Only one evidence-based evaluation of a systems approach in pharmacy education was identified. Planas and Er[11] used a systems approach to progressively develop the communication skills of student pharmacists and then demonstrated the effectiveness of the approach by documenting improvements in assessment scores. Also, in the 2009 Rho Chi lecture, Manasse called for the creation of interdisciplinary and interprofessional educational experiences for pharmacy students and applied a systems approach to suggest a means by which his proposal could be implemented.[12]

What Matters in Applying the Systems Approach to Pharmacy Education? The Four Pharmacy Education Scenarios

The remainder of this chapter is organized around the application of the systems approach to four educational scenarios of increasing complexity: a single class, a course, the development of a content theme across the curriculum, and a review of the doctor of pharmacy curriculum for your institution. Within each scenario, you will be guided through the analysis of each situation using a systems approach.

But how can each be considered a system? Isn't a system supposed to be viewed holistically? Meadows and Wright, in their book *Thinking in Systems: A Primer*, say "There are no separate systems. The world is a continuum. Where to draw a boundary around a system depends on the purpose of the discussion."[13] So, for purposes of this discussion, the holistic world of pharmacy education will be viewed as a series of nested concentric circles or systems set within an internal environment (inside your institution) and an external environment (outside your institution) (see **Figure 3–1**). A boundary is first drawn around a class, and it is treated as a system. Classes form a course, courses are grouped within a semester, semesters form a year, and the classes across all years constitute the curriculum. Each successive layer pushes out the system boundary and redraws it around the next more complex level. Remember that each of the previous systems now becomes an element within the progressively larger system. To the overall pharmacy education system, all of this can be influenced by factors internal to the university, such as institution-specific curriculum requirements as well as external factors, such as the healthcare system, accreditation standards, state board of pharmacy requirements, and other policies and regulations.

But there is one cautionary note as we examine each of our scenarios: what is *internal* and what is *external* to a system is relative; it is very much dependent in which system you stand. For example, if you are teaching biopharmaceutics (a system at the course level), what is taught in physical chemistry is an important external influencer on your course. But if you are examining the overall PharmD curriculum system, then both of these courses are internal to your systems approach.

Scenario 1: The Class

You are a new clinical faculty member and have been asked by the therapeutics coordinator to give a lecture on diabetes pharmacotherapy in next semester's therapeutics class. You have completed a PGY1 pharmacy practice residency, and last year you completed a PGY2 ambulatory care residency. You feel very qualified to present the class but also see it as a challenge. You ask yourself, Where do I start?

Reflective Exercise

Stop now and jot down some answers to the following three questions in **Table 3.1**:

1. What is the aim of the class (the system of Scenario 1)?
2. From a holistic perspective, what are the elements (the component parts) of the class? At this point, complete only the left-hand column for this question.
3. How are the elements connected and how do they interact?

Table 3–1 Systems Approach Work Sheet for Planning a Single Class

1. What is the aim of the class? (In this scenario, the system is the class.)

2. From a holistic perspective, what are the elements (the component parts) of the class?

3. How are the elements connected and how do they interact?

	Input	Process	Output

4. Select two of your elements and map their interconnections with other elements in your list.

What Is the Aim of the Class?

Did you have trouble with this question? Do you think the therapeutics coordinator's request lacked specificity? If you answered yes, you are right.

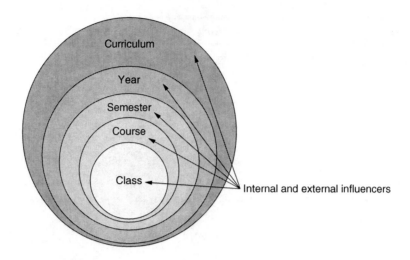

Figure 3–1 Systems Set Within Internal and External Environments

Note: Class content is part of a course that is presented in a semester during a year within the doctor of pharmacy curriculum. All components of the curriculum influence one another and in turn are influenced by internal and external factors.

What does "give a lecture on diabetes pharmacotherapy" mean? Are you to cover all medications across all patient age ranges for all types of settings and for all forms of diabetes? What does "cover" mean—just the drugs or also their mechanisms of action? Are you to develop the topic from a historic perspective or focus only on current pharmacotherapeutic agents? What about drugs that are in the drug approval pipeline? Are adherence–persistence, psychosocial–economic, and cultural–ethnic issues to be included?

You could determine the aim of the class by yourself, but as you know from a systems approach, your class is nested within the therapeutics course. What you do in your session can have an impact on other parts of the system. You could talk to the faculty member who gave the class last year, but what if the course coordinator changed the flow and content of this year's course? A better strategy would be to talk to the course coordinator directly and, based on your expertise and the coordinator's overall course aims, the two of you can mutually determine the specific aims for your therapeutics session. With these aims firmly established, you can proceed with planning the class. If you have more questions during your planning process, be sure to ask the coordinator for further clarification.

From a Holistic Perspective, What Are the Elements (the Component Parts) of the Class?

Now that you have the aims established, naturally the first thing you want to do is to start planning the subject content of the class and determining

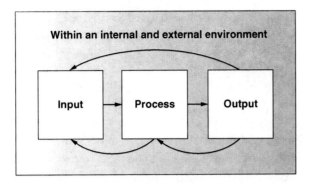

Figure 3–2 Initial Elements of a Systems Approach to Education

how you will organize its flow. But from a systems approach, you also realize that the content is only part of the system. Whether or not the aim of the class is achieved is dependent on such factors as student characteristics, classroom arrangement, technology availability, and other factors. You decide to use the two months before your class to apply some systems thinking to identify these factors and understand their interconnections. With a holistic understanding of the system in place, you can then plan the content of your class and improve the effectiveness of the learning–teaching process.

Let us consider more of these elements and organize them into the three phases of your class: its input, process, and output. **Figure 3–2** summarizes the concept that inputs of the class affect the processes used in class, and those processes affect the outputs—all three components are interconnected and interrelated. Feedback is an important feature of the system; information about one component of a system can serve as feedback to prompt revisions in another component.

Reflective Exercise

Look at the elements you identified in Table 3–1. Now indicate in the right-hand table columns whether you would classify each as an input, process, or output. Can you identify more elements that you need to consider as you plan your class? If so, enter them in Table 3–1 and indicate the type of the input element. You will refer back to this table as you compare these responses to additional examples in the sections that follow.

Phase One: Input   As you plan your class and identify *input* elements, consider how they could influence the content and approach you could use during the class session. Seven examples follow:

1. *Previous content*: What is the background of the students? Based on the diabetes-related content that students have received from this and previous courses, will they have sufficient preparation for your class and the content you wish to cover? Will you need to present new preparatory material? Will you need to review previous content?

2. *The course*: How is the course organized? Does the course have a combined reading pack, or are instructors responsible for their own assignments and readings? If you want a preclass assignment, is this possible? How do you communicate this to the students? How long is your class? Is there sufficient time for the content you initially want the student to learn? Is there a scheduled break in the class? Will that affect the flow of the material? What is the content in the therapeutics class before and after yours? Is a seminar or practice laboratory session associated with the course? Is a diabetes case or exercise scheduled for those sessions?

3. *Students*: How many students are in the class? Given what you learned from Chapter 2, what characteristics of Millennial students need to be considered as you plan your class?

4. *Physical space*: How large is the classroom? How are the seats organized? Are they fixed seats, or are the chairs moveable? If you want to have time for small groups to discuss a case during the class session, is that possible within your classroom? Is distance learning involved?

5. *Available technology*: What type of technology is available? Do you need a microphone, and is one available? Are a computer and an attached projector present for visuals? If audience response systems ("clickers") are used in the course, do you know how to use the technology? Is audio recording equipment available if you decide to have the lecture component available via podcast? If you want to assign preclass readings, is there a way to electronically communicate the assignment to the class?

6. *Learning and teaching strategies*: Your understanding of various strategies to improve the student-centered, learning–teaching process is an important element as you design your class. What teaching and learning strategies are appropriate and can be used in this course? What strategies have been used in previous sessions of this course? Have you used interactive engagement (IE) strategies?

7. *Currency of content for the class*: What are the current practice guidelines for type 2 diabetes treatment as recommended by the American Diabetes Association (ADA)[14] and the American Association of

> The use of IE or high-tech methods, by themselves, does not ensure superior student learning.
> R.R. Hake

Clinical Endocrinologists (AACE)[15]? Are new therapies expected in the future? Are there any controversies in clinical approaches?

Phase Two: Process   In the next phase, how you organize and present the class content (the *process* elements) is dependent on what you learned from the input phase. The systems approach has helped you identify these inputs, and now you can consider them as you proceed. This helps you better plan a student-centered class that is appropriate, given the students' characteristics and prior learning, the structure of the course and its physical setting, the available technology, and the currency of the class content.

Let us identify several *process* elements and then consider how each interconnects with what you have learned from the input phase. Also see Chapter 5 (large classroom), Chapter 6 (technology), and Chapter 7 (small group discussion) as well as Chapter 2 (student-centered learning); they will be valuable as you plan your class.

Class Content   Based on the specific aims of your class, you have tailored the class content given such inputs as your review of diabetes-related content in the students' previous courses and the time constraints of this class.

For this therapeutics course, the course coordinator does not use an integrated course pack; instructors are responsible for their own assignments and handouts. You do have access to a Web-based student notification system. Therefore, two weeks before your class, you e-mail the students the reading assignments, the objectives of your class, and a copy of the PowerPoint slides. You include a list of questions to help the students focus on the important content of the readings and the PowerPoint slides. You consider giving a Web-based pretest, but because students have not had such an assignment before, you decide not to do it.

Learning–Teaching Methods   The course, which consists of two 50-minute halves with a 10-minute break, has 160 enrolled students. The course is held in an amphitheater with 180 fixed seats, designed primarily for a lecture-type presentation. A distance learning component is not present with this course. The room is equipped with a computer and an attached projector. A student response system has not been used in this course, and students do not have the individual response pad technology. This is an example of the interconnectedness of elements; the unavailability of technology (an input) prevents your use of this type of learning and teaching strategy in your class (the process). However, other types of interactive engagement strategies are still possible.

Given Bloom's cognitive learning taxonomy, the learning characteristics of Millennial students, the classroom arrangement, and available technology, what processes would you use in your class? For example, you could use the 100-minute time block to divide the class into two 50-minute parts and use different learning–teaching processes with progressively more active learning as the class progresses. In the first half of the class you could use a lecture to gradually build the subject content, following the stages of Bloom's Taxonomy (understand, apply, analyze, and evaluate). To encourage active learning, as you develop the content and scaffolding for more complex learning, you could insert questions into your PowerPoint slides. After the break, again to encourage active learning, you could direct the students to pair up with a student in an adjacent chair, and based on your lecture have them create a summary chart of the classes of antidiabetic agents, their primary uses and mechanisms of action, and the advantages and disadvantages of each. To help them get organized, you could project an empty chart of the categories on the screen. After the pairs have worked for 20 minutes, you could bring the collective class together, and in a group activity they could assist you as you complete a projected version of the chart. Finally, using a third learning–teaching process, you could end the class with the student pairs determining the appropriate medication therapy management strategy of several patients with diabetes, followed by a collective wrap up. See Chapter 5 for further development of what matters in large classroom instruction.

Reflective Exercise

For the previous input and process examples, list the ways in which information from the analysis of the inputs influenced the learning–teaching processes. One example is provided: the lack of a technology (input) prevented the use of a learning–teaching strategy (a process). Also look at the elements you identified in Table 3–1. Can you identify interrelations between some of your identified input and process components? Are they supportive or restrictive relationships?

_____

_____

_____

_____

Phase Three: Output   What is the *output* of this systems approach to planning and presenting the pharmacotherapy of diabetes to your class? What are some output elements that you can include to determine if you have met the aims, goals, or objectives of the class? What other outcome elements or measures are important to you?

First, consider it from your point of view. Immediately after the session, take some time to write your reflections of the session. Was the coverage of content appropriate for the time of the session? Did the students read the assigned readings before class? What seemed to work in the processes you selected for the class? Did the students appear to be engaged? Did they take the two in-class exercises seriously? When you brought the class back together and had the collective class discussion, did the students have appropriate answers to your follow-up questions? If you are responsible for this class again, what would you change about the class, and why?

Second, consider asking the course coordinator to attend your class and provide feedback to you. Before the class, you could ask the coordinator to critique specific aspects of the class, or you could ask the individual to provide holistic feedback.

Third, consider asking the students to complete a brief survey at the end of class. Ask them the same questions that you asked yourself, but give them a Likert scale set of responses. This will give you the students' perception of how well the class went.

Fourth, we know that the students' learning needs to be objectively measured to determine whether they have achieved the aims of the class. Be sure that the aims, the class content, and the evaluation methods are aligned. Appropriate test questions should evaluate the content and level of learning that was included in the learning–teaching process, which in turn was based on the aims of the class.

Finally, an ideal long-term output measure would be to determine if students can apply the content to patients in an advanced pharmacy practice experience (APPE). A survey of APPE preceptors could provide this information.

The systems approach to learning–teaching now requires that you perform one more step—the *feedback* step. This is illustrated by the feedback arcs in Figure 3–2. You can use the results from various output measures to improve characteristics of the input elements as well as modify the processes within the class. For example, suppose that students indicated that they liked the in-class discussions and that the process helped them apply the concepts from the class. However, they indicated that a more structured collection of their individual responses to questions in the first half of the class would be helpful. This feedback directs you to consider if, the next time you present this class, audience response systems (input elements) would be helpful in improving the learning–teaching experience (process elements).

At first reading, planning a class from a systems approach may appear to be quite complex. But the implicit input scan you presently use when planning a class is likely to be insufficient to identify the many interactions among the numerous factors that you need to consider when planning a learning–teaching experience. And most likely, you are conducting it from a faculty-centered, not a student-centered, perspective. The use of the systems approach and systems thinking, guides you to see the complex interconnections, interrelations, and interactions among the elements of this system we have defined as an instructional class. With clarity of aims for the class; identification of input, process, and output elements and their interactions; and application of feedback information, you have a holistic approach to the learning–teaching system and to the education of a student pharmacist.

Scenario 2: The Course

You have been a pharmaceutical science faculty member at your school of pharmacy for the last four years. In planning your faculty load for next year with your department chair, she asks you to assume teaching the first in the two-course sequence of pharmacology courses. Given your doctoral work and postdoctoral research fellowship in endocrine pharmacology, you are well qualified for this assignment. Also, although another faculty member has been the coordinator of this course for the last two years, you are currently teaching 40 percent of the classes and have been using the systems approach as you plan, present, evaluate, and revise your sessions. Now you ask yourself, Where do I start preparing for assuming responsibility for the course? What do I have to do now that I am in charge of the course?

> A course is more than a collection of class sessions.

A course is more than a collection of class sessions, and applying a systems approach to a course involves more than planning a series of classes. Your systems boundary is now defined as the *course*; all its input, process, and output elements are now something for you to consider. In this section the primary focus is on the input elements for a course. Further development of the processes involved in large classrooms will be found in Chapter 5 and assessment issues are presented in Chapter 4.

Reflective Exercise

Reflect upon the differences between presenting several lectures in a class and assuming responsibilities for a course. Using a systems approach, identify three input elements that you need to consider in the design and presentation of the course that you would generally not need to include when planning only several classes.

_____

_____

_____

_____

Before we examine the course inputs, let us consider the aim of the course, or because your course is a part of a two-course sequence, why not develop the goals and objectives for the complete two-part pharmacology package with the other course instructor? This would provide a good opportunity to involve faculty in both pharmacology courses and other courses for which pharmacology is a prerequisite. When the overall pharmacology goals are set, then the content can be parsed between the two courses and sequenced within each.

With the course goals in place, let us now examine seven categories of inputs given in this scenario:

1. *Operations*: This is a catchall category for all things that affect the physical operations of your course and the teaching–learning environment. What are the characteristics of the assigned *classroom*? Given that you are a strong proponent of active learning activities, will the classroom accommodate this approach? Are small-group discussions possible? What type of *technology* is available in and out of the classroom? Is the room equipped for audience response systems? For your computer and projection needs? Is software available for site-of-action drug simulations? Will you be able to communicate with students and post material via Blackboard or similar systems?

2. *Course schedule*: Although you generally do not have control over the assigned class times, you do have control over the dates of tests and major projects. Consider a student-centered approach and meet with other faculty who are teaching in the same semester. Coordinate the class schedules so that the student stress points are spread apart as much as possible. Also, if the subject matter permits, consider asking each course instructor to cross-reference and make connections with content in other courses that students are taking that semester. For example, consider a semester when students are taking both pharmacoeconomics (PE) and therapeutics. One week, the therapeutics topic is depression and associated treatment modalities, and in PE the students are learning about cost-effectiveness analysis (CEA). This would be an ideal time for the PE instructor to illustrate CEA concepts by using examples from the depression CEA literature. Survey results from unpublished PE course surveys indicate that students appreciate seeing this type of linkage between concurrent courses (Barr, 2008, Northeastern University).

3. *Syllabus*: The syllabus for your course is your contract with the students. It is a public document and conveys to your students, fellow faculty members, and the administration the organization of your course, your policies, your assignments and deadlines, your expectations of the students, and their responsibilities. Many universities

have lists of required elements that must be included in a syllabus. An excellent syllabus development tutorial is provided on the Web by the Center for Teaching and Learning at the University of Minnesota.[16]

4. *Textbook*: The course book is an important input; its selection requires a balancing of several factors. The book that contains the most information may be so dense that the format impedes student learning. Remember that different students have different learning styles (see Chapter 2); visual appeal and page layout would be important considerations for visual learners. Other factors to consider in the textbook selection include currency of content, inclusion of learning exercises and other study aids for students, availability of instructor teaching aids, and price.

5. *Faculty*: Will you be the only faculty member, or will you be the coordinator of several faculty members who are each responsible for different subject content and classes? Obviously, there is less administrative work if you are the sole instructor; however, there is more course preparation and organization. If you are the course coordinator, you need to consider your faculty as inputs to the course. Identify what elements of the learning–teaching process you would like to have consistent across all classes in the course and communicate that to the participating faculty. This could be as simple as a standard PowerPoint template or as complex as consistent learning–teaching strategies. Consider inserting forms of interactive engagement (IE) in as many classes as possible.

> The use of IE strategies can increase the effectiveness of conceptually difficult courses well beyond that obtained by traditional methods.[8]
>
> R.R. Hake

Assist faculty who may need development in some of these areas. For example, if you would like all faculty to include in-class active learning experiences, you may want to ask the staff in your campus learning and teaching center to offer a session on active learning and instructional engagement strategies to the faculty participating in your course.

6. *Students*: Pharmacology is scheduled relatively early in the professional years of the curriculum. Although you have taught this course for the last two years, now is an excellent time for you to consider if the course is designed at the appropriate level given the students' intellectual development and level of reflective judgment. Based on the content of Chapter 2, what types of learning and teaching strategies and evaluative approaches would be appropriate for students in this class?

7. *Previous content*: Given the aims of the class and your identification of the objectives for the course, do the students have the appropriate content and level of preparation from previous classes? Because you will assume the course next year, is the prerequisite course being offered now? Can you talk with its instructor about subject

content that would be valuable to students to master so that the bridge is stronger for entry into your course?

These are several of the additional inputs that need to be considered as you plan a course. Additional factors will be considered in the chapters on large classrooms (Chapter 5), teaching with technology (Chapter 6), and laboratory-based courses (Chapter 7).

Scenario 3: Topic-Specific Longitudinal Curricular Content

You have been a preceptor in an ambulatory diabetes clinic for 10 years and have taught the diabetes lectures in the therapeutics sequence for the last six years. Over the last four years you have worked with the pharmacology and pathophysiology faculty to develop an interconnected coverage sequence of diabetes content across these three courses. Also, for the last three years you have served on the pharmacy curriculum committee. This year the chair of the curriculum committee asked you to head a task force to make recommendations for updating the longitudinal diabetes content across the curriculum. You are excited about the assignment and feel prepared given your clinical experience, content expertise, work with the pharmaceutical science faculty, and experience on the curriculum committee. Now you ask yourself, Where do I start?

What an exciting opportunity to look across courses and develop a longitudinal diabetes curriculum! Now your system boundary has been drawn across content within courses throughout a curriculum, rather than a single course. The members of your task force are representative; they are faculty members who teach diabetes-related content in pharmaceutical sciences, social and administrative sciences, clinical practice, and experiential courses. Your first thought is to work with the members on the task force, and with them and other affected faculty, to start to define the goals of the diabetes content curriculum project. What are the diabetes-specific knowledge, skills, and attitudes that student pharmacists need to be able to achieve by graduation? What are the diabetes-specific, abilities-based outcomes (ABOs), and what enabling content will the students need to achieve these ABOs?

However, identifying the diabetes-specific ABOs at this time is likely to be premature. Preparatory work is needed before that step. The task force needs to collect information from both internal and external sources and educate itself; it needs to identify the necessary inputs to do its business. First, consider conducting an internal diabetes-specific curriculum mapping project.[17] What diabetes-specific content is presently covered and in what courses? Conduct a brief survey of all faculty and ask them to identify in which course (if any) they cover diabetes content or include diabetes-related examples. Map the progressive development of the present content longitudinally across the curriculum.[18] The identification of what is currently present in the curriculum provides a baseline of the content and is a vital input to your progress.

Second, conduct an environment scan by collecting inputs from external sources. This will help you identify what is new or under development in the field. Perform literature searches, interview experts, consult patient advocacy groups, and review policy statements of pharmacy, medical, and public health organizations. Identify promising research findings as well as controversies in the field. Think broadly during this phase and examine topics from the pharmaceutical sciences to population and public health. In addition to traditional scientific and clinical fields, examine the diabetes objectives in Healthy People 2020[19] as well as explore the broad pharmacy education and practice implications found in such resources as the educational underpinnings of Healthy People 2020 in the Clinical Prevention and Population Health Curriculum Framework,[20] the Centers for Disease Control and Prevention Health Systems Dynamics Project,[21] and the National Academies of Practice call for interdisciplinary practice.[12,22] This approach provides the potential for the proposed curriculum to be as inclusive and futuristic as possible.

Third, examine the information you have collected from internal and external sources. Critically review your inputs and, using a work sheet similar to **Table 3–2**, make an exhaustive list of the curricular elements that your task force thinks could be included in the coverage of diabetes-related topics. Indicate if the topic is presently covered and in which courses, or determine if it is a proposed new topic.

Table 3–2 Work Sheet for Curriculum Content Identification and Course Mapping: Selected Examples from Social Administrative Sciences Content Area

Curricular Elements	Covered Now?	What Course?	New Content	Retain Topic Y/N	In What Course?
Adherence/persistence issues					
Stages of change (example)					
Diabetes-related impact on quality of life					

Cultural issues related to:
   Food selection
   Health beliefs					

Socioeconomic status					
Environmental and community issues					
Medicare coverage of diabetes supplies					

Now it is time to define the diabetes-specific ABOs. Your task force has examined the internal and external inputs, identified possible diabetes-related content, and organized these topics. You have the needed information to develop ABOs that will be relevant and contemporary. With your ABOs clearly stated, you can proceed in the work sheet and determine whether each of the curricular content elements contributes to the student achievement of one or more of the new ABOs. Through an iterative process, determine whether each content element should be retained, and if so, in what course your task force would recommend that it be placed. As you do this, be realistic about what new content the curriculum can absorb, but also be strategic to reduce duplication across the curriculum while maintaining linkages among courses for longitudinal content development. Last, consider placement of content in different settings; for example, how can diabetes content be covered in a didactic course on campus, reinforced in an introductory pharmacy practice experience, and then followed up with more advanced content when the student returns to campus.

Reflective Exercise

Select a disease state. What resources, professional organizations, or other bodies would you contact for external inputs as you identify relevant disease-specific content? What disease-specific curricular elements would you list? What broader topics, such as cultural competence and motivational interviewing, are needed for your selected disease state as well as across many disease states?

_____

_____

_____

_____

Scenario 4: Comprehensive Curriculum Review

You have been an active faculty member in the school of pharmacy for the last 10 years. You have fulfilled the three responsibilities of a tenure-track faculty—you taught several courses in the doctor of pharmacy curriculum, received external funding and published your research, and served on the curriculum and several other committees. After you received tenure, the dean asked you to chair the curriculum committee, and given that the school's self-study for the Accreditation Council for Pharmacy Education (ACPE) is due in two years, she asked the curriculum committee to conduct a thorough review of the curriculum and make recommendations for improvements. You are excited about such an opportunity, and now you ask yourself, Where do I start?

Books have been written about goals and processes for curriculum development and review, so it is presumptuous to think that a section of a chapter can be anything more than an introduction—and a focused introduction it will be. Remember that this chapter started with identifying the overall goal of our system (the doctor of pharmacy program at your institution)—the preparation of pharmacists for current and future pharmacy practice. As in the previous scenario, you must start your process with collecting information to determine what are current and future pharmacy practices, refining your current programmatic ABOs based on your internal and external scans, identifying content needed to achieve these ABOs, and mapping the ABOs to content in specific courses.

Pharmacy-Specific Sources of Information

This section is focused on five important sources of external information (the inputs) that are important for you to review in this process. Over the last 20 years, a number of pharmacy organizations have issued reports or policies that have defined and then redefined the practice of pharmacy. Within a few years, as systems theory predicts, these reports influenced changes in curriculum content recommendations, accreditation standards, and licensure examinations. Of most relevance for a current review of a doctor of pharmacy curriculum would be those that have been issued since 2004. Several of these reports are briefly reviewed in the following discussion; their contents should provide the foundation upon which a contemporary doctor of pharmacy curriculum can be built. All reports and sources were current as of late 2009. As mentioned, in this system of interrelated elements, a change in the position or report from one source is likely to prompt changes in other positions, policies, and requirements. Therefore, you are cautioned to check for more recent updates as time passes.

The year 2004 was a busy one for pharmacy education and practice statements. In anticipation of the movement to the all PharmD curriculum, in May 2004 the American Association of Colleges of Pharmacy's (AACP) Center for the Advancement of Pharmaceutical Education (CAPE) issued the 2004 CAPE Educational Outcomes.[23] This document identified three sets of educational outcomes that pharmacy graduates should achieve for entry to practice: (1) provide pharmaceutical care to patients and populations, (2) manage various types of resources and medication use systems, and (3) promote public health, cooperate in interdisciplinary teams, and develop public health policy. The 2005–2006 AACP Educational Outcomes and Objectives Supplement Task Force produced detailed curriculum supplements in 10 disciplinary areas to support the broad statement of the 2004 CAPE Educational Outcomes. These curriculum guides are a rich source of content detail and are valuable for curriculum review purposes. The AACP provides the 2004 CAPE Educational Outcomes document and each of the 10 discipline-specific supplements on its Web site.[23]

In July 2004, a coalition of 11 pharmacy organizations issued a collective position paper called "Medication Therapy Management Services: Definition and Program Criteria."[24] This statement is an itemized description of a more proactive form of patient-specific pharmacy practice in all types of settings. In medication therapy management (MTM), the pharmacist goes beyond the general dispensing and education functions and actively consults with a specific patient and other care providers as needed, to enable the patient to achieve optimal medication therapy and therapeutic outcomes. Nine (nondispensing) activities and responsibilities are identified as constituting MTM services; each summarizes a different method by which pharmacists can manage and improve medication therapy. The identification of these activities, and the knowledge and skills necessary to perform them, provides inputs to consider during the curriculum review process. Incidentally, an important component of this position paper is the statement that an MTM service should receive payment for these services regardless of whether dispensing services were provided.

Three months later the Joint Commission of Pharmacy Practitioners (JCPP), which consists of many of the same organizations that developed the MTM statement, published its collective view of the preferred type of pharmacy practice 10 years in the future. Its report, "Future Vision of Pharmacy Practice," envisions that by 2015, pharmacists will (1) provide patient-centered care, population-based care, and wellness and health prevention support; (2) have the authority and autonomy to be responsible for the management of drug therapy; and (3) be recognized and appropriately compensated for services, including consultation.[25] Again, the goal is for pharmacists to provide optimal medication therapy management and to receive appropriate compensation for such services. However, realizing that the achievement of the MTM model of pharmacy practice will require changes in the underlying pharmacy business model, insurance coverage policies, state and federal legislation, and attitudes of patients and other healthcare professionals, JCPP issued an action plan in 2008 to implement its vision.[26] This 86-page document provides an excellent view into the financial, political, power, and policy issues that affect the future world of pharmacy practice. As such, it is an important input in the curriculum of future practitioners.

In this milieu of envisioned changes in professional pharmacy practice, between 2003 and 2006 the ACPE revised the standards for pharmacy education programs, making the doctor of pharmacy degree a requirement for pharmacy education programs starting in 2007. Central to the new requirements published in *Accreditation Standards and Guidelines for the Professional Program in Pharmacy Leading to the Doctor of Pharmacy Degree*[27] are expanded clinical course work and patient care experiences. Embedded within the 30 accreditation standards are numerous direct and indirect references to curriculum content requirements and expectations. The attainment of problem solving and critical thinking skills and the development of

> A good hockey player plays where the puck is. A great hockey player plays where the puck is going to be.
> Wayne Gretzky

leadership and professionalism are also emphasized. The elements of the scientific content that ACPE identified as necessary for the development of pharmacists is provided in Appendix B of their report. The 30 ACPE standards, particularly the curriculum standards (standards 9–15), and the curriculum elements in Appendix B are important inputs into the systems approach to conducting a curriculum review of the PharmD program.

Another input to pharmacy curriculum development is the Blueprint and Competency Statements of the North American Pharmacist Licensure Examination (NAPLEX). This document guides the composition and complexity of questions in the NAPLEX examination. In late 2009, after an analysis of the contemporary changes in pharmacy practice and the level and type of knowledge that is now needed for practice, the National Association of Boards of Pharmacy updated the NAPLEX Blueprint, effective for the March 2010 examination.[28] According to the Blueprint, the NAPLEX examination consists of three parts. The majority of the test items (approximately 56 percent) will "assess pharmacotherapy to assure safe and effective therapeutic outcomes." Questions related to assurance of "safe and accurate preparation and dispensing of medication" constitute approximately 35 percent of the test, and items covering information related to the provision of healthcare information and promotion of public health constitute 11 percent. The Blueprint, which contains more content detail within each of these three sections, provides additional input information for curriculum development and review.[28]

Although the five sources previously discussed are all formal documents and policy statements of organizations, they are subject to change as the profession and its practices evolve. For example, change is already underway within the AACP. In September 2009, the association sponsored the AACP Curricular Change Summit to examine issues of critical importance in redefining the professional curriculum. Five white papers were commissioned to stimulate thought and debate during the summit.[29] Although the thoughts in the papers and the debate at the summit represent individual opinions, the process has been started to revise the association's curriculum-related documents, such as the CAPE outcomes statements.[23] Jungnickel et al.'s white paper for the summit, "Addressing Competencies for the Future in the Professional Curriculum," proposes revision to pharmacy practice competencies and "the development of five cross-cutting abilities: professionalism, self-directed learning, leadership and advocacy, interprofessional collaboration, and cultural competency."[30] As you consider the PharmD curriculum for present and future practice, the review of this set of white papers, particularly the Jungnickel paper, will prepare your task force for future curriculum considerations and changes.

For those who are interested in including inputs from even further projected alternative futures, consider the report of the 2007–2008 Argus Commission[31] that examined the implications to pharmacy education of

> Change is constant.
> Benjamin Disraeli

the Institute for Alternative Futures report, "The 2029 Project: Achieving an Ethical Future for Biomedical R&D."[32]

Cross-Disciplinary, Interprofessional Curriculum Projects

Pharmacists are members of the healthcare team, and as such, pharmacy education should consider broader health education issues that cross disciplinary boundaries. National curriculum projects have developed curriculum objectives and content for cross-disciplinary instruction in such topics as health promotion and disease prevention,[20] interdisciplinary delivery of health care,[22] cultural competence,[33] and genetics.[34] From ACPE accreditation standards[27] and several pharmacy-specific curricular recommendations,[12,23,30,31] it is clear that these interprofessional topics are important components of pharmacy practice. These documents provide content guidance during the curriculum review process.

Reflective Exercise

You feel comfortable with how you will organize and incorporate pharmacy-specific scientific and clinical curriculum elements identified by the five sources in the previous sections. But even after you identify interprofessional curriculum content that you want to retain, how do you incorporate it into your pharmacy-specific curriculum? You could embed it in pharmacy-only courses, but is that meeting the broader intent of the recommendations? What are at least two recommendations (one embedded in an on-campus activity or course and one during clinical experience) that the task force could make to enable the students in the professions to learn together before they practice together?

_____

_____

_____

_____

Other Inputs

As described earlier, the doctor of pharmacy program is a series of nested classes and courses set within a curriculum that itself is shaped by external pharmacy-specific recommendations and regulations. But to be true to the holistic nature of the systems approach to curriculum review, the environmental scan needs to examine inputs such as the following:

- Requirements of your own institution
- Institutional resources
- State-specific licensure or practice requirements or regulations of your state board of pharmacy

- Requirements and regulations of regional education accreditation boards
- Requirements and regulations of the U.S. Department of Education
- Policies of third-party payers
- Policies of your experiential sites
- Trends in the organization of, and payment for, pharmacy-specific healthcare services
- Other inputs that affect the ones mentioned

These are only a few of the influencers that are present in the internal and external environments as shown in Figures 3–1 and 3–2. Although a faculty member who is preparing a class is unlikely to consider these higher-level influencers, they should be part of a comprehensive environmental scan during the curriculum review process. Remember what Meadows said: "There are no separate systems. The world is a continuum. Where to draw a boundary around a system depends on the purpose of the discussion."[13]

Summary

Our journey to apply a systems approach to the pharmacy curriculum has led us through a comprehensive examination of the world of pharmacy education. You have used a holistic systems approach to travel through a class, a course, a stream of topic-specific content across a curriculum, and a comprehensive curriculum review assignment. Each time you have defined the boundaries of the system, defined the systems' aims and goals, and identified and analyzed the inputs specific to that system. You have seen how the elements within a system interconnect and how the various levels of a system interact and interrelate.

This chapter has primarily helped you consider the *inputs* as you moved through progressively more complex educational systems. The output component and its assessment are covered in the next chapter. The process components, specific to various types of teaching and learning situations, will then follow. Enjoy your journey!

References

1. von Bertalanffy L. *Problems of Life*. New York, NY: Harper Torchbooks; 1960.
2. von Bertalanffy L. 1968. *General Systems Theory: Foundations, Development, Applications*. New York, NY: George Brazelier Inc; 1968.
3. Deming, WE. *The New Economics for Industry, Government & Education*. Cambridge: Massachusetts Institute of Technology Center for Advanced Engineering Study; 1993.
4. Senge P. *The Fifth Discipline: The Art and Practice of the Learning Organization*. New York, NY: Doubleday; 1994.
5. United Nations Educational, Scientific and Cultural Organization. *A Systems Approach to Teaching and Learning Procedures: A Guide for Educators*. Paris, France: UNESCO Press; 1981.

6. Cromwell RR, Scileppi J. A systems approach to education. http://www. eric.ed.gov/ERICWebPortal/custom/portlets/recordDetails/detailmini.jsp?_ nfpb=true&_&ERICExtSearch_SearchValue_0=ED392151&ERIC ExtSearch_SearchType_0=no&accno=ED392151. ERIC No. ED392151. Published 1995. Accessed December 15, 2009.

7. Kaufman RA. A system approach to education: derivation and definition. *Educ Technol Res Dev*. 1968;16:415–425.

8. Hake RR. Lessons from the physics education reform effort. *Ecol Soc*. 2002; 5(2):article 28. http://www.ecologyandsociety.org/v015/iss2/art28/inline.html. Accessed December 26, 2009.

9. Westra R, Boersma K, Waarlo AJ, Savelsbergh E. Learning and teaching about ecosystems based on systems thinking and modeling in an authentic practice. In: Pintó R, Cousa D, eds. *Contributions from Science Education Research*. New York, NY: Springer; 2007:360–374.

10. Hake RR. 2009. Over two-hundred annotated references on systems thinking. http://www.physics.indiana.edu/~hake/200RefsSystems2c.pdf. Accessed December 26, 2009.

11. Planas LG, Er NL. A systems approach to scaffold communication skills development. *Am J Pharm Ed*. 2008;72(2):article 35.

12. Manasse HR. 2009 Rho Chi lecture–interdisciplinary health education: a systems approach to bridging the gaps. *Am J Pharm Ed*. 2009;73(5):article 90.

13. Meadows DH. Wright D, ed. *Thinking in Systems: A Primer*. White River Junction, VT: Chelsea Green Publishing; 2008.

14. Nathan DM, Buse JB, Davidson MB et al. Medical management of hyperglycemia in type 2 diabetes: a consensus algorithm for the initiation and adjustment of therapy. *Diabetes Care*. 2009;32:193–203.

15. Rodbard HW, Jellinger PS, Davidson JA et al. Statement by an American Association of Clinical Endocrinologists/American College of Endocrinology consensus panel on type 2 diabetes mellitus: an algorithm for glycemic control. *Endoc Pract*. 2009;15:540–549.

16. University of Minnesota Center for Teaching and Learning. Syllabus development. http://www1.umn.edu/ohr/teachlearn/tutorials/syllabus/. Accessed December 19, 2009.

17. Kelley KA, McAuley JW, Wallace LJ, Frank SG. Curricular mapping: process and product. *Am J Pharm Ed*. 2008;72(5):article 100.

18. Barr JT, McIntosh J, Gonyeau M et al. Mapping population/public health competencies across the doctor of pharmacy curriculum. Poster presented at: AACP Annual Meeting; July 20–23 2008; Chicago, IL

19. Office of Disease Prevention and Health Promotion, US Department of Health and Human Services. Developing Healthy People 2020 draft, Diabetes. http://www.healthypeople.gov/hp2020/Objectives/TopicArea.aspx?id=16& TopicArea=Diabetes. Accessed December 3, 2009.

20. Association for Prevention Teaching and Research. Official clinical prevention and population health curriculum framework—2009 Revision. http:// www. atpm.org/CPPH_Framework/index.html. Accessed December 3, 2009.

21. ASysT Institute. CDC's health systems dynamics project [video]. http://asysti.org/ videopresentations.aspx. Accessed December 29, 2009.

22. Brashers VL, Curry CE, Harper DC, McDaniel SH, Pawlson G, Ball JW. Interprofessional health care education: recommendations of the National Academies of Practice expert panel on health care in the 21st century. *Issues Interdiscip Care: Natl Acad Pract Forum*. 2001;3:21–31.

23. American Association of Colleges of Pharmacy. CAPE educational outcomes. http://aacp.org/resources/education/Pages/CAPEEducationalOutcomes.aspx. Accessed June 12, 2009.

24. Academy of Managed Care Pharmacy; American Association of Colleges of Pharmacy; American College of Apothecaries et al. Medication therapy management services: definition and program criteria. http://www.pharmacist.com/AM/Template.cfm?Section=MTM&TEMPLATE=/CM/ContentDisplay.cfm&CONTENTID=4577. Accessed December 29, 2009.

25. Joint Commission of Pharmacy Practitioners. Future vision of pharmacy practice. http://www.ascp.com/advocacy/coalitions/upload/JCPP%20Future%20Vision%20for%20Pharmacy%20Practice-2004.pdf. Published November 10, 2004. Accessed June 12, 2009.

26. Joint Commission of Pharmacy Practitioners. An action plan for implementation of the JCPP future vision of pharmacy practice. http://www.ascp.com/advocacy/coalitions/upload/JCPP-FinalReport.pdf. Published November 2007. Revised January 31, 2008. Accessed June 12, 2009.

27. Accreditation Council for Pharmacy Education. Accreditation standards and guidelines for the professional program in pharmacy leading to the doctor of pharmacy degree. http://www.acpe-accredit.org/pdf/ACPE_Revised_PharmD_Standards_Adopted_Jan152006.pdf. Published 2006. Accessed June 12, 2009.

28. National Association of Boards of Pharmacy. NAPLEX blueprint. http://www.nabp.net/programs/examination/naplex/naplex-blueprint/. Accessed June 7, 2010.

29. American Association of Colleges of Pharmacy. White Papers for AACP Curricular Change Summit. http://www.aacp.org/meetingsandevents/othermeetings/curricularchangesummit/Pages/MeetingMaterials.aspx. Accessed January 6, 2010.

30. Jungnickel PW, Kelley KW, Hammer DP, Haines ST, Marlowe KF. Addressing competencies for the future in the professional curriculum. *Am J Pharm Ed*. 2009;73(8):article 156.

31. Wells BG, Beck DE, Draugalis JR et al. Report of the 2007–2008 Argus Commission: what future awaits beyond pharmaceutical care? *Am J Pharm Ed*. 2008;72(suppl):article S8.

32. Institute for Alternative Futures. The 2029 project: achieving an ethical future for biomedical R&D. http://www.altfutures.com/2029.asp. Accessed March 7, 2010.

33. Georgetown University Center for Child and Human Development. National Center for Cultural Competence. http://www11.georgetown.edu/research/gucchd/nccc/index.html. Accessed December 26, 2009.

34. National Coalition for Health Professional Education in Genetics. Preparing health professionals for the genomics revolution. http://www.nchpeg.org/. Accessed December 26, 2009.

Additional Resources

1. *Summarizing CDC's Health Systems Dynamics Project*, a 2008 award-winning, 19-minute video from the Centers for Disease Control and Prevention that applies the systems approach to their public and population health planning and its new health protection mission is provided online at http://asysti.org/videopresentations.aspx.

2. Two early books on designing educational programs using the systems approach are as follows:

> Ford CW, ed. *Clinical Education for the Allied Health Professions.* Saint Louis, MO: CV Mosby; 1978.
>
> Ford CW, Morgan MK, eds. *Teaching in the Health Professions.* Saint Louis, MO: CV Mosby; 1976.

3. A workbook that applies a systems approach to education and program planning is as follows:

> Watson M. *Systems Approach to Education and Program Planning.* Sudbury, MA: Jones and Bartlett; 2010.

CHAPTER 4

What Matters in Assessment?

Katherine A. Kelley, PhD

Introduction

If we are to focus on a learner-centered model of pedagogy (as presented in Chapter 1), how can we measure our success as teachers? How do you know that you have been successful in the classroom? Did the students learn? Did they achieve the course objectives? How do you know that they learned? The answer is through assessment of student learning and through assessment of teaching.

Assessment helps us show the outcomes of our teaching efforts; in other words, assessment can be used to document student learning. By determining what students have learned as a result of instruction, we can identify whether the objectives of an assignment, lecture, or course have been achieved. Assessment can be viewed as fulfilling two important purposes: improvement and accountability. Outcomes data can be used to help us improve our teaching, curricula, or student learning outcomes, but we can also use assessment data to answer to external reviewers or stakeholders, such as alumni, parents, or accrediting bodies.

Assessment of learning can be focused at the individual, course, or program and curricular levels. Although there will be some information on assessing courses and curricula in this chapter, the main focus will be on assessing student learning and assessing individual teaching.

Before you read this chapter, take a few minutes to examine where you are as a teacher. Are you a prospective faculty member, a graduate student or pharmacy resident serving in the role of teaching assistant, or an experiential copreceptor? Are you a new faculty member hired to teach one or two lectures and precept students in experiential education? Are you an existing faculty member responsible for teaching your own course? No matter which scenario describes your teaching role, one of the tasks you must initially undertake is to write a set of learning outcomes for your teaching assignment. The easiest way to approach this task is to ask yourself, What do I want students to take away from my teaching (lecture, rotation, or course)? When you have decided what students should be able to learn from your teaching, you have essentially defined your learning outcomes.

There are many resources that can help you hone your skills for writing learning objectives; two of the author's favorites are provided in the reference section at the end of this chapter.[1,2] This process of beginning with the end in mind is known as backward design and is a key concept in the assessment of student learning.[3] It is the same as defining the aim of the system in the systems approach (see Chapter 3) and then designing the input, process, and output. Backward design means that we first write the outcomes that we wish our students to achieve, and then we design the learning experiences that will enable the students to achieve those outcomes (lectures, clinical experiences, courses). In other words, we design our curriculum backward and deliver it forward.[3]

Reflective Exercise

Spend a few minutes reflecting on, and then writing down, an answer to the following question: How do I currently determine that students have learned what I intended for them to learn as a result of my teaching?

_____

_____

_____

_____

This chapter is divided into three sections. The first section provides an overview of the language of assessment by covering definitions of common assessment terms and fundamental concepts. The second section reviews and provides examples of some commonly used assessment tools and strategies for assessing student learning. And finally, the last section provides an overview of how to use the information gathered in the second section to improve student learning, courses, or curricula. By focusing on assessment in the context of the teaching and learning environment, this chapter will attempt to provide some answers to the following questions:

- How do I know if learning has been achieved as a result of my teaching?
- What kinds of tools are available to help me collect assessment data?
- How can I use assessment to improve student learning?
- How can I use assessment to improve my teaching?

What Are the Terms and Concepts Associated with Assessment?

As in any area of inquiry, assessment has its own theories, concepts, and language. The following is a very brief review of some key concepts, theories, and definitions. In the area of the scholarship of assessment, there are many scholarly books and works; however, you may find that some of these works define the same terms differently. Given this somewhat frustrating state of affairs, the assessment terminology used in this chapter will first be defined. As a reminder, when working with others on assessment matters in the future, you are encouraged to clearly and mutually define key terms and concepts to avoid any potential misunderstandings.

What Is Assessment?

Palomba and Banta define *assessment* as "the systematic collection, review, and use of information about educational programs undertaken for the purpose of improving student learning and development."[4] This definition is very appropriate within the context of this book due to its emphasis on using data to improve student learning and development. Now that we have a working definition of assessment, what are some of the reasons we undertake assessment? Or alternatively, what is the purpose of assessment? Assessment activities can be used for formative or summative activities. Formative assessment is typically undertaken to provide feedback to improve something.[4] For example, when students are required to turn in a draft outline of a project, they are provided with critical feedback or a formative assessment but not a grade. Summative assessment, on the other hand, is that which is undertaken to provide a judgment about the quality of something.[4] In the aforementioned example, the summative assessment would be the final grade for the project. Therefore, assessment can be conducted to fulfill two different purposes: improvement and accountability.

A pharmacy school could also collect assessment data via a survey tool that asks students about their experiences with the curriculum. These data could be used as a formative assessment strategy to make changes to or improve the curriculum. Assessment data could also be collected for a summative assessment to measure the degree to which students enrolled in a program successfully counseled a patient on a new medication at a given point in the curriculum. These data could be used to demonstrate that the program is meeting its learning objectives and to demonstrate accountability (summative assessment) to external bodies, such as the pharmacy accrediting agency (Accreditation Council for Pharmacy Education [ACPE]).

Another important consideration for educational assessment is the idea of the level of assessment. In science, the unit of analysis is similar to the level of assessment. As faculty members, we are probably most familiar

Fact or myth: Assessment of student learning is just a fancy way to describe written exams.

What role will assessment play in my overall philosophy of teaching?

What are the differences between formative and summative assessments?

with assessment that occurs at the student level. This would be assessment of individual students' knowledge, skills, or attitudes. But we can also look at course-level assessment. Examples of course-level assessments are the percentage of students who achieved a stated course outcome or students' perceptions about the delivery of a specific course. These examples illustrate that within course-level assessment or classroom assessment we can look at measures of student learning as well as measures of teaching effectiveness. Another level of assessment occurs at the program or institution level.[5] The percentage of students who pass the national pharmacy licensing exam could be a program outcome, and the percentage of graduating students who secure offers of employment could be an institution-level outcome.

> Direct measures of assessment are tangible; indirect measures are proxy signs that students are probably learning.[6]
> L. Suskie

There are two basic types of assessment measures: direct and indirect. Direct evidence of student learning is "tangible, visible, self-explanatory, and compelling evidence of exactly what students have and have not learned."[6] Examples of direct evidence of student learning are scores from the national licensing exam and preceptor evaluations. Indirect evidence "consists of proxy signs that students are probably learning."[6] Student self-assessments of achievement and the numbers of honors or awards received by students are examples of indirect measures of student learning.

Now that you know some of the terminology relative to assessment, how do you go about deciding what to assess? Assessment should focus on determining whether students have achieved the intended goal; these are the outcomes or objectives of the learning activity (course, lecture, etc.). Other terms that educators use to describe what students are supposed to learn are *competencies, proficiencies,* or *ability-based outcomes.* These terms are often used interchangeably and are sometimes defined differently. The following are some common definitions and distinctions among these terms:

- A *goal* is a statement of what you intend to achieve.[6] For example, a pharmacy management professor may have a goal that her students learn about the Medicaid system.
- An *objective* is a detailed aspect of the goal. Objectives are the "tasks to be accomplished to achieve the goal or the *process* used to achieve the goal."[6] In the previous example, the management professor may have an objective that her students apply the criteria of state Medicaid prescription coverage to patient cases. Numerous objectives are typically developed to describe the process by which a goal is achieved.
- An *outcome* refers to "the destination instead of the path taken to get there."[6] Outcomes are related to the final product, not the process used to achieve that product. For example, if the students meet the goal of learning about the Medicaid system, they may be asked to demonstrate this learning by directly assisting patients with their Medicaid drug benefits. The outcome would be described as a

demonstration of their learning in any of the domains of learning (i.e., cognitive or knowledge-based, psychomotor or skills-based, and affective or attitudinally based learning). As described in Chapter 2, the various levels of each of these domains can help instructors define their intended learning outcomes as well as strategies for measuring the achievement of these outcomes.[7]

- *Competency* and *proficiency* are often used synonymously with outcomes or objectives. However, they typically should be used to describe skills rather than knowledge or attitudes.[6]
- An *ability-based outcome* is an explicit statement describing what students will be able to do as a result of the *integration* of knowledge, skills, and attitudes gained from their instructional experiences.[8] An example of an ability-based outcome is "PharmD graduates will be able to assess a patient's response to therapeutic interventions."[9]
- A *standard* or *benchmark* is the "specific target against which we gauge success in achieving an outcome."[6] The ACPE has standards by which PharmD programs are accredited.[10] An example of a benchmark would be a PharmD program that set a criterion of 100 percent of third-year pharmacy students being able to counsel a patient on a new medication.

Understanding the basic terms and definitions used in the assessment literature is a critical first step in learning about the assessment of learning outcomes. To understand the interrelationships among outcomes, courses, and curricula, as well as the external or environmental influences on these relationships, see **Figure 4–1**.

Now that you understand the terminology, you next need to consider which model or framework will be used to conceptualize how you will go about planning your assessment activities. Just as you would not typically report a patient's therapeutic outcomes in the absence of relevant patient data and drug information, so too you should strive to report student learning outcomes within the context of the learning environment and the personal characteristics of the learners. This is the context for Astin's IEO (inputs, environment, outcomes) model.[11] Assessment data are more meaningful if you know relevant information about the learners and the environments to which they have been exposed. The students' prior academic performances and attitudes toward learning or the subject are examples of inputs. The environment is what they experience in the program, and outcomes are measured in terms of student performance. A classroom-based example using this model might involve the following: A faculty member is interested in demonstrating that a new learning strategy leads to higher exam scores. She implements the new strategy in one section of the class and teaches the other section using the standard technique. The new strategy versus the old technique is the environment.

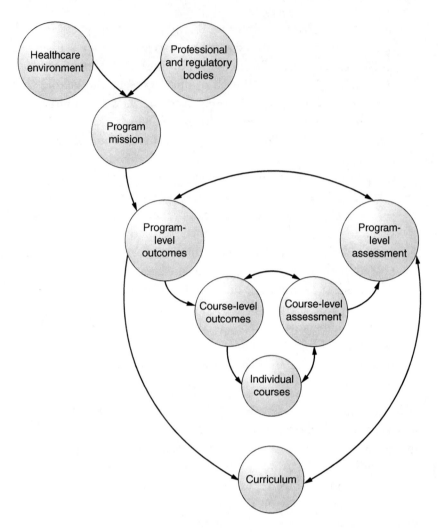

Figure 4–1 Concept Map of the Relationship Between Outcomes, Courses, and Curricula

Source: Courtesy of Kelley KA, McAuley JW, Wallace LJ et al. *Am J Pharm Educ.* 2008; 72(5):article 100.

She would measure the students' prior learning at the beginning of each section of the class. This is the input. Then she would measure their learning at the end of the class with a posttest. The posttest is the outcome.

A second framework is presented by Walvoord's three steps of assessment.[12] Step one is to articulate the goals for your students. Step two is to gather evidence about how well students are meeting these goals. And step three is to use the evidence collected for the purpose of improvement. A similar model is given by Maki's assessment cycle or assessment loop[5] shown in **Figure 4–2**. This model is often referred to in the assessment

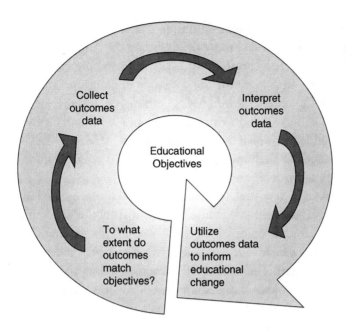

Figure 4–2 The Assessment Cycle

Source: Courtesy of Maki PL. *Assessing for Learning: Building a Sustainable Commitment Across the Institution*. Sterling, VA: Stylus Publishing; 2004.

literature when authors are describing the use of assessment results for improvement known as "completing the assessment loop" or "completing the loop."[5] For example, you collect information concerning your students' perceptions about a course project via a survey, combine the survey results with an assessment of the projects' quality and an assessment of student performance on the project overall, then use all of these sources of information to improve the students' projects the next time the course is delivered.

What Techniques and Tools Are Used in Assessment?

There are many assessment techniques and tools that can help you gather needed evidence to determine whether students are meeting your educational goals and outcomes. The following is a small set of tools to begin building your assessment toolbox. These tools can be divided into three groups: direct measures of student learning, indirect measures of student learning, and tools for evaluating your instruction or the course itself.

Direct Measures

Remember that direct assessment measures focus on what students know or what they can do with what they know. The most common type of direct measure, one that we have all been on the receiving end of, is the examination. There are two basic types of exams: free response and forced choice, such as the ubiquitous multiple-choice (MC) and true–false exam. In general, you will spend more time grading the first type and writing the second type. There is a real art and science to writing effective MC questions. Bloom's Taxonomy for the cognitive domain provides a useful way to link learning outcomes with MC questions.[7] Haladyna and colleagues[13] reviewed the literature on writing MC test questions and formulated a best practices guideline, which has been reproduced in **Table 4–1**. The National Board of Medical Examiners has also produced a handbook for constructing written test questions.[14]

A second and very useful assessment tool that can be used in a number of situations is the rubric. A rubric is a scoring tool that lays out the specific expectations for the completion, and therefore the grading, of an assignment.[15] Rubrics have four basic elements. The first is a description of the task or assignment. The second is a scale for grading the assignment. The third is the dimensions of the assignment or the specific items on which the student will be graded, and the fourth is a description of what constitutes each level of performance on the scale.[15] **Figure 4–3** is a sample rubric from an assignment in a pharmacy management course with each of these four characteristics labeled. Rubrics are very useful assessment tools in that they help an instructor to articulate the specific expectations of many assignment types by dividing the assignment into its component parts (dimensions) and designating acceptable and unacceptable performance levels (scale and levels of performance).[15] Rubrics are also described by Walvoord and Anderson[16] in a technique called Primary Trait Analysis.

The third tool for your toolbox is a performance assessment. Performance assessments are examinations in which the student is faced with a simulated task or problem and must solve the problem or complete the task by performing specific elements. Consider a pharmacy professional practice laboratory where a student is asked to counsel a standardized patient (i.e., an actor who is playing the role of a patient in a consistently predetermined way). The student is then graded on whether he or she successfully completed required elements of the patient encounter. (A rubric would be useful here.) When several different performance assessments are conducted as part of the same examination session, the result is known as an objective structured clinical exam (OSCE)[17,18] and is further described in Chapter 8.

A portfolio is another tool for assessing student performance. Portfolios are collections of a student's work to demonstrate his or her accomplishments.[19] Portfolios can also be reflective in nature, whereby the student includes writings that critically analyze the contents.[20] One of the main advantages of a portfolio over other types of direct measures of assessment mentioned here is that the portfolio includes a variety of types of evidence gathered over time instead of evidence from a single measurement collected at one specified time. The element

Table 4–1 A Revised Taxonomy of Multiple-Choice (MC) Item-Writing Guidelines

Content concerns:

1. Every item should reflect specific content and a single specific mental behavior, as called for in test specifications (two-way grid, test blueprint).
2. Base each item on important content to learn; avoid trivial content.
3. Use novel material to test higher-level learning. Paraphrase textbook language or language used during instruction to avoid testing for simply recall.
4. Keep the content of each item independent from the content of other items on the test.
5. Avoid overly specific and overly general content.
6. Avoid opinion-based items.
7. Avoid trick items.
8. Keep the vocabulary simple for the group of students being tested.

Formatting concerns:

9. Use the question, completion, and best answer versions of the conventional MC, the alternate choice, true–false (TF), multiple true–false (MTF), matching, and context-dependent item and item set formats, but *avoid* the complex MC (Type K) format.
10. Format the item vertically instead of horizontally.

Style concerns:

11. Edit and proofread items.
12. Use correct grammar, punctuation, capitalization, and spelling.
13. Minimize the amount of reading in each item.

Writing the stem:

14. Ensure that the directions in the stem are very clear.
15. Include the central idea in the stem instead of the choices.
16. Avoid window dressing (excessive verbiage).
17. Word the stem positively; avoid negatives such as *not* or *except*. If you use negative words, use them cautiously and always ensure that they appear capitalized and boldface.

Writing the choices:

18. Develop as many effective choices as you can, but research suggests that three choices are adequate.
19. Make sure that only one of the choices is the correct answer.
20. Vary the location of the correct answer according to the number of choices.
21. Place the choices in logical or numeric order.
22. Keep the choices independent; choices should not overlap.
23. Keep the choices homogeneous in content and grammatic structure.
24. Keep the length of the choices about equal.
25. *None of the above* should be used carefully.
26. Avoid *all of the above*.
27. Phrase choices positively; avoid negatives such as *not*.
28. Avoid giving clues to the right answer, such as the following:
    a. Specific determiners, including *always, never, completely,* and *absolutely*
    b. Clang associations (choices identical to or resembling words in the stem)
    c. Grammatic inconsistencies that cue the test taker to the correct choice
    d. Conspicuous correct choice
    e. Pairs or triplets of options that clue the test taker to the correct choice
    f. Blatantly absurd, ridiculous options
29. Make all distractors plausible.
30. Use typical student errors to write your distractors.
31. Use humor if it is compatible with the teacher and the learning environment.

Source: Courtesy of Haladyna TM, Downing SM, Rodriquez MC. A review of multiple-choice item-writing guidelines for classroom assessment. *Appl Meas Educ.* 2002;15(3):309–334.

Pharmacy 673: News and Views Presentation Rubric

Student:_____

Article title: _____

Date presented: _____

Assignment: Select one current event from popular media sources (i.e., not journal articles) to present to the class. Articles are required to be relevant to the course content (i.e., Medicare or Medicaid, pharmacist roles, healthcare provider roles, distribution of pharmaceutical products, healthcare coverage, etc.).

Key to rubric contents:

Column 1: the dimensions of the project

Cells in the rubric table: the performance descriptors

Grading scale: points 1 through 4 across the top of the rubric

Points

	4	3	2	1	
Body language	Movements seemed fluid and helped the audience visualize	Made movements or gestures that enhanced articulation	Very little movement or descriptive gestures	No movement or descriptive gestures	_____
Eye contact	Holds attention of entire audience with the use of direct eye contact	Consistent use of direct eye contact with audience	Displayed minimal eye contact with audience	No eye contact with audience	_____
Introduction and closure	Student delivers open and closing remarks that capture the attention of the audience and set the mood	Student displays clear introductory or closing remarks	Student clearly uses either an introductory or closing remark but not both	Student does not display clear introductory or closing remarks	_____
Pacing	Good use of drama, and student meets apportioned time interval	Delivery is patterned but does not meet apportioned time interval	Delivery is in bursts and does not meet apportioned time interval	Delivery is either too quick or too slow to meet apportioned time interval	_____
Poise	Student displays relaxed, self-confident nature about self, with no mistakes	Makes minor mistakes, but quickly recovers from them; displays little or no tension	Displays mild tension; has trouble recovering from mistakes	Tension and nervousness is obvious; has trouble recovering from mistakes	_____

Figure 4–3 Sample Rubric (*Continued*)

Voice	Consistent use of fluid speech, complete sentences, correct English, and no fillers (*um, uh, and stuff*)	A few instances of nonfluid speech, or incomplete sentences, or incorrect English, or fillers	Significant issues with one of the defined elements (fluid speech, complete sentences, correct English, and no fillers)	Consistent issues with two or more of the defined elements (fluid speech, complete sentences, correct English, and no fillers)	＿＿＿
	3			**0**	
Topic	Topic selected is related to the course content and is summarized for the class			Topic selected is not appropriate or does not conform to the criteria required	＿＿＿
Discussion questions	Discussion questions related to the article are presented, and the class members are encouraged to respond			No questions are posed	＿＿＿

Figure 4–3 Sample Rubric

of reflection as a part of a portfolio makes it both an assessment process and a product.[21]

Indirect Measures

One of the most commonly used indirect measures of student learning is the survey. In terms of assessing student learning, the survey can be used to gather student self-reports of outcomes achievement.[22] The advent of online survey tools has increased the popularity of this form of assessment; however, the ease of use of these tools does not negate attention to good practices in survey development and deployment. Draugalis et al.[23] have reviewed the elements of good survey research; and Fink[24] provides a user-friendly guide to creating your own surveys.

Other indirect measures of student learning are quantitative in nature, such as the numbers of students engaging in research with faculty or the numbers of students participating in health screenings or health fairs.

When designing assessment plans or assembling data for decision-making purposes, it is generally a good idea to include data from different categories or methods. This process is known as triangulation or gathering corroborating evidence.[6] Consider an assessment committee of a PharmD program that is currently reviewing the curriculum as it relates to the development of student professionalism. The committee would review students' self-reports of their achievement of professionalism outcomes, preceptor survey data regarding the professionalism of students, and findings related to students' performance on the professionalism component of the experiential evaluations. As described, the committee would review the triangulated evidence dealing with professionalism prior to making changes to the curriculum.

Tools for Evaluating Your Instruction and Course

Obtaining information about how your course is going and students' perceptions of their own learning, as well as their perceptions of the course, provides valuable feedback for you to use to improve your teaching process. Evaluation of your instruction can be as formal as a standardized university-wide student evaluation at the end of the term or as informal as the adjustment you make to your lecture on the fly because you notice there are several puzzled looks among your students. The first set of techniques presented in this section will help you gather information about what students are learning and provide you with feedback about how your instruction is going. In this section, the use of clickers, peer evaluations of teaching, and supplemental assessments of instruction and courses will also be discussed.

Angelo and Cross[25] have written a much-referenced book, *Classroom Assessment Techniques*, that contains a set of tools for gathering student feedback in the classroom. These classroom assessment techniques (CATs) can help monitor learning throughout the course. CATs are formative in nature and help the learner and the teacher determine the extent of learning that is taking place. Just two of the many CATs are the *minute paper* and the *muddiest point*. In the minute paper technique, the instructor directs the students at the end of a class session to answer two questions: (1) What was the most important thing you learned today? and (2) What questions still remain uppermost in your mind as we conclude this class session? The muddiest point is a similar technique where students are asked, What was the muddiest point in my lecture today? These exercises are intended to help you obtain immediate information about what students are learning and what they are struggling with while the course is ongoing. Checking student learning in a formative way at various points during the term helps both students and instructors assess learning in an ongoing manner.[25]

> Think of a course you are currently teaching. How could you integrate the minute paper into this course to acquire feedback from students?

Audience response systems, often referred to as *clickers*, are small remote control devices that are programmed to allow students to respond to multiple-choice questions during a lecture or presentation. Besides encouraging active learning, these devices can be used to quiz students and check for understanding and comprehension of material during class time. This technique can help students and teachers focus on areas needing further explanation or development.[26]

Peer evaluation of teaching is another means of gathering feedback about your teaching. Several examples of peer evaluation of teaching models in pharmacy have recently been published.[27-29] In general, this type of assessment can be conducted by another faculty member in your department or by someone from the university teaching and learning center. Many campuses have centers for teaching that provide consultation and assessment services for their faculty. This can be a valuable resource for obtaining information as well as one-on-one assistance with classroom issues of many types, including assessment.[1]

Summative measures of course or instructor evaluations are tools that are generally used at the end of the course to assess the instructor and the course (e.g., student evaluations of a course). Often these assessments are required components of formal dossiers of teaching performance used for promotion and tenure purposes. As a new instructor, it is a good idea to identify the required assessment tools and processes for your courses and determine how the data will be reported and used. When the data are reported, it is also important to keep copies of these evaluations for your teaching portfolio and your dossier for promotion and tenure. These required assessments are typically general in nature due to their widespread use across many different types of courses. Supplementing these general evaluations with more course-specific questionnaires can really help instructors obtain detailed feedback on what was successful in a course and where to focus improvement efforts. You can start simply by asking your students two questions: (1) What was the most valuable aspect of this course? and (2) Please provide an honest, thoughtful critique of the course; I am genuinely interested in the process of continuous improvement. Additionally, if you have specific areas that you wish to probe, the use of Likert-scaled questions can be added to these two open-ended questions. For example, you may wish to know some specific information about the exams in your course. You could ask several Likert-scaled questions about the degree of difficulty of the questions and whether the questions tested application versus memorization.[1] There is a particularly useful online tool that lists Likert-scaled and open-ended questions for use on course evaluations. Simply enter any name and e-mail address to enter the tool at http://buckeyelink1.osu.edu/fyi/.

Reflective Exercise

Which of the preceding techniques could you incorporate into one of your courses or teaching assignments? Take a few minutes while the ideas are fresh to brainstorm where and how you will incorporate at least one of these techniques.

_____

_____

_____

_____

How Do I Use Assessment Information to Improve My Teaching, My Courses, and the Curriculum?

Now that you know a bit about assessment, its role, and the tools you can use to gather feedback, we need to consider how to use the data to make informed changes to your teaching, courses, and the curriculum. How can you successfully use the information you have gathered about your teaching to better facilitate learning? Often in assessment it is helpful to start small and continue to build. I like to call this process capitalizing on small wins. Here is a strategy for using the data collected from the supplemental evaluations described in the previous section. First, read through the feedback gathered from the students several times. Next, make a list of the common themes that you see in the comments and answers to your questions from your students. Choose two or three themes upon which to create an action plan for the subsequent academic year. This action item list can be shared with a teaching mentor or department chair. After the following year, assess and report on the implementation of the action items. This process is a continuous improvement process that empowers you to choose what to improve about your course based on data you collect from your students.[25]

One comment about student feedback: you need to be empowered and take charge of your reaction to these comments. Often student feedback is given anonymously, which tends to enable students to hide behind the mask of anonymity and make inappropriate, unhelpful, or worse—hurtful—comments. Here are two suggestions to help you with this situation. First, tell students in advance to be professional and provide helpful, constructive feedback. Before you collect data about your teaching, let your students know that their feedback matters and what you intend to do with the information (i.e., improve the course). Inform them that although comments like "management stinks" may be cathartic for them, these comments do not help you narrow down what about the management course frustrated them. Also reinforce that these types of comments fall short of demonstrating the professionalism that is required of top-notch pharmacy professionals. A second suggestion is to let go of unhelpful comments. Although the veil of anonymity may make students feel free or entitled to provide derogatory or hurtful feedback, you are also free to ignore such comments.

The following is a case example about improving examination quality in a course. Several years ago, I chose to work on my exam writing skills based on my analysis of the responses to my open-ended questions on the supplemental evaluations of the course. Students were telling me that my exams were not an effective means of judging their learning in this course. My action plan consisted of working on my exam skills via various methods. After a subsequent delivery of the course, I surveyed my students about exams again, this time with both Likert and open-ended questions. I repeated the cycle several more times, each time asking students for feedback at the end of the course while at the same time continuing to learn about and improve my exam writing skills. Eventually, the student feedback began to show a trend of improvement.

Reflective Exercise

Write down one question you have about your teaching, and outline how you will collect data to answer the question.

_____

_____

_____

_____

The next level of assessment occurs at the course and curricular or program level. Assessment data derived using the techniques and tools presented in this chapter can be used to assess whether a sequence of courses or the entire curriculum is meeting its intended outcomes. An assessment plan is a document outlining the means and methods that will be used to show how a program is meeting its outcomes or goals.[12] Student learning outcomes are an essential part of the assessment plan. Being able to show with student learning data that a program is successfully achieving its intended outcomes is an essential element of the ACPE accreditation process. And more importantly, data on student learning outcomes provide an evidence-based approach to changing the curriculum. The following is an example of how assessment data were used to improve a sequence of courses.

A group of three professors in a management sequence of courses conducted a series of supplemental course evaluations. A number of common themes were discovered, including the length of the sequence and overlap of content. In addition, the college's process of curricular mapping (i.e., process of linking courses with required content as well as program outcomes) had also uncovered a few gaps as well as overlaps in course content among these three courses. The three faculty members decided to revise this course sequence. The student feedback, the curriculum mapping process, and the students' exam performances served as inputs to the revision process. The course sequence was revised to include all the required content with no overlaps in two instead of three courses. Subsequent student course evaluations showed an increased satisfaction with the revised sequence, and the courses were better aligned with the required content according to ACPE.[10]

Curricular assessment at the program level functions similarly to the previous example for courses. The keys are to have an assessment plan that outlines how you will show that the program outcomes are being achieved by your students and to measure student learning outcomes in a variety of ways. Another very important point to keep in mind is to complete the assessment loop. Assessment data should always be collected with the intent of using that data to provide feedback and answer questions about the curriculum and make decisions based on the analysis of these data. Simply collecting the data on student outcomes is not sufficient. The data must be analyzed and shared with the appropriate stakeholders.

ACPE has a set of 30 standards with accompanying guidelines that describe the required elements of doctor of pharmacy education. Once every six years, PharmD programs engage in a mandatory process known as the self-study. The self-study process gives programs an opportunity to evaluate themselves based on these standards. Assessment plans, analyses of data, and data-driven approaches to curricular change are all integral, and in fact required, in this process.[10]

Assessment may seem to be a large and overwhelming task. Assessment is like many other areas of scientific inquiry that are built upon purposefully gathering data or information to answer pertinent questions. So if you start small and build upon your successes, you will soon be using an evidence-based approach to guide the improvement of your teaching and the effectiveness of your program.

Reflective Exercise

Moving forward, how will you use assessment techniques to help you determine what students have learned from your teaching?

_____

_____

_____

_____

References

1. Ohio State University. Assessing teaching. http://ucat.osu.edu/read/teaching/assessing/assessment.html. Accessed July 8, 2009.

2. Schultheis NM. Writing cognitive educational objectives and multiple-choice test questions. *Am J Health-Syst Pharm.* 1998;55:2397–2401.

3. Huba ME, Freed JE. *Learner-Centered Assessment on College Campuses: Shifting the Focus from Teaching to Learning.* Boston, MA: Allyn and Bacon; 2000.

4. Palomba CA, Banta TW. *Assessment Essentials: Planning, Implementing, and Improving Assessment in Higher Education.* San Francisco, CA: Jossey-Bass; 1999.

5. Maki PL. *Assessing for Learning: Building a Sustainable Commitment Across the Institution.* Sterling, VA: Stylus Publishing; 2004.

6. Suskie L. *Assessing Student Learning: A Common Sense Guide.* 2nd ed. San Francisco, CA: Jossey-Bass; 2009.

7. Clark DR. Bloom's Taxonomy of learning domains: the three types of learning. http://www.nwlink.com/~donclark/hrd/bloom.html. Published June 5, 2009. Accessed August 6, 2009.

8. Zlatic TD. Abilities-based assessment within pharmacy education: preparing students for practice of pharmaceutical care. *J Pharm Teach.* 2000;7(3/4):5–27.

9. Ohio State University College of Pharmacy. Program-level, ability-based outcomes for PharmD education. http://www.pharmacy.ohio-state.edu/academics/assessment/documents/Outcomes_for_PharmD.pdf. Accessed July 8, 2009.

10. Accreditation Council for Pharmacy Education. Accreditation standards and guidelines for the professional program in pharmacy leading to the doctor of pharmacy degree. http://www.acpe-accredit.org/pdf/ACPE_Revised_PharmD_Standards_Adopted_Jan152006.pdf. Accessed July 9, 2009.

11. Astin AW. *Assessment for Excellence: The Philosophy and Practice of Assessment and Evaluation in Higher Education.* New York, NY: Maxwell Macmillan; 1991.

12. Walvoord, BE. *Assessment Clear and Simple: A Practical Guide for Institutions, Departments and General Education.* San Francisco, CA: Jossey-Bass; 2004.

13. Haladyna TM, Downing SM, Rodriquez MC. A review of multiple-choice item-writing guidelines for classroom assessment. *Appl Meas Educ.* 2002;15 (3):309–334.

14. Case SM, Swanson DB. *Constructing Written Test Questions for the Basic and Clinical Sciences.* 3rd ed. Philadelphia, PA: National Board of Medical Examiners; 2002. http://www.nbme.org/publications/item-writing-manual-download.html. Accessed July 2, 2009.

15. Stevens DD, Levi AJ. *Introduction to Rubrics.* Sterling, VA: Stylus Publishing; 2005.

16. Walvoord BE, Anderson VJ. *Effective Grading: A Tool for Learning and Assessment.* San Francisco, CA: Jossey-Bass; 1998.

17. Harden RM. What is an OSCE? *Med Teach.* 1988;10(1):19–22.

18. Austin Z, O'Byrne C, Pugsley J, Munoz LQ. Development and validation processes for an objective structured clinical examination (OSCE) for entry-to-practice certification in pharmacy: the Canadian experience. *Am J Pharm Educ.* 2003;67(3):article 76.

19. Larson RL. Using portfolios to assess the impact of a curriculum. In: Banta TW, ed. *Portfolio Assessment: Uses, Cases, Scoring and Impact.* San Francisco, CA: Wiley & Sons Inc; 2003:7–10.

20. Plaza CM, Draugalis JR, Slack MK, Skrepnek GH, Sauer KA. Use of reflective portfolios in health sciences education. *Am J Pharm Educ.* 2007;71(2):article 34.

21. Zubizarreta J. *The Learning Portfolio: Reflective Practice for Improving Student Learning.* 2nd ed. San Francisco, CA: Jossey-Bass; 2009.

22. Kelley KA, Demb A. Instrumentation for comparing student and faculty perception of competency-based assessment. *Am J Pharm Educ.* 2006;70(6): article 134.

23. Draugalis JR, Coons SJ, Plaza CM. Best practices for survey research reports: a synopsis for authors and reviewers. *Am J Pharm Educ.* 2008;72(1):article 11.

24. Fink A. *How to Conduct Surveys: A Step by Step Guide.* 4th ed. Thousand Oaks, CA: Sage Publications Inc; 2009.

25. Angelo TA, Cross PK. *Classroom Assessment Techniques: A Handbook for College Teachers.* San Francisco, CA: Jossey-Bass; 1993.

26. Bruff D. *Teaching with Classroom Response Systems: Creating Active Learning Environments.* San Francisco, CA: Jossey-Bass; 2009.

27. Schultz KK, Latif D. The planning and implementation of a faculty peer review teaching project. *Am J Pharm Educ.* 2006;70(2):article 32.

28. Hansen LB, McCollum M, Paulsen SM, et al. Evaluation of an evidence-based peer teaching assessment program. *Am J Pharm Educ.* 2007;71(3):article 45.

29. Trujillo JM, DiVall MV, Barr J et al. Development of a peer teaching-assessment program and a peer observation and evaluation tool. *Am J Pharm Educ.* 2009;72(6):article 147.

What Matters in Learning and Teaching Settings?

CHAPTER 5

What Matters in Large Classroom Teaching?

Judith T. Barr, ScD, MEd

Introduction

You have reached a new stage in your journey. You have examined the teacher within, traveled across the developmental stages and learning styles of your students, passed through the systems approach with all of its inputs and processes, and explored the purpose and value of assessment.

It has been quite an adventure—some would say an odyssey.

But now it is time to travel on to the next stage—that of application. What better place to start applying the lessons you have learned than to the teaching and learning opportunities that exist in large-enrollment classes? First, let us examine the characteristics of the traditional, uninterrupted lecture, when it may be appropriate to use such an approach, and then suggest some basic ways to make even the passive lecture more student centered. But let us be clear—although it is possible to improve the traditional passive lecture, this is not the way to create a student-centered classroom and maximize student learning. We will review the active learning transformation, the scientific support of active learning, and the evidence-based findings from classroom research. We will examine the disconnect between those findings and what happens in the teacher-centered lecture. The bulk of the chapter will then present a series of ever-more intensive methods to refocus the experiences in large classes to incorporate active learning experiences during both in-class periods (with and without technologic enhancements) and out-of-class individual and collaborative learning projects.

This chapter will help you answer the following questions:

- What is the role and place of the traditional passive lecture? How can basic methods to include some active learning opportunities be incorporated into the traditional lecture?
- What does cognitive neuroscience and evidence-based classroom research tell us about ways that students learn?
- What are the implications of this information for large-enrollment classes?
- What are methods that you can implement to provide progressively more active learning activities in large classes?
- What type of out-of-class assignments can increase higher-level cognitive skills and complement large classroom-based content coverage?

The sources for this chapter on teaching and learning in large classes are many and include summaries of scientific results from developmental psychology, cognitive psychology, and neuroscience fields; reports from national surveys of college students and faculty; evidence-based results and recommendations from studies of national curricular revisions; evidence-based, observational, and descriptive studies based on institutional-level experiences of faculty and students; recommendations from organizational policy statements and accreditation standards, as well as commentaries and editorials from individuals and committees; and personal experiences of the author during 40 years of trying to include active learning experiences in large class courses. As you can see from this list, conclusions and recommendations from different sources come with varying degrees of rigor.

What Matters in the Traditional Passive Lecture? What Are Some Suggestions for Beginning to Move into Active Learning?

Why include a section on the traditional lecture method to begin a chapter on student-centered, active learning in a large classroom setting? Well, it is the way that many of us were taught, and hence, it is the default method that many of us comfortably fall back on. We focus on "presenting" the content, getting the facts across, giving a test, and then moving on to the next topic that needs to be covered. Remember the overused description, "Faculty are the sage on the stage?" We use our expertise to organize and package the content material (the sage part), and then in a type of performance, we convey the content to the students during the lecture process (the stage part). Our emphasis in this approach is on the teaching part of this learning–teaching continuum. But are there ways, even in the lecture, to improve student learning? Although there are not evidence-based classroom studies on the improvement of the lecture approach (as there are in the implementation of active learning strategies), there is empirical evidence

> The lecture came into prominence when it was assumed that . . . students' minds are empty vessels into which instructors pour their wisdom.[1]
> D.W. Johnson, R.T. Johnson, K.A. Smith

on how learning occurs. Based on this evidence, suggestions can be made to improve the passive lecture method.

First, let us describe our image of a traditional passive, faculty-centered lecture. You will need this definition as a baseline as you consider progressively adding more student-centered forms of classroom engagement and learning. In our view of the basic lecture approach, instructors organize their content into self-contained, logical, and sequential blocks of information. They "deliver" the organized and structured knowledge to the students, stopping for questions during the class, but commonly leaving questions for a question-and-answer period at the end of the class. In parts of the lecture, they may elaborate on the assigned readings, but rarely is the student held accountable to have mastered the readings prior to class. Instead, this basic lecture is prepackaged in its final form and does not rely on any type of interaction with, nor engagement of, the students.

Given this description, what are some appropriate uses for a lecture? According to Johnson and colleagues, there are at least five[1]:

1. To disseminate a large amount of material to many students in a short period of time, especially when the material needs to be presented in a particular order or is on a low level (alternatives are presented later in the chapter)
2. To present material that is not available elsewhere
3. To expose students to content in a brief time that might take them much longer to locate on their own
4. To arouse students' interest in a subject
5. To teach students who are primarily auditory learners

These authors further qualify the place for the lecture: "Lecturing at best tends to focus on lower-level cognition. When the material is complex, detailed, or abstract, when students need to analyze, synthesize, or integrate the knowledge being studied, or when long-term retention is desired, lecturing is not a good idea."[1] However, on the extreme negative end of the spectrum concerning the value of lecture classes, Felder and Brent argue that "much of what happens in most classes is a waste of everyone's time. It is neither teaching nor learning. It is stenography. Teachers recite their course notes; students do their best to transcribe them, and the information does not pass through anyone's brain."[2]

Is there a middle ground? Can we acknowledge that the traditional passive lecture is an efficient method of transmitting content, generally at lower cognitive levels? However, if you are using this method, you can create opportunities to improve your present lecture delivery while moving to incorporate strategies to increase student engagement and active learning. Let us explore some of these.

Reflective Exercise

Think about a lecture that you recently attended. Was the content well organized? Did the presenter convey mastery of, and interest in, the topic? Did the lecture appeal to auditory and visual learners? Were handouts available before or at the session? Did the presenter hold your attention? For how long? Reflect on what you can learn from that lecture (the good and the bad) for the next time you give a lecture.

_____

_____

_____

_____

Improving the Passive Lecture: Basic Steps to Incorporate Active Learning

Let us start at the basics. As was mentioned in Chapter 3, at the course level you need a well-organized, detailed syllabus that describes the organization, structure, content, and expectations of the course. Clear course goals must be in place before the course starts. The same is true for a specific class or lecture; clear and measurable objectives are necessary, preferably with reading assignments, prior to the lecture. Consider writing objectives in a form that parallels the progression of cognitive levels captured by Bloom's Taxonomy (Chapter 2). For example, Level One knowledge content, such as definitions, is presented first, followed by content related to Level Two comprehension, and so forth. This will help the student see the organization, structure, and progression of the content. Also, although you will include *nice to know* material in the session, the objectives help direct the students to what you consider to be the important *need to know* parts of the lecture.

Next, let us focus on the lecture itself. This section combines recommendations from several sources[1,3–7] as well as the author's experiences. Suggestions are provided for methods that you can use to strengthen your traditional lecture presentation; these are teacher-centered approaches directed to help you, the teacher, improve your teaching. In addition, suggestions are made for ways that you can further strengthen some of these methods by adding active learning components; they can be considered active learner-centered approaches that engage students and improve student learning. These examples are summarized in **Table 5–1**. For additional recommendations specific to your own institution, consult the learning and teaching center on your campus.

Let us consider the traditional 50- or 90-minute lecture that consists of three parts: the introduction, the body, and the conclusion. In the first

Table 5–1 Teacher-Centered Strategies to Strengthen Lecture Presentations and Extensions to Provide Learner-Centered Active Learning Opportunities

Examples to Strengthen Teacher Presentation of Lecture *Teacher Centered*	Examples for Teacher to Build on Each to Create Active Learning Experiences *Learner Centered*
Provide lecture objectives.	Have students write questions to test their mastery of the objectives.
Assign preclass readings.	Provide questions to guide reading assignments. Provide questions to be completed before class.
Provide handouts.	Provide space for students to take notes. Leave some of the slides partially blank for students to complete as the lecture progresses.
Make links to past learning.	Ask students to identify past learning that has relevance to the new topic.
Describe the underlying structural organization of the content.	Have students assign examples of new content to the underlying structural organization.
"Chunk" the content into digestible segments of no more than 20 minutes.	Introduce a problem-solving activity to enable students to work with the chunk of content.
Give concrete examples to illustrate topics.	Ask students to form pairs and identify additional examples.
Summarize the important points.	Ask students to summarize the most important thing they learned or identify the part of the lecture that was most difficult for them to understand.[10]

five minutes, establish where students have been and where you plan to take them. Briefly review what has been covered in a previous class or course that relates to the new topic. This helps students explicitly see how the content of the present lecture is building upon prior work. Tell students why the content is important and how it will be followed up in future experiences. Review the lecture objectives, and highlight the major topics to be covered. This alerts students to the structure and important content of the lecture.

Concerning the body of the lecture, here are several topics for you to consider as you prepare the lecture. First, let us consider the progression of content within your lecture. After the introduction and description of objectives, try to include a bridge for students to link and transfer what they have already learned and now apply it to this new content. Evidence indicates that activating prior learning facilitates the acquisition of new knowledge[6,7]; the prior learning is the scaffolding upon which new learning is constructed. You could even pause in the lecture and provide an opportunity for the students to examine knowledge that they possess and apply it to your new content. As you progress within the lecture, include methods to guide students in understanding the structural organization of the subject; this helps them to "support their abilities to remember"[7] and "guides the cognitive processes during learning."[6]

Second, providing handouts for the lecture is an excellent way to guide students as you develop the content of your subject. Handouts can be included in a course package, obtained via uploaded material available to students on Web sites, or distributed in class. You can easily use narrative handouts or slide sets to engage the students and provide simple active learning opportunities. In both forms of handouts, you can provide a column, parallel to the content, for students to take notes.[8] To encourage students to pay attention to the lecture, you can occasionally leave a list, diagram, or definition incomplete and have the student insert the missing content as the class progresses. This would also be a good prompt for you to stop and involve students by having them identify their own concrete examples to illustrate the topic that you mentioned. Again, organize the lecture so that students explicitly see the structure of the content.[7]

Appropriately designed PowerPoint presentations provide an organizing structure and can be especially helpful to visual learners. Three brief comments about a PowerPoint slide set are as follows: First, it should serve as an organizing structure, not a verbatim transcript of your presentation. If all the content is on the slide set and you do not provide any additional explanation or examples, why should the student come to class? Second, as summarized by Bransford and colleagues, studies indicate that "comparisons of people's memories for words with their memories of pictures of the same objects show a superiority effect for pictures."[6] Therefore, try to include pictorial representations of objects, topics, and concepts whenever possible. Third, do follow PowerPoint format guidelines. Small fonts, overly busy slides, and distracting special effects interfere with the students' ability to follow the subject content. Consult your teaching and learning center, and review guidelines and examples of appropriately formatted slide sets.

A third topic concerning the body of the lecture is the need to consider the attention span of the students. Middendorf and Kalish summarized several studies and described college students' attention span as being between 15 and 20 minutes.[5] That was in 1996, before attention spans may have declined further as a result of increased television viewing, currently with 11 minutes of programming between commercials, and YouTube videos shorter than two minutes. Varying the intensity and pace of the lecture as well as providing concrete examples to illustrate concepts can help improve the learning process. You can "chunk" content into 15- to 20-minute blocks and organize them in a logical and meaningful sequence,[5] pausing between blocks to illustrate the concepts with metaphors, concrete examples, or other means to make the content come alive. At this point you could even ask the class to form pairs and have them identify examples that would further illustrate the topic. This allows students to become actively engaged in the learning process. After the brief discussion, you can pull the class back together by asking for examples that were identified during the exercise consolidating the examples, and then transitioning to the next point in the lecture. This process could be used several times during a class period, thus helping to reset the attention span clock and maintain interest in the topic.

In the third and final part of the lecture, you can summarize the main points, review the objectives, indicate how the present content will link with future content, and ask for questions. However, realize that few students typically ask questions in large lectures, even if the instructor encourages questions, because many students are intimidated by the large class.[1] In one study, more than 50 percent of questions in large classes came from 2 to 3 percent of the students.[9] To initiate some learner-centered activities in this part of the lecture, you could ask students to summarize the most important thing they learned that day or which part of the lecture was the most difficult (the *muddiest point*) for them to understand.[10] You can use this feedback to modify your presentation for future classes.

> Lecturing by its very nature impersonalizes learning.[1]
> D.W. Johnson, R.T. Johnson, K.A. Smith

Reflective Exercise

Consider a lecture that you are scheduled to present. What are some teacher-centered methods that you can use to guide the cognitive process and improve student learning? If you want to include a learner-centered component in the lecture, which method would you try first? Why that one?

_____

_____

_____

_____

The Transformation from Teaching to Learning

There has been a transformation within the academy from an emphasis on improving teaching to an emphasis on improving and, more recently, assessing student learning. The roots of this learner-centered interest extend back to ancient times when Socrates encouraged students to learn through questioning, and ancient Chinese approaches are summarized in the proverb, "I hear, and I forget. I see, and I remember. I do, and I understand." In more modern times, thinkers such as Dewey advocated learning by doing, and Piaget provided insight into the cognitive development process, encouraging the learner to be active and engaged in real learning.

In this section, we will concentrate on three sources of important milestones in the learning–teaching transformation that have occurred within the last 25 years. First, are the roots of the modern movement that developed from national descriptive studies of what practices were associated with outstanding undergraduate education. Next are empiric, classroom-based studies in the disciplines that provided an experimental validation of the active learning, student-centered approach. Third, are the most recent findings from neuroscience and developmental and cognitive psychology that provided additional scientific understanding of the learning process.

Institutional Good Practices

> Learning is not a spectator sport.[11]
> A.W. Chickering,
> Z.F. Gamson

As mentioned in Chapter 1, a major catalyst in this transformation was Chickering and Gamson's 1987 article in the *AAHE Bulletin* (American Association for Higher Education), "Seven Principles for Good Practice in Undergraduate Education."[11] Synthesizing research on effective university teaching and learning practices that had been collected during a 50-year period, they proposed seven principles central to the promotion of undergraduate student learning. These principles have been a touchstone to the realignment of higher education practices in general and have lessons that can be applied to large classes in particular. In 1991, Chickering and Gamson published a book containing comprehensive analysis of their findings.[12] Given the value of these principles in structuring the learning–teaching processes in large classes, they are again listed in **Table 5–2** with several suggestions for integrating each into a large classroom environment.

Table 5–2 Chickering and Gamson's Seven Principles for Good Practice in Undergraduate Education with Applications to Large Class Courses

Seven Principles for Good Practice in Undergraduate Education[11]	Applications to Large Class Courses
Encourages contact between students and faculty	Establish office hours and communicate through e-mail
	Set up electronic discussion boards
Develops reciprocity and cooperation among students	Provide opportunities for in-class small-group discussions and peer–cooperative learning
Encourages active learning	Provide in-class and out-of-class activities and assignments that emphasize active learning (further developed in the following sections)
Gives prompt feedback	Promptly turn around evaluations
	Use in-class student response system (clickers)
	Provide practice sets with student access to answer key
Emphasizes time on task	Help with time management
	Provide guidelines and suggested timetable for projects
Communicates high expectations	"Expect more and you will get more,"[11] but be sure that you provide clear objectives and helpful guidelines
Respects diverse talents and ways of learning	Provide pictures and words in visuals (see Chapter 2)

Source: Adapted from Chickering AW, Gamson ZF. Seven principles for good practice in undergraduate education. *AAHE Bull.* 1987;39:3–7. http://honolulu.hawaii.edu/intranet/committees/FacDevCom/guidebk/teachtip/7princip.htm. Accessed December 28, 2009.

Also published in 1991 was Pascarella and Terenzini's 20-year study, *How College Affects Students.*[13] The authors concluded that their strongest finding was that "the greater the student's involvement or engagement in academic work or in the academic experience of college, the greater his or her level of knowledge acquisition and general cognitive development."[13]

With Chickering and Gamson's[11,12] and Pascarella and Terenzini's[13] findings as a foundation, work was begun on an objective alternative to college rankings as an indication of good educational practices in higher education across the country. A battery of questions, rooted in the seven principles, became the National Survey of Student Engagement (NSSE) that was first administered in spring 2000 to 75,000 first-year and senior students at 276 institutions.[14] Over the years, results from NSSE reports provided support for the value of active and collaborative learning as powerful aids of student learning. Asking questions in class, engaging in peer instruction, and working on group projects in and out of class all contributed to enhanced student achievement.[15] Among results from the many studies reported on the NSSE Web site,[16] further evidence indicates that the degree of active learning activities, as reported by students on the NSSE survey, had a positive correlation with an index developed by the RAND Corporation to measure critical thinking and other college-level learning.[17]

Although it is not evidence based, arguably the most impactful call for the transformation from teaching to learning was Barr and Tagg's 1995 *Change* article "From Teaching to Learning—A New Paradigm for Undergraduate Education."[18] This essay directed the academy to transform its mission and move from delivering instruction to producing learning and measuring learning outcomes. Although their call for transformation was targeted at higher education in general, two components of their call for a comprehensive paradigm shift had particular import to large class courses. In the new learning paradigm, (1) classes should not be constrained by the traditional 50-minute class blocks nor by the learning environment, and (2) learning is active, student centered, and constructed. Over time, these and other elements of the paradigm shift have prompted faculty to design innovative changes in educational structures and learning strategies. In such student-centered activities as collaborative learning projects and in-class, student-led, small-group discussions, students are "active discover[er]s and constructors of their own knowledge," and faculty content experts are "designers of learning methods and environments."[18]

Discipline-Specific Scientific Teaching

Prompted by national calls, such as the one from the National Research Council,[19] to apply what is known about learning to science curricula, numerous reform efforts have started to take hold in math, biology, chemistry, engineering, and physics. In a 2004 Policy Forum article in the journal *Science,* Handelsman and colleagues describe the results and value of several science education reform efforts. These reforms, based on scientific teaching (the use of scientific results from programs that have systematically tested the impact of active learning strategies on students in the process of teaching science), indicate that active participation "helps students develop the habits of mind that drive science."[20] Although the time devoted to active learning and inquiry-based activities was found to reduce some coverage of previous content, empirical evidence indicated that learning is enhanced and knowledge acquisition, as measured by standardized tests, is retained.[21]

However, Handelsman does express frustration. Why are these methods not more widely incorporated into the undergraduate science curriculum? Scientific evidence establishes that student involvement and active learning increases and improves learning. Why are the scientists not following the science? Noting that "most scientists do not read these reports (of effectiveness of active learning techniques in applied or education journals), but do read *Science,*"[20] the authors provide a guide to science faculty and administrators to help implement scientific teaching in the science lecture halls in higher education. An online supplement to their article with examples from university-based science programs is provided.[22] Several of these innovative approaches will be included in later sections.

Insights from Neuroscience, Cognitive Psychology, and Developmental Psychology

Concurrent with these research studies and calls for reform in the higher education enterprise, the fields of neuroscience, cognitive psychology, and developmental psychology produced studies that began to provide a scientific understanding of how learning occurs. In 1999, the National Academy of Science (NAS) synthesized the research findings from these fields in a book, *How People Learn: Brain, Mind, Experience and School.*[6] This is a meaty distillation of learning-based research. The book also fulfills an another extremely valuable function by linking the scientific findings to recommendations for change in the classroom and in student learning strategies. *How People Learn* is available free online at http://www.nap.edu; it is highly recommended.

Five excerpts from *How People Learn* that are of particular relevance to this chapter are as follows:

1. The new science of learning is beginning to provide knowledge to improve significantly people's abilities to become active learners who seek to understand complex subject matter and are better prepared to transfer what they have learned to new problems and settings.[6]

2. One of the simplest rules (in understanding the structure of the brain) is that practice increases learning and there is a corresponding relationship between the amount of experience in a complex environment and the amount of structural change in the brain. Learning changes the physical structure of the brain. Structural changes alter the functional organization of the brain; in other words, learning organizes and reorganizes the brain.[6]

3. A knowledge-centered perspective on learning environments highlights the importance of thinking about designs for curricula. To what extent do they help students learn with understanding versus promote the acquisition of disconnected sets of facts and skills? Curricula that are a "mile wide and an inch deep" run the risk of developing disconnected rather than connected knowledge.[6]

4. A focus on the degree to which environments are learner centered is consistent with the evidence showing that learners use their current knowledge to construct new knowledge and that what they know and believe at the moment affects how they interpret new information. Sometimes learners' current knowledge supports new learning; sometimes it hampers learning.[6]

5. Because many new technologies are interactive, it is now easier to create environments in which students can learn by doing, receive feedback, and continually refine their understanding and build new knowledge.[6]

Additional scientific evidence can be found in primary research reports in the fields of neuroscience, cognitive psychology, and developmental psychology. Recent books are also available that update the scientific understanding and practical implications of the science of learning and provide a rich variety of evidence-based suggestions to improve the teaching–learning process. Two examples from 2008, are Jensen's *Brain-Based Learning: The New Paradigm of Teaching*[23] and Mayer's *Learning and Instruction*.[7]

In summary, you can improve student learning with your teaching strategies and how you structure your large class experiences. Based on research findings, you can help students maximize their learning by providing examples to support the subject content, assisting students to make connections to other areas of learning, structuring opportunities for them to practice and develop expertise, and then applying their problem solving and critical thinking processes to new situations. This is deep learning, not surface learning. This is the type of learning that students will take with them; learning that has been structurally created in the brain as they actively use, reinforce, and then apply their new knowledge in new situations.

Reflective Exercise

What are the ways *you* learn best? Do you try to create structure within the subject content—a coherent cognitive structure? Do you make explicit connections between what you had previously learned and the new material? Do you actively create relationships and internal connections among topics and ideas to enhance the retention of conceptually relevant information? Do you try to apply new principles and information to concrete examples? How do you make sense of new material? Research indicates that all of these strategies promote learning and help transfer learning to new situations.[7] What strategies can you use to help students get involved with their own learning and achieve this enhanced learning?

_____

_____

_____

_____

What Matters in Increasing Active Learning Experiences: Getting Ready for Inclusion of Active Learning Activities in Your Large Class

Let us start this section with another reflective exercise; this time one developed by Weimer in her 2002 book, *Learning-Centered Teaching*.[24] She recommends that prior to selecting new teaching strategies, the instructor should "start with a complete and accurate understanding of the instructional self." She continues with prompts to guide this self-reflection:

- How much do you know about how you teach?
- Can you accurately and in detail describe what you do to promote learning?
- Can you explain the connections that exist among the proclivities of your style (what you believe you do well), the configuration of content in your discipline, and the learning style of your students?
- Can you identify the assumptions inherent in the particular set of policies, practices, and behaviors you use in the classroom?
- Do you know what you believe about teachers, learners, content, and context and their respective roles, responsibilities, and contributions to the educational enterprise?

In the sections that follow, you will gradually move from learning–teaching strategies that require a low threshold for incorporation into your large class to those that require a complete course redesign. That progression begins with teacher-centered approaches and evolves with more emphasis on active learning strategies that progressively emphasize a more student-centered method. As Sylvia argues in Chapter 1, there is a strong and necessary interaction between the approaches directed toward teachers in the teacher-centered side of the equation and those directed toward students in the learner-centered camp. For both teachers and students who are not familiar with the new roles and responsibilities required in a student-centered approach, a gradual, rather than radical, transformation with a progressive shift in focus is a reasonable course of action. But as you will see in the discussion that follows, even though active learning is at the center of this transformation, active learning strategies by themselves, without appropriately planned assignments and faculty-planned learning activities, may not create the improvements that you seek. Although various active learning activities will be the focus in the remainder of this chapter, the transformation in learning requires more than the introduction of active learning strategies alone. It requires a reexamination of the roles of the faculty and the student, the scope and depth of content, and attention to the development of independent thinkers across the doctor of pharmacy curriculum.

> The real challenge in college teaching is not covering the material for the students; it's uncovering the material with the students.[25]
> K.A. Smith,
> S.D. Sheppard,
> D.W. Johnson,
> R.T. Johnson

Now (hopefully) you are a true believer in the value of student-centered, active learning experiences. You have read the evidence and are convinced that student engagement and active involvement will improve student learning in your course. You have conducted your own teaching style inventory and feel comfortable with adding or expanding the use of active learning in your large class. Where do you start implementing this approach in your large class?

Where you start very much depends on where you sit. If you have primarily used the traditional lecture approach and your students are acculturated to being passive learners, you may want to start with some teacher-directed student-engagement activities (low threshold). If students have participated in active learning activities in previous courses and you have experience with the approach, you could consider a progressively more student-centered assignment.

Here are some words of advice to those of you who are just starting to teach with active learning exercises (see **Table 5–3**). As you consider the

---

Table 5–3 Summary of Active Learning Implementation Steps

1. Start gradually and incrementally.
2. Start early in the semester to establish that active learning activities are the standard operating procedure for your class.
3. Match your active learning strategies with the environment—the content of the course, the physical structure of the classroom, the availability of technology, students' prior experience with active learning, and your experience with using active learning strategies.
4. Expect student push back (covered at the end of this chapter).

examples that follow, be selective. Start small and select one or two active engagement strategies that are appropriate for your class content and with which you feel comfortable. Introduce one early in the semester and repeat it during several sessions so that students adjust to this new course expectation. Reflect upon the impact of the first strategy you used, and consider adding another during the semester. But do not try to do too much too soon. That will just lead to frustration for your students, if they are not accustomed to active learning, and disappointment for you. If you are part of a multiple-instructor course, perhaps the course coordinator could hold a meeting prior to the beginning of the semester during which the collective instructors agree to incorporate one active learning strategy that remains consistent across all lectures. As you gain experience and confidence (and as the students adjust to the shift of responsibility), consider varying the method and incrementally move the class from teacher-centered teaching to student-centered learning.

Active Learning in Action in Large Classes: Pedagogies of Engagement

Let us establish a continuum of active learning experiences, or as Edgerton called them, "the Pedagogies of Engagement."[26] On one end is the passive lecture with minimal opportunity for students to raise questions. On the other end, is problem-based learning where students, with faculty serving as guides, construct their own learning that is needed to understand the problem. For the purposes of this chapter, we will exclude both of these extremes. It is assumed that the reader who has gotten this far in the book would reject the former and the latter, which generally requires a small-group format, and will be discussed in Chapter 7.

The journey that you will take through the Pedagogies of Engagement, and the stops that you will make along the continuum, is not exhaustive, but it is representative. You will start with low-threshold strategies that involve small (and then progressively more impactful) changes in the class and its content. The next stage of sophistication is the technology-enhanced class with course content supplemented and reinforced with, and at times directed by, student-response systems (clickers). Blended learning is also briefly visited at this stop. The third and last stop in your journey is the cooperative–collaborative learning activities that range from in-class small-group discussions to out-of-class group projects. Although these three types of strategies are initially presented as three distinct categories, in actuality there are many overlapping areas along the continuum.

Many tour guides were available to the author as she planned your journey. From "Twenty Ways to Make Lectures More Participatory," a brief online document from the Derek Bok Center for Teaching and Learning at Harvard University,[27] to Angelo and Cross's encyclopedic tome *Classroom*

Assessment Techniques: A Handbook for College Teachers[28] (a wonderful collection of assessment tools with step-by-step procedures that can be used as in-class and out-of-class prompts to engage students in their learning and provide feedback concerning their progress), to Fink's *Creating Significant Learning Experiences: An Integrated Approach to Designing College Courses*,[29] all provide excellent examples (albeit primarily not technology-based) of places we can stop and methods you can consider. These and many other ideas are included in the following sections.

Low-Threshold Strategies for Active Learning

By far the most examples illustrating active learning are at this end of the continuum. They are useful first steps as methods to introduce active learning to both students and instructors. Some of these strategies were mentioned in an earlier section of this chapter but are included here for completeness. Most can be classified as teacher directed and learner centered.

Remember that with any instructor-prompted question-and-answer period or group discussion, there is a natural lag between the instructor's question and the student's answer. As you pose the question, try moving out from behind the lectern and move into the class. Let your body language be encouraging. For thoughtful, meaty questions that cannot be answered with simple yes or no answers, provide time for students to process the question, mentally scan their previous knowledge, review the new content, determine their response, and then decide whether or not to share their thoughts with the instructor and the class. Two suggestions may prove helpful in these types of exercises. First, have the students jot down some thoughts about the questions.[27] That gets their thought process activated. Second, feel comfortable with silence in the classroom while you are waiting for student responses. Do not rush in and fill the silence with your answer to the question. Wait at least 10 seconds (singing "Happy Birthday" under your breath is a good approximation). Restate the question, and generally by that time, some of the students feel uncomfortable with the silence and will offer their responses. Be supportive of both correct and incorrect responses. To keep a discussion going, deflect both correct and incorrect responses by asking the class, or a specific member of the class, if they agree with the previous response and why.

Several examples in the sections that follow suggest the use of in-class discussions that can be characterized as either teacher centered or student centered. When the instructor poses the question and orchestrates a class-wide discussion, it can be described as a teacher-centered discussion. When the teacher initiates a question, and the discussion is internal to a small number of students, it can be described as a learner-centered discussion. After small-group discussions, the faculty member is likely to draw the entire class back together for a summary discussion.

However, the formative discussion that has occurred is internal to a small group of students. Think–pair–share and small-group discussions are examples of student-centered discussions and are included as a separate category. Brookfield and Preskill's book *Discussion as a Way of Teaching: Tools and Techniques for Democratic Classrooms* is a comprehensive examination of this teaching method.[30]

Preclass Assignments

One approach to introduce active learning is to provide directed readings and study questions to guide preassigned readings (the daily dozen reading questions).[31] The preassigned study questions could be modified to be items on quizzes and tests. Also, students could be assigned to develop their own questions for quizzes and exams based on the reading. These can be combined into student study guides, and some could be incorporated into the actual test.[32]

You can also provide question prompts about the lecture content for students to consider before class.

In-Class, Teacher-Centered, Student Active Engagement (Nontechnology-Enhanced)

End-of-Lecture-Summaries　End-of-lecture summaries are one example of this form of engagement and at least three types of these written summaries could be used. Students could be asked to spend the last two or three minutes of the class (1) writing a summary of the important points of the lecture, (2) identifying the most important thing they learned today, or (3) describing the muddiest part of the lecture—an area they did not understand.[10]

The advantage of this approach is that it creates little disruption with the usual flow of your class. However, there are two major disadvantages in placing the only active learning activity at the end of the lecture. Remember that it is at *the end* of an uninterrupted class when students are at their nadir and are using "take leave behavior" to get to their next class. You should have low expectations that any high-level, active thinking is occurring during these summaries. If you use any of these techniques, combine them with other higher-order strategies that are inserted within the body of the lecture.

Bookending the Lecture　Bookending the lecture[25,33] is a second example of this category. In this method, the faculty member starts the lecture with a structured question-and-answer period related to the lecture topics (perhaps the previously discussed preclass question prompt). At the end of the class (the other end of the bookend), the instructor concludes with summary questions asking students to apply the content to a new situation. To expand upon engaging students only at the beginning and end of the session, you can insert structured, probing questions periodically during the session to prompt class discussion and to reengage the student (remember the attention span issue).[4]

Insert an Activity to Engage A third example of this category is to insert an activity within the class to engage students. Two of many possible ways are presented to illustrate this method. I call the first *Tell me a story*. Rather than explaining the conclusions of a figure or table that you use during the lecture, provide a copy to the class and, through a class discussion, ask the students to "Tell you the story," that is, what are the implications or conclusions that can be drawn from this artifact? For example, copy a table or graph from a journal article that is important to your lecture topic. Rather than telling them the conclusions, ask the students to apply their knowledge of statistics and research methodology to draw their own conclusions.[27]

A second way to provide in-class engagement is to pause after you have presented a new concept and provided examples, then ask the students to take a few moments and think of several of their own examples to illustrate the concept.[28,34] This helps the students to package and insert the new concept upon their own knowledge scaffolding. If appropriately prompted, the students will be prompted by the question to make connections to prior learning and transfer the information to similar situations.[28,34] Then ask for volunteers to share their examples; use this process to generate class discussion and comment about the appropriateness of the examples. An alternative approach is to collect the students' examples prior to the classroom discussion. This will provide you with an indication of class-wide understanding as well as individual student progress while still facilitating a classroom discussion.

In-Class, Student-Centered, Small-Group Discussions (Nontechnology-Enhanced)

Two representative types of student-centered, small-group discussions are the think–pair–share exercise[28] and small-group discussions. In the *think–pair–share* activity, the instructor prompts the students to *think* (and perhaps briefly write) about an aspect or application of a new topic, *pair* with another student, and then *share* and discuss their mutual ideas, first with each other, and then with the larger class. The mechanism to share with another classmate what each student has individually thought about the topic serves to (1) keep students on task by being accountable to the other member of the pair and (2) share and learn from another member of the class.[28]

There are many formats for the second type—small-group discussions. The physical arrangement of the classroom can affect the number of students in each group, and the instructor's objective for the discussion can influence the frequency and duration of the session. One format that the author has used in a large health care systems course is to assign three students to a discussion group at the beginning of the semester. The three-student configuration, where one member of the group sits in the middle with the other two students on either side, works well in fixed-seat large classrooms. To create some heterogeneity for discussion of the course's topics, the students are assigned to groups of three in which at least one student has had introductory pharmacy practice experience (IPPE) in a community pharmacy and one has had IPPE in a hospital pharmacy. Eleven of the 28 class sessions have 20- to 30-minute small-group discussions when students must apply the topic that was presented in that day's class to a new situation or analyze the implications of the topic for their future practice. The group summarizes its discussion on a structured work sheet that is collected, graded, and collectively becomes 20 percent of the students' course grade. As you can see, rather than the think–pair–share approach where the selection of a pair is an ad hoc event, this type of small-group assignment can be done purposefully. The students in each group benefit from both the IPPE experiences and perspectives of each member; thus the small-group discussions serve as a link between the students' past experiences and their increased understanding of the new content.

Several other features of this specific type of small-group discussion format are noteworthy. Not only do students discuss the topic within their group, but they gain experience in three functional roles: (1) leading the group, (2) keeping track of time so that they complete the assignment within the allotted time, and (3) summarizing the discussion and completing the work sheet. These three functions are rotated among the members of the group during the course of the semester. Also, the group discussion topics provide an opportunity for the students to think of a topic from different perspectives. For example, when the class topic is financial incentives in healthcare delivery, the group discussion assignment has each student assume a different perspective, for example, managed care administrator, a hospital director, and a pharmacist to examine incentives inherent in different payment systems.

Postclass Assignments for Individual Students

In-class active learning strategies are helpful to engage students with the content at the moment of the class. However, many in-class activities are of short duration and may not engage in deeper understanding. Thoughtful postclass assignments can provide the structure around which students can reflect upon the new content and build their own understanding of the topic.

Rewriting lecture notes and postclass application assignments are two such strategies. Research indicates that students who rewrite their lecture notes in their own words (rather than copying or restating the instructor's words) retain information longer. Students can create a new version of the lecture information that has now been organized in personally meaningful ways that are more likely to be retained, learned, and used.[7,23,35] They have now written the notes in their own words, and in the process, they encoded it into something that lasts longer.[35]

Postclass assignments can be designed to guide students in making connections among the new concepts and meaningful situations and examples. For example, you can ask the students to write a paragraph connecting your lecture and a recent clinical situation. Or you could ask them to describe how a clinical case would be altered by changes in the pharmacokinetic parameters that were the topic of today's class. Helping students make the linkages between what they see in class and what they will see in clinical practice will aid them, and you, in developing effective learning experiences.[35]

> You can help students see connections between your offerings and their future work.

Medium Threshold for Active Learning: Technology-Enhanced Classroom

One form of technology that is being used to encourage student participation and active learning is classroom response systems, or clickers. A clicker is an electronic response pad that transmits a response to a multiple-choice question to a receiver that collects and then displays the response distribution. Based on a 2010 survey of 550 faculty from a representative sample of 4,500 U.S. and Canadian universities, nearly 25 percent of the faculty have used clickers.[36] A rich literature includes descriptive information of their use and evaluative evidence of their effectiveness; a January 2010 bibliography of clicker articles lists 253 citations.[37]

Chapter 6 presents a comprehensive discussion of the issues that are facing faculty as they consider whether or not to introduce technology into their classrooms. As you read the section that follows, consider the social, educational, and economic logistics of incorporating such a system in your class, as well as what type of resources and technologic support is available at your institution to assist you in the introduction and maintenance of the technology. This is a medium-threshold activity, but it does require that if you decide to incorporate clickers into your course that you adapt your pedagogical style so that they become an integrated, rather than add-on, feature.[38]

Student Response System Used to Engage Students with the Lecture Content

Clickers have been introduced into classes, particularly large lecture classrooms, as a means to actively engage students during the class session. Questions strategically placed throughout the lecture can help students actively construct their learning by considering and then responding to the questions. The collective answers of the class can then be displayed graphically, either with or without the correct response. The display of the response distribution without the answers disclosed is useful feedback to the instructor, who can use the information as a prompt for further discussion with members of the class to justify their answers.

The literature describing and evaluating the use of clickers is from many fields. A particularly useful reference is a 2007 special feature series in *CBE Life Sciences Education*.[39–41] Caldwell's article contains a section of tips for best practices for the use of the clickers, as well as writing appropriate questions.[40] A 2008 special article in the *American Journal of Pharmaceutical Education* (*AJPE*) contains a primer on audience response systems.[42] Two other *AJPE* articles assess the effectiveness of clickers; the first is in a physiological chemistry–molecular biology course,[43] and the second is in a drug information course.[44]

The overall results are variable. Although students have a positive attitude toward the system, is this due to novelty or real value? Some studies report overall grade improvement[45]; others indicate that higher grades were achieved only by those who were more active participants.[46] As more faculty adopt the use of clickers to more fully engage students during the class session, it is important that the focus be kept on students and improvement of student learning rather than the technology.[47] Our goal is a student-centered, not a technology-centered, approach.

Student Response System Combined with Peer Instruction and Small-Group Discussion

Two articles in the January 2, 2009 issue of *Science* announced the arrival of clickers to mainstream science instruction in higher education.[48,49] In both cases, the report involved the use of clickers combined with peer instruction and group discussion. Smith and colleagues asked an average of five clicker questions in a 50-minute genetics course.[48] Students were encouraged to talk with their peers about their answers. The results indicated that students performed better on the subject content that was reinforced with clicker questions and peer discussion.

Mazur goes one step further. In his physics class at Harvard, he assigns his students readings that are to be completed before class.[49] During class, he uses clickers as the vehicle to ask short, conceptual multiple-choice questions that are then discussed by students in small groups. Interspersed between these clicker question-prompted discussions, he makes brief presentations to illustrate or clarify the content. As Mazur states, "Instead of teaching by telling, I am teaching by questioning."[49] This combination of technology-mediated learning enhanced with small-group discussion and peer instruction has transformed the typical large lecture class.

Blended Learning

At a more technologically sophisticated level, blended learning combines the traditional face-to-face teaching and classroom interactions with online capabilities to expand the boundaries of the classroom beyond the physical space. Online material can be accessed by students at times that fit their schedules. Course content can be shared across institutions, and institutions have the ability to tailor aspects of the content and the assignments for their unique needs and objectives. This blended approach has the potential to increase the efficiency of the educational process while at the same time increasing the effectiveness of student learning.[50,51] Several examples of blended learning in pharmacy include a Web-based assignment in nonprescription medicines,[52] Internet-facilitated student learning in a large therapeutics course,[53] a self-paced pharmaceutical mathematics course using Web-based databases,[54] and interactive digital images in pharmaceutics.[55] Also, podcasts of lecture content have been blended with further development of the content through reflective assignments and seminar case studies.

High-Threshold Activity: Formal Cooperative Learning Groups

Studies indicate that student-to-student interaction, whether during in-class sessions or out-of-class assignments and study groups, has a positive effect on learning.[1,25,56] However, in group work, care must be taken to ensure equitable distribution of workload and transparency in group grading.[57] Informal learning groups, such as think–pair–share and small-group discussions, were included in an earlier section of this chapter. Collaborative learning activities[58] and group capstone projects are examples of learning within groups. However, cooperative learning, one of the more structured types of group learning, appears to be particularly effective in increasing student learning. Smith and colleagues describe cooperative learning as follows:

> Cooperative learning is the instructional use of small groups so that students work together to maximize their own and each others' [sic] learning. Carefully structured cooperative learning involves people working in teams to accomplish a common goal, under conditions that involve both *positive interdependence* (all members must cooperate to complete the task) and *individual and group accountability* (each member individually as well as all members collectively accountable for the work of the group). . . . Cooperative learning requires carefully structured individual accountability, while collaborative learning does not.[25]

Extensive studies of the use of cooperative learning in engineering programs indicate that students who participated in these groups performed higher than traditional students in academic achievement (knowledge acquisition, retention, accuracy, creativity in problem solving, higher-level reasoning), increased the quality of their relationships with other students and their *spirit de corps*, and improved their psychological health and their attitudes toward the college experience. Academically, based on effect sizes, Johnson and colleagues estimate that "students who would score at the fifty-third percentile when learning individually will score in the seventieth percentile when learning cooperatively."[1]

Cooperative learning does require the instructor to devote time and energy to creating the environment for positive interdependence among group members while retaining individual students' accountability. Putting a group together or letting students self-select their own groups and then telling them to work on a project is not sufficient. The instructor does need to prepare the class for this type of interdependent learning by covering interdependency, teamwork skills, and group-processing methods. Methods to assess individual accountability must be developed. Time needs to be structured into early class sessions to facilitate the human dynamics of this approach, and time could be reserved during some regular class sessions for group meetings. Generally, students are also expected to continue their group work in out-of-class sessions.

Cooperative learning is frequently targeted toward course content mastery and academic achievement. But perhaps the more creative and expanding role for group learning is through the assignment of a course project or capstone activity. In that situation, the student groups apply their collective knowledge to an original effort. Faculty need to prepare the students for the group activity and develop suggested timetables and guidelines, but after that the role of the instructor is to step back, watch the learning take hold and the creativity develop, and be available as a resource when needed. Group projects can be powerful opportunities for learning and application.

Lessons from Undergraduate Physics Education Reform Efforts

You might ask, What can I learn from physics education reform in higher education? Much! Why? Because for the last 15 to 25 years, the higher-education physics community has benefited from two national standardized student assessment tests: (1) the Mechanics Diagnostic (MD) test of conceptual understanding of Newtonian mechanics and (2) the Force Concept Inventory (FCI). By having gold standards against which traditional lecture methods and innovative teaching–learning strategies can both be measured, the physics education community can examine the comparative effectiveness of various strategies.[58]

Since 1992, Hake has collected national test scores from pre- and posttest administration of these standardized tests from physics courses that used traditional as well as interactive engagement (IE) pedagogies.

Based on 62 introductory physics courses with 6,542 enrolled students that covered the same material, Hake reached the following conclusion: the interactive engagement (IE) classes performed significantly higher than the traditional classes. Nearly all of the IE groups scored higher than the traditional classes.[58]

What is important about these findings is not only that they affirm previously cited studies, but they do so with such scientific rigor and such statistical power. The evidence is substantial that incorporating interactive engagement of students with their subject—small-group discussions, use of student response systems, collaborative learning, or other methods—improves and retains learning. As you consider where you can start to incorporate active learning/interactive engagement strategies in your teaching, use the following exercise to get you thinking about the many opportunities.

Reflective Exercise

Consider the methods in **Table 5–4**. Which of them are you presently using? Which additional ones would you consider? What would you need to do to implement a new teaching strategy? (VanAmburgh and colleagues[59] provide a representative list of active learning strategies that can be used as a scorecard to inventory the type of active learning strategies that are included in courses.)

Be Prepared for Student Push Back

There is a disconnect between the pedagogy of engagement and our traditional students. They are acculturated to passively sit in class and have you deliver information to them in bite-size pieces. But ironically, when you adopt a *student-centered* pedagogy of engagement, depending on the developmental state of your students (see Chapter 2), the students may become angry.[2] Now you are telling them that they need to work for new knowledge, that they need to take responsibility for their learning. They can turn hostile and demanding, saying "I'm paying all this tuition. Why aren't you doing your work? Why aren't you lecturing? I have to spend all this time in my group trying to figure things out, but you could save us a lot of grief if you would just tell us the answer. You call this student centered?"

Do not give up. Work with other interested faculty members to form a faculty learning community. Develop a strategy to incrementally introduce progressively more engaging active learning elements across the curriculum. Give guided directions to students for preclass readings. Hold them accountable for completing the readings before class so that the class session can be devoted to further content development. Prepare the class for small-group and collaborative learning so that interpersonal and

Table 5–4 Selected Active Learning Strategies

Active Learning Strategy	Have You Used?	Would You Consider Using?
Students complete directed readings prior to class.		
Students respond to questions inserted during the lecture.		
Students complete an in-class summary of the lecture's main points.		
Students identify the muddiest point at the end of the lecture.		
Students rewrite the lecture in their own words.		
Students complete application assignments.		
Students discuss the topic in the think–pair–share format.		
Students participate in small-group discussions during class.		
Students use clickers to supplement the lecture.		
Students use clickers in a class emphasizing discussion overlecture format.		
Students use a blended format of in-class lectures with online learning.		
Students participate in cooperative learning for content mastery.		
Students participate in a cooperative learning project.		

communication problems within the groups can be minimized. Contact your institution's learning and teaching center for assistance and read some of the cited references.

And while we are likely to get push back from the students, we do know two things: (1) active learning is good for the students, and (2) it is required by the American Council for Pharmacy Education for accreditation of the doctor of pharmacy program.[60]

One Last Consideration

You have created a student-centered, active learning environment for your students that includes interactive lectures with group discussions, clickers in the classroom, collaborative learning, and group projects. You included many of Chickering and Gamson's seven principles[11] in the design of the learning activities in your large classroom. What else can you do to facilitate student learning?

According to Jensen, in his book *Brain-Based Learning: The New Paradigm of Teaching*, you can attend to the *nonconscious*, the term he uses to describe "something that we do not pay attention to in the moment."[23] We exert much conscious effort in planning the structure and flow of the content and in designing the strategies to actively engage students and facilitate learning, but how much attention do we give to the microenvironment that surrounds the actual moment of the learning–teaching effort? In the moment, do we actively pay attention to the way we come across to students? Are we so caught up in the moment that we do not consciously consider the impact of our enthusiasm (or lack thereof), our attitude, our empathy, our posture, even our clothes, on our students? Our encouragement and conversely our venting of frustration, all have effects on student learning. In his chapter "The Nonconscious Learning Climate," Jensen summarizes research, which indicates that students do unconsciously pick up on clues that we as instructors convey during the instructional effort. As implied, students do not consciously feel these behaviors at the moment, but they are integrated into and do become part of their total learning experience. Whether our persona has a positive or negative effect on learning depends, in part, on how well we pay attention to creating the right learning moment, with all its surrounding attention to our verbal and nonverbal clues and behaviors.

> Much of what impacts learning is not in a teacher's lesson plan. Rather, it is in the hundreds of microvariables present in every learning environment.[23]
>
> E. Jensen

The two-part take-home message for this chapter is (1) create student-centered, active learning engagement activities that are an integral part of your large class, but (2) pay attention to the moment by attending to the nonconscious microvariables so that they do not interfere with or cancel all the effort you have devoted to improving student learning.

References

1. Johnson DW, Johnson RT, Smith KA. *Cooperative Learning: Increasing College and Faculty Instructional Productivity*. Washington, DC: George Washington University, School of Education and Human Development; 1991. ASHE-ERIC Higher Education Report No 4.
2. Felder RM, Brent R. Navigating the bumpy road to student-centered instruction. *Coll Teach*. 1996;44:43–47.
3. Davis BG. Preparing to teach the large lecture course. http://teaching.berkeley.edu/bgd/largelecture.html. Accessed January 15, 2010.
4. Cantillon P. Teaching large groups: ABCs of learning and teaching in medicine. *BMJ*. 2003;326:437–440.
5. Middendorf J, Kalish A. The "change-up" in lectures. *NTLF*. 1996;5(2). http://www.ntlf.com/html/pi/9601/article1.htm. Accessed January 5, 2010.
6. Bransford JD, Brown AL, Cocking RR, eds. *How People Learn: Brain, Mind, Experience and School*. Washington, DC: National Academies Press; 1999. http://www.nap.edu/openbook.php?record_id=6160. Accessed December 23, 2009.
7. Mayer RE. *Learning and Instruction*. New York, NY: Pearson Merrill Prentice Hall; 2008.
8. Pardini EA, Domizi DP, Forbes DA, Pettis GV. Parallel note-taking: a strategy for effective use of webnotes. *J Coll Read Learn*. 2005;35:38–55.

9. Karp DA, Yoels WC. The college classroom: some observations on the meaning of student participation. *Sociol Soc Res.* 1976;60:421–439.

10. Mosteller F. The "muddiest point in the lecture" as a feedback device. *On Teach Learn.* 1989;3. http://isites.harvard.edu/fs/html/icb.topic58474/mosteller.html. Accessed January 15, 2010.

11. Chickering AW, Gamson ZF. Seven principles for good practice in undergraduate education. *AAHE Bull.* 1987;39:3–7. http://honolulu.hawaii.edu/intranet/committees/FacDevCom/guidebk/teachtip/7princip.htm. Accessed December 28, 2009.

12. Chickering AW, Gamson ZF. *Applying the Seven Principles for Good Practice in Undergraduate Education.* San Francisco, CA: Jossey-Bass; 1991.

13. Pascarella ET, Terenzini PT. *How College Affects Students: Findings and Insights from Twenty Years of Research.* San Francisco, CA: Jossey-Bass; 1991.

14. Kuh GD. Assessing what really matters to student learning. *Change.* 2001; 33(3):10–17, 66.

15. Kuh GD, Kinzie J, Schuh JH, Whitt EJ. *Assessing Conditions to Enhance Educational Effectiveness: The Inventory for Student Engagement and Success.* San Francisco, CA: Jossey-Bass; 2005.

16. National Survey of Student Engagement. Publications and presentations. http://nsse.iub.edu/html/pubs.cfm?action=&viewwhat=Journal%20Article, Book%20Chapter,Report,Research%20Paper. Accessed January 15, 2010.

17. Carini RM, Kuh GD, Klein SP. Student engagement and student learning: testing the linkages. *Res High Educ.* 2006;47:1–32.

18. Barr RB, Tagg J. From teaching to learning—a new paradigm for undergraduate education. *Change.* November–December 1995:13–25. http://ilte.ius.edu/pdf/BarrTagg.pdf. Accessed December 28, 2009.

19. National Research Council, Committee on Undergraduate Science Education. *Transforming Undergraduate Education in Science, Mathematics, Engineering, and Technology.* Washington, DC: National Academy of Science; 1999.

20. Handelsman J, Ebert-May D, Beichner R et al. Scientific teaching. *Science.* 2004;304:521–522.

21. Ebert-May D, Brewer C, Allred S. Innovation in large lectures—teaching for active learning. *Bioscience.* 1997;47:601–607.

22. Handelsman J, Ebert-May D, Beichner R et al. Scientific teaching. Online supplement with references demonstrating effectiveness of scientific teaching/active learning in sciences. http://0-www.sciencemag.org.ilsprod.lib.neu.edu/cgi/data/304/5670/521/DC1/1. Accessed December 15, 2009.

23. Jensen E. *Brain-Based Learning: The New Paradigm of Teaching.* Thousand Oaks, CA: Corwin Press; 2008.

24. Weimer ME. *Learner-Centered Teaching: Five Key Changes to Practice.* San Francisco, CA: John Wiley and Sons; 2002.

25. Smith KA, Sheppard SD, Johnson DW, Johnson RT. Pedagogies of engagement: classroom-based practices. *J Engin Ed.* 2005;94:1–15.

26. Edgerton, R. *Education White Paper.* Washington, DC: Pew Charitable Trusts, Pew Forum on Undergraduate Learning; 2001.

27. Derek Bok Center for Teaching and Learning. Tips for teachers: twenty ways to make lectures more participatory. http://isites.harvard.edu/fs/html/icb.topic58474/TFTlectures.html. Accessed November 20, 2009.

28. Angelo TA, Cross KP. *Classroom Assessment Techniques: A Handbook for College Teachers.* 2nd ed. San Francisco, CA: Jossey-Bass; 1993.

29. Fink LD. *Creating Significant Learning Experiences: An Integrated Approach to Designing College Courses*. San Francisco, CA: Jossey-Bass; 2003.

30. Brookfield SD, Preskill S. *Discussion as a Way of Teaching: Tools and Techniques for Democratic Classrooms*. San Francisco, CA: Jossey-Bass; 1999.

31. Ambruster P, Patel M, Johnson E, Weiss M. Active learning and student-centered pedagogy improve student attitudes and performance in introductory biology. *CBE Life Sci Educ*. 2009;8:203–213.

32. Bean JC. *Engaging Ideas*. San Francisco, CA: Jossey-Bass; 1996.

33. Allen D, Tanner K. Infusing active learning into the large-enrollment biology class: seven strategies, from simple to complex. *Cell Bio Ed*. 2005;4: 262–268.

34. Angelo TA. A "teacher's dozen": fourteen general, research-based principles for improving higher learning in our classrooms. *AAHE Bull*. April 1999:3:3–13.

35. Jason H. Becoming a truly helpful teacher: considerably more challenging, and potentially more fun, than merely doing business as usual. *Adv Physiol Educ*. 2007;31:312–317.

36. Primary Research Group. *The Survey of Higher Education Faculty: Use of Educational Technology*. New York, NY: Primary Research Group; 2010.

37. Bruff D. Classroom response system ("clickers") bibliography. http://www. vanderbilt.edu/cft/resources/teaching_resources/technology/crs_biblio.htm. Accessed January 21, 2010.

38. Trees AR, Jackson MH. The learning environment in clicker classrooms: student processes of learning and involvement in large university-level courses using student response systems. *Learn Media Technol*. 2007;32:21–40.

39. Barber M, Njus D. Clicker evolution: seeking intelligent design. *CBE Life Sci Educ*. 2007;6:1–8.

40. Caldwell JE. Clickers in large classrooms: current research and best-practices tips. *CBE Life Sci Educ*. 2007;6:9–20.

41. Preszler RW, Dawe A, Shuster CB, Shuster M. Assessment of the effects of student response systems on student learning and attitudes over a broad range of biology courses. *CBE Life Sci Educ*. 2007;6:29–41.

42. Cain J, Robinson E. A primer on audience responses systems: current applications and future considerations. *Am J Pharm Ed*. 2008;72(4):article 77.

43. Cain J, Black E, Rohr J. An audience response system strategy to improve student motivation, attention, and recall. *Amer J Pharm Ed*. 2009;73(2):article 21.

44. Liu F, Gettig JP, Fjortoft N. Impact of a student response system on short- and long-term learning in a drug literature evaluation course. *Am J Pharm Ed*. 2010;74(1):article 6.

45. Mayer RE, Stull A, DeLeeuw K et al. Clickers in college classrooms: fostering learning with questioning methods in large lecture classes. *Cont Ed Pysch*. 2009;34:51–57.

46. Gauci SA, Dantas AM, Williams DA, Kemm RE. Promoting student-centered active learning in lectures with a personal response system. *Adv Physiol Educ*. 2009;33:60–71.

47. Mayer RE, Almeroth K, Bimber R et al. Technology comes to college: understanding the cognitive consequences of infusing technology in college classrooms. *Educ Technol*. 2006;46:48–53.

48. Smith MK, Wood WB, Adams WK et al. Why peer discussion improves student performance on in-class concept questions. *Science*. 2009;323:122–124.

49. Mazur E. Farewell, lecture? *Science*. 2009;323:50–51.

50. Blouin RA, Joyner PU, Pollack GM. Preparing for a renaissance in pharmacy education: the need, opportunity, and capacity for change. *Am J Pharm Ed.* 2008;72(2):article 42.

51. Blouin RA, Riffee WH, Robinson ET et al. Roles of innovation in education delivery. *Am J Pharm Ed.* 2009;73(8):article 154.

52. Nykamp D, Marshall LL, Ashworth L. An active-learning assignment using nonprescription medicines. *Am J Pharm Ed.* 2008;72(1):article 20.

53. Crouch MA. Using the Internet to facilitate student learning in a large therapeutics course: a three-year perspective. *Am J Pharm Ed.* 2001;65:7–13.

54. Bourne DWA, Davison AM. A self-paced course in pharmaceutical mathematics using Web-based databases. *Am J Pharm Ed.* 2006;70(5):article 116.

55. Fox LM, Pham KH, Dollar M. Using interactive digital images of products to teach pharmaceutics. *Am J Pharm Ed.* 2007;71(3):article 58.

56. Springer L, Stanne ME, Donovan SS. Effects of small-group learning on undergraduates in science, mathematics, engineering, and technology: a meta-analysis. *Rev Educ Res.* 1999;69:21–51.

57. Austin Z, Boyd C. Development of a sequenced strategic thinking assignment syllabus for a senior-level professional practice course. *Am J Pharm Ed.* 1998;62:392–397.

58. Hake RR. Lessons from the physics education reform effort. *Ecol Soc.* 2002; 5(2):article 28. http://www.ecologyandsociety.org/vol5/iss2/art28/inline. html. Accessed December 26, 2009.

59. VanAmburgh JA, Devlin JW, Kirwin JL, Qualters DM. A tool for measuring active learning in the classroom. *Am J Pharm Ed.* 2007;71(5):article 85.

60. Accreditation Council for Pharmacy Education. Accreditation Standards and Guidelines for the Professional Program in Pharmacy Leading to the Doctor of Pharmacy Degree. The Accreditation Council for Pharmacy Education Inc. http://www.acpe-accredit.org/pdf/ACPE_Revised_Pharm.D._ Standards_Adopted_Jan152006.pdf. Accessed July 9, 2009.

Additional Resources

1. A library of examples for using the seven principles enhanced by technology is provided online by the Teaching, Learning, and Technology (TLT) Group at http://www.tltgroup.org/seven/Library_TOC.htm.

2. Publications and presentations of the National Survey of Student Engagement are provided online at http://nsse.iub.edu/html/pubs.cfm?action=& viewwhat=Journal%20Article,Book%20Chapter,Report,Research%20Paper.

3. Periodicals related to college teaching for general readership are provided online by Professional Organizational Development Network in Higher Education at http://www.podnetwork.org/resources/periodicals.htm.

4. Quotations for college faculty are provided online by Western Kentucky University, Faculty Center for Excellence in Teaching at http://www.wku. edu/teaching/db/quotes/.

5. A global listing of teaching and learning centers is provided online by the University of Kansas, Center for Teaching Excellence at http://www.cte.ku.edu/ cteInfo/resources/websites.shtml.

CHAPTER 6

What Matters in Applying Technology to Teaching, Learning, and Assessment?

Evan T. Robinson, RPh, PhD

Introduction

There are a variety of ways to be innovative in teaching, learning, and assessment; however, listing each of these innovative methods in this chapter would serve little purpose. With time, the newest and greatest strategies or innovations change, and some have been shown to fall short of their claims. The central premise to educational innovation is the attainment of the *intended educational outcomes* at the *appropriate level* and in a *manner* that creates a *positive learning environment*. Specific examples include enhancing student engagement, fostering collaborative or self-directed learning, linking theory and practice for the learner in an applied manner, and finally (and not to be forgotten), making the learning environment more fun and welcoming.

One particular innovation in teaching, learning, and assessment—the use of technology—will be the focus of this chapter. To frame this discussion, you are directed to the work of Ralph W. Tyler. In *Basic Principles of Curriculum and Instruction*, Tyler posited that there are four key questions to consider in the development of a curriculum and the planning of an educational experience.[1] The four questions are as follows:

1. What educational purposes should the school seek to attain?
2. How can learning experiences be selected that are likely to be useful in attaining these objectives?
3. How can learning experiences be organized for effective instruction?
4. How can the effectiveness of learning experiences be evaluated?

133

> If we teach today as we taught yesterday, we rob our children of tomorrow.
>
> John Dewey

Tyler used these four questions as the framework for curricular and instructional decision making. One could argue that the spirit of educational innovation could be identified by answering the same four questions with the intent of enhancing the learning environment. Later in this chapter, Tyler's questions will be used to help explore why faculty might consider the adoption of technology to enhance their teaching and the potential for student learning. To meet this end, this chapter will begin by answering the following questions:

- What is the role of technology in teaching, learning, and assessment?
- What are the considerations for adopting technology?
- Why should you consider applying technology to enhance teaching, learning, and assessment?
- How should technology be integrated with your teaching and assessment strategies?

To begin our discussion, please meet Gabrielle, a junior faculty member. Gabrielle has been an assistant professor for a little more than two years. She has been team teaching with her colleagues but has had very little course ownership. However, next semester she will have prime responsibility, and be the instructor of record, for a core course in the PharmD curriculum. Gabrielle would like to enhance the student learning experience by increasing the use of technology in the course, and she will use the next few months to determine how best to accomplish this.

Where does she start? Refer back to scenario 2 from Chapter 3 and focus specifically on how technology would affect the systems involved in designing a course. What are the characteristics of the inputs, processes, and outcomes that would influence the role and function of the use of technology to enhance student learning?

Let us first consider several inputs. Gabrielle has been assigned a new, technologically advanced classroom in a new building on campus. This room could be considered a classroom in one sense, albeit it in a traditionalist view, because it has seats, walls, and is a place students congregate to hear from a faculty member. In another sense, and from Gabrielle's perspective, the room is a very intimidating, high-tech, and futuristic environment due to the technology available to both the faculty member and the students. An additional concern for Gabrielle is that the students in her class have expectations to learn both with and about technology and are extremely technologically savvy. So a central question for Gabrielle is how to appropriately choose from the myriad of available technologic options, software and hardware alike, to identify a means of enhancing the learning environment in a manner in which she feels comfortable.

The challenges Gabrielle faces in determining the appropriate inclusion of technology to enhance teaching, learning, and assessment will provide the basis for the rest of this chapter. As different sections are presented, each will represent a question that Gabrielle needs to consider as she determines how to integrate technology into her class and her role as a faculty member.

> Any growth requires a temporary loss of security.
> Madeline Hunter

Reflective Exercise

Think of the first time you used technology (software or hardware) in the classroom. This could include PowerPoint, prerecorded materials, audience response systems, or even integrating podcasts into the learning environment. What were the reasons for your choice? What challenges did you need to overcome? Make notes of your answers to these questions and think about them as you continue through the chapter and plan for your next class.

_____

_____

_____

_____

What Is the Role of Educational Technology?

As Gabrielle researches the use of technology in the classroom and talks about technology with colleagues and mentors, she comes to the conclusion that technology by itself does not ensure that the educational outcomes will be achieved or that the learning environment will be enhanced. Technology represents a mechanism by which the learning environment, and the corresponding educational outcomes, can either be positively or negatively affected. As with anything introduced into the learning environment, technology needs to be considered with respect to how it benefits the learner and the environment. It should not be introduced for any other possible reasons. This then begs the question, When is it most appropriate to integrate technology into the learning environment? The answer to this question is not easily determined due to the variety of considerations that go into technology integration. In the following sections you will follow Gabrielle as she explores the different issues that relate to the use of technology to enhance teaching, learning, and assessment.

Before discussing the learning environment from the faculty member's perspective, it is important to consider it from the learner or potential learner's perspective. In some instances, students do not ask about the availability of technology and its access (wireless as one example), not because they are not interested in technology, but because they view it as a given. The Millennial generation thinks of pervasive technology in their environment much like previous generations thought of having a telephone in a dorm room or a pay phone on the corner. Times, and expectations, have changed.

> Do not confine
> your children to
> your own learning
> for they were born
> in another time.
>
> Chinese proverb

And it should be noted that any planning made for tomorrow's learner will most likely become dated as a result of the expectations of the learner who arrives the day after tomorrow.

A discussion as to whether technology has a positive or negative impact on teaching, learning, and assessment starts with the perspectives of the learner and teacher. First, do the participants in the educational process—the teacher and learner—have an appreciation for technology? What is the perceived value of technology on both of their parts? Is its potential impact on the learning environment appreciated by the faculty member and the learner? The answer to the latter question is challenging in that it has as much to do with the *perception* of the impact of technology as it does with the actual impact of technology. For example, consider the comprehensive multimedia classroom with state-of-the-art technology available to Gabrielle. This classroom may be perceived as a dynamic learning environment by both the teacher and the learner. However, if the technology in this classroom is not appropriately applied to foster the achievement of educational outcomes, then it could be perceived to negatively impact the learning environment, or at the very least not improve it. Now consider a second example of a classroom with some technology, but not the newest and greatest, that is appropriately applied to the course instruction. In this classroom, assume that the educational outcomes are attained. In both situations, the technology could be associated with the outcomes, but this would not be a completely correct assertion. It is the *appropriate* application of technology that is to be associated with the educational outcomes. Integration of the right technology to achieve the desired outcome will foster learning. And this can only happen if faculty members know what to do and how to do it when creating their educational materials.

Technology in the Learning Environment

So where does Gabrielle start in terms of learning about the available technology? Her first stop was the university's office of educational technology (EdTech), an office that is available on most campuses. She took several of their faculty development workshops and gained a comfort with the use of some of the available technology. The EdTech staff also guided her to online resources that are continuously updated and provide valuable links to quality books, journals, conferences, and learning communities, including the following:

- The Sloan Consortium (http://www.sloan-c.org/)
- Educause (www.educause.edu)
- *The Chronicle of Higher Education* (http://chronicle.com)
- United States Distance Learning Association (www.usdla.org)
- *Online Journal of Distance Learning Administration* (http://www.westga. edu/~distance/ojdla/)

- *American Journal of Pharmaceutical Education* (www.ajpe.org)
- American Association of Colleges of Pharmacy (www.aacp.org)

Although the different options, issues, and considerations involved in the application of technology to the learning environment may be overwhelming, the EdTech staff helped Gabrielle examine her options. They suggested that she categorize the technology considerations in terms of hardware versus software, then in terms of who is actually applying it (faculty, students, both) to teaching, learning, and assessment.

To be clear, hardware without software does not necessarily work, so the examples provided are in some ways oversimplified. The point is that in some instances hardware is the point of enhancement, and in other instances the software or Web-based application is the point of educational enhancement as long as minimal technology requirements are met. Although this topic may seem out of context in a chapter that examines technology-enhanced teaching, it is the author's contention that some innovations either succeed, stumble, or fail as a result of a lack of awareness regarding the infrastructural pieces that support the educational endeavor. All too often innovation is recommended, but a systems understanding of achieving that innovation is lacking. This is not for the purposes of turning faculty into technology experts, but instead to create just enough awareness to help them seek advice from the appropriate individuals.

> Teachers need to integrate technology seamlessly into the curriculum instead of viewing it as an add-on, an afterthought, or an event.
>
> Heidi-Hayes Jacobs, Educational Consultant

What Are the Considerations to Implementing Technology Initiatives?

The key to using technology is to be sure that it is applied appropriately. To accomplish this, it is important to have the necessary resources to make these experiences flow smoothly and allow for the use of technology that promotes not only enhanced teaching and learning, but does so in a manner that empowers the student and faculty member alike. To foster this level of success, Gabrielle must consider a variety of contributing factors including, but not limited to, technology support of hardware and software, infrastructure issues, faculty development, and student development. The absence of any of these components can lead to a less than satisfactory outcome and subsequently diminish the possibilities for future use of technology as an enhancement to the learning environment.

Resource Considerations

The application of technology to enhance teaching, learning, and assessment requires, as one might guess, working technology. Although Gabrielle now feels comfortable with the technology and has the support of the EdTech staff, other faculty must realize that without the infrastructure and support, the applications that benefit the learning environment may be limited in

Any teacher that can be replaced by a computer deserves to be.

David Thornburg

scope or even problematic to use. Unfortunately, implementation problems can result in discontinued use of technology or failure to adopt innovations in the future.

Wired classrooms and ubiquitous access to technology infrastructure are becoming more common as higher education becomes a wired and wireless domain. To this end, there is a need for a wired classroom available to the faculty member as he or she facilitates the learning experience. To define a wired classroom would date this material, so for the purposes of this discussion, in general it means a classroom in which sufficient hardware and software exists to support the appropriate integration of technology into the learning environment. This could include but not be limited to presentation software, audio and video presentation and recording media, audience response systems, and a wireless environment.

To put these resources in place is not inexpensive, nor is it a one-time expense. Technology integration is a longitudinal expense that has a significant amount of recurring personnel costs associated with it. A vast array of literature has been devoted to the topic of technology infrastructure and support and could by itself be an entire topic of discussion. To identify the literature, which changes almost daily, Gabrielle was referred to the Web sites for the *Chronicle of Higher Education* (www.chronicle.com) and Educause (www.educause.edu). It suffices to say that the more complicated a system becomes, the more planning, consideration, and education must take place to facilitate success. In the case of technology-mediated education, the facilitation of success requires an up-to-date infrastructure (not necessarily state-of-the-art), appropriately trained support staff, and faculty and students who are appropriately educated on how to use the technology. Again, none of these things can be accomplished without sufficient planning and resource allocation.

However it is implemented, there must be some form of centralized accountability and communication to ensure that programmatic issues are being addressed and that one aspect of technology enhancement does not jeopardize other aspects of the educational program. The question is how centralized accountability works into the planning and implementation process and the different considerations. For example, cost is the obvious consideration to get any plan started. What about annual license renewal fees or program upgrade costs (if applicable), hardware and software compatibilities, long-term support, and continued faculty development as either the product changes or new faculty join the program?

Considerations for the Faculty

No application of technology will take place to enhance student learning unless the faculty are comfortable with its application. This can be as uncomplicated as using PowerPoint to as complicated as virtual reality, simulations, and social networking media. Unless the faculty member is comfortable in both the how and why of using technology, it will not be successfully implemented. The how can be defined as what the technology is and what is necessary to make it work, which can be as simple as turning it on to as complicated as how to create an avatar or a simulated scenario with multiple outcomes.

Gabrielle now considers how the available hardware and software would impact her teaching and role as a faculty member. One could argue that the inception of technology occurred far before the computer with the introduction of the overhead projector. Prior to the overhead, technology was chalk and blackboards. And yet today, overheads and chalkboards (or whiteboards) still exist. To fast forward to today and the Millennial learner's environment, the technology of the day is a computer in the classroom integrated to some smart device that facilitates the use of technology that permits faculty members to do as much or as little as they would like.

So what were some of Gabrielle's findings as related to the hardware and software at her disposal as she considered what to do within her classroom? Gabrielle thought it would be a good idea to start a list of the hardware and software and was surprised by all the things she found. Her list included the following:

- Smart classroom technology (computer, video presentation, screen editing and capture, document camera, etc.)
- Smart classroom extenders that facilitate a classroom to become distance-learning enabled
- Audio and video capture systems that allow for synchronous and asynchronous use of the materials
- Audience response systems that enable formative and summative assessments anonymously and can also be used as an engagement strategy
- Online assessment programs that enable testing via myriad mobile technologies ranging from laptops and tablets to smart phones
- Simulation and gaming programs that help the student to engage with the content (e.g., permit a student to virtually be inside the heart to see blood flow and an occlusion as opposed to seeing a picture of the heart)
- Social networking media that create virtual online communities, permitting synchronous and asynchronous exchanges of information, knowledge, and interactions
- Virtual reality environments that provide a means for learning or interaction to take place in a technology-mediated manner, similar to a real-world encounter
- Animatronic simulations that allow students to interact with physical-simulated situations, such as patients who can breathe, talk, and have pulses, thus creating a host of physiological challenges

Hardware and software in the educational environment are always evolving; there will always be something newer and greater to consider.

- Portable technologies that are commonly available to students, like laptops, cell phones, and other devices
- Learning management systems like Blackboard that provide one-stop shopping for the students

The lesson Gabrielle took away from her assessment became crystal clear—although she has attended several technology workshops, the hardware and software in the educational environment is always evolving, and there will always be something newer and better to consider. She also realizes that what is more important is whether the technology that is present is appropriate for the given situation and whether it will benefit teaching, learning, and assessment.

Reflective Exercise

Consider a recent class you taught in which you felt you could have done a better job facilitating learning or creating an excited learning environment due to the complexity of the course material or topic being taught. Could technology-mediated teaching and learning have helped you with your class design and delivery? What type of technology? Think about the list Gabrielle provided as a possible starting point.

_____

_____

_____

_____

Considerations for Students

At this point in Gabrielle's preparation, she realizes she has spent time considering the applications of technology to enhance teaching, learning, and assessment mostly from the perspective of the faculty member. But to be effective, she also has to consider it from the perspective of the students.

The technology being applied by the Millennial learner is used not only to receive and interact with information, but also to find information and create new knowledge. And much like the technology used by the faculty, the technology used by the student has evolved from the desktop computer, to the laptop, to the tablet PC, and to the smart phone, iPod, iPad, and audience response system (personal response station). The type of technology is a function of the connectedness the student seeks to attain with his or her peers and the learning environment. And the Millennial student is more connected than ever before in all forms and facets.

From the perspective of the learner, the applications and opportunities created by innovative software are truly unique. Although there are software applications that can be linked to the student, many more are considered classroom extenders or facilitators between the faculty member and the learner. Software can help the student learn and facilitate success in learning.

Why Consider Applying Technologic Innovations?

To this point in her research, Gabrielle had answered a number of interesting questions, but one thing still nagged her—finding the answer to the question why. Gabrielle realized that when it came to the challenges of integrating technology into the classroom, it was important to leave supposition out of the consideration and focus on the facts. If some aspect of technology is being considered because someone thinks it might have value, then significant possible problems could ensue. This is not to say that all innovation requires empirical research, and in many instances, advances in teaching, learning, and assessment have to start somewhere and could be based upon a hunch. But in times of tight resources and ever more complex educational systems, it is important to go beyond *think* to at least *know*, especially in light of the fact that the evidence to prove the effectiveness of an innovation may not exist. In summary, decisions to implement technology initiatives, albeit large or small, necessitate an evidence-based approach to ensure that decisions are based on fact and not supposition.

As we return to Gabrielle, she identified seven *why* questions to answer that she felt would help her determine the best reasons and the best technologies to enhance teaching, learning, and assessment. As you review the seven why statements that follow, take time to answer each for yourself—why let Gabrielle do all the work!

The First Why: The Student

Gabrielle learned that according to a national study of college students regarding technology use, "students preferred a moderate use of IT in their courses and expect faculty to use technology well."[2] In addition, "the primary benefit of technology in courses is convenience, followed by connectedness," and 41 percent of the students said they preferred their professors to use information technology moderately in class.[2] Students in the survey most commonly said that convenience was the primary benefit to the use of technology in courses and that virtual connectivity was second. The same survey also found that students brought technology other than computers to college with them.[2] The purpose and intent of the students bringing the technology, which included cell phones, mobile music devices, and PDAs, was due more to societal integration and it becoming a part of their social fabric than for teaching and learning. The key is for institutions of higher education to take advantage of the technological prowess and interest of the Millennial generation.

This why statement represents an interesting challenge in that satisfying it for the right reasons will elevate teaching, learning, and assessment. Satisfying this why statement for the wrong reasons, like meeting student expectations without the ability to integrate the technology into the fabric of the educational processes, is a dangerous proposition. This could result in expectations that will not be met because there is no more reason to have the technology than to not have it. By virtue of this, the technologic version of keeping up with the Jones's, the institution will spend vital capital on resources without a coherent plan to use the technology to benefit the learner, faculty, or institution.

As we find Gabrielle mulling over this question, she comes back to the same issue. Will the student who uses technology in her class leave the better for it? Will it improve the student's learning? She finds that talking with her peers and the EdTech staff, reviewing educational innovations in the literature, and participating in online learning communities, much like her students do, help provide her with sound examples to consider. When she is armed with ideas, she then takes them to the EdTech staff on campus to see if her ideas can be implemented.

The Second Why: Learning Occurs Anywhere and Everywhere

When Gabrielle decides she has a handle on why technology benefits students, she then decides to try to tackle the question of where. The issue of where learning can occur is truly puzzling to Gabrielle in that she is coming to the realization that even though her classroom is technology-laden, there may not be walls to her classroom anymore. She is faced with the fact that her students could either be in her classroom, in class some of the time, not in the classroom, or not even interacting with her in real time and still be learning. It is the author's belief that one perspective on teaching and learning is that learning occurs anywhere and almost in the fashion of just-in-time learning. Experiences and discussions outside of the traditional classroom lead to teachable moments (planned and self-derived), and subsequent learning leads to a constantly evolving growth both in terms of the learner's personal database as well as his or her ability to apply that database in the real world. It is important to realize that mechanisms are in place to facilitate teaching, learning, and assessment anywhere, irrespective of location or time (real or elapsed). Mobile learning technologies in the form of handheld devices, cell phones, iPods, etc., have created a means by which information acquisition and interactivity occur easier than ever before. With this growth in mobile devices and virtual connectedness, however, comes the risk of enhanced levels of expectation that are not attainable by either the learner or the educational institution.

The topic of distance learning is one that Gabrielle explored through her reading and research and with the EdTech staff. Although it might seem possible for Gabrielle to make the decision herself to deliver her course via some form of distance learning methodology, it is not likely that she would do so without it being a program-based decision due to the resources required by the college or university as well as by the learner. According to a 2002 report from the Council for Higher Education Accreditation, of the 5,635 accredited institutions in the United States, approximately 35 percent (1,979) offer some form of distance education.[3] Not all of these distance learning programs are online distance learning, but a significant portion of the growth in higher education today is coming from online education, and the resources necessary to accommodate that growth may be different than those needed to deliver a traditional curriculum. Distance education represents a means of changing the location for teaching, learning, and assessment from one point to another via fixed technology, like point-to-point teleconferencing and Web-based distributive learning models that go to many learners in many places. Distance education also changed the model from all teaching, learning, and assessment being at the same time (synchronous) to models of distributed teaching, learning, and assessment that can take place at any time (asynchronous).

In a survey of schools of pharmacy conducted in 2006, 93 percent of the respondents indicated that their universities provided course work via distance education, and 50 percent of respondents indicated that the school of pharmacy provided course work via distance education.[4] The basis for the decision of what technology should relate to where learning should take place is addressed in more detail in the sixth why statement.

The Third Why: Lifelong Learning and the Learner's Database

The appropriate use of technology within the learning environment has the wonderful benefit of fostering lifelong learning abilities because it helps foster technology literacy and hopefully information literacy and intellectual curiosity. The ability to foster lifelong learning is important to Gabrielle and is one of the reasons why she is interested in technology integration. Applied technology used by the learner can create a situation in which the learner can continuously revise and update his or her personal database. Using the practice of pharmacy as an example, consider the frequency with which new medications or indications are added and how quickly patient-care protocols can change. In this dynamically changing environment, the ability to find and apply new information should be seamless. Pharmacy, similar to many other disciplines within higher education, faces the challenge of a continuously increasing body of knowledge and only a finite amount of time in which to prepare the learner. It is no longer possible to prepare the learner only for content mastery; the speed with which things change in health care and pharmacy necessitates a lifetime of learning. The use of technology within the learning environment can help facilitate the development of lifelong learning skills by giving the learner the opportunity to practice finding and applying information within different courses or curricula. The challenge is that to accomplish this, the technology must be in the hands of the learner, not necessarily the faculty. One simple learning example is a laptop program in which all students have a laptop, course content is available via the Internet in some manner, and students are expected to gather, interpret, and apply information to predetermined problems. In this example, the student has the technology, and the faculty member creates the learning context that facilitates the student use of technology. This example could just as easily have been a handheld device or cell phone. The key is that this will only work if the learner has the technology and knows how to use it, and the faculty member creates learning experiences that require the student to reach beyond known resources to find the answer.

Facilitating lifelong learning abilities within the student should be a curricular outcome, but it may or may not be a part of the public plan. If lifelong learning via technology is a part of the stated planned curriculum, then it is identifiable as a curricular outcome and is mapped to unique courses to ensure it is attained. The ability could also be a part of the hidden curriculum, in which it could be a stated curricular outcome, but instead of being mapped into specific courses it is accomplished in a more subdued, low-key manner within the curriculum. For example, each course has to have some outcomes related to lifelong learning, but the outcomes are scattered across a large number of courses. In this manner, it should still be measureable but not as evident.

The Fourth Why: What Educational Purposes Should the School Seek to Attain?

Tyler's first question, "What educational purposes should the school seek to attain?,"[1] points to the issue of the educational outcomes or curricular outcomes for the school of pharmacy. To address this why statement, Gabrielle needs to consider the bigger picture within her school of pharmacy and how her course supports the mission of the program. How does the introduction of technology help facilitate the achievement of one or more of the curricular outcomes? If, for example, problem solving and critical thinking are curricular outcomes, then does the technology help students successfully attain this outcome? To further expand upon this example, let us consider the use of mobile learning devices within a program. What is gained by incorporating these devices into the learning environment? Well, students have instant access to online resources and can bring them into discussions dynamically. Faculty can now ask students to find answers to ill-defined problems during class time, knowing that they can search and bring the information into the discussion. The students have a means by which information retrieval and application can be used irrespective of location, albeit within the didactic or experiential portions of the program. But what is the outcome being sought, and does the why statement justify the costs and challenges of getting there?

The other consideration when answering Tyler's first question is the collateral benefits that can result for the student but are not explicitly stated either within the curricular outcomes or whatever is driving the consideration. In the previous example of the mobile learning device, would students also be increasing their technological literacy; could its exposure help faculty, preceptors, and practitioners better understand the applications of technology; and could it provide a catalyst for change on campus? Given the interconnectedness of components of the educational system, how does the introduction of new technology affect other parts of the system? No innovation occurs within a vacuum, and even though these examples represent indirect benefits, they are benefits, nonetheless, that can prove very helpful when trying to justify adopting innovative technology. But there is a caution: remember to base your justification on more fact than supposition, as stated earlier.

Admittedly, addressing this why statement is bigger than the self and requires the faculty member to be knowledgeable of the program needs and then link to them. Using the systems approach, Gabrielle realizes that it is vital to know the program's mission, curricular outcomes, technology plan, and assessment plan and to consider how these components interrelate to one another. This process also helps Gabrielle gain a much better appreciation of what her faculty colleagues are doing within their respective courses.

The Fifth Why: How Can Learning Experiences Be Selected That Are Likely to Be Useful in Attaining These Objectives?

Tyler's second question asks us to consider how the technology will be used within the learning environment and what types of activities need to be created to ensure the appropriate use of technology to achieve the outcomes. Gabrielle considers the integration of mobile learning devices and how to design her course to achieve the desired effect. First, classroom management and guidelines might have to change to create a more facilitative, student-centered environment where the student is more empowered to find, discuss, and constructively disagree with other students and the faculty member. This not only requires identifying means within the learning environment to accomplish this, but also may necessitate a reeducating of the student to function and learn in a new environment. Faculty development programs may be needed to ensure that faculty members are comfortable in this new role. Depending on the current role definitions held by the student and faculty, these changes could be very easy or very difficult to make. It is important to remember the end user in these instances and, as pointed out before, to make sure the end user is involved in any discussions regarding technology introduction, innovation, or change.

Through this research and reflection, Gabrielle realizes that she should try to address some general questions before deciding what, if any, technology should be integrated into the classroom. Some of her questions include, but are not limited to, the following:

- How will teaching, learning, and assessment be enhanced?
- How will my class and course objectives be met, or enhanced, as a result of integrating technology?
- How much time prior to class will it take to plan for appropriate technology integration?
- What is the reason to implement technology (i.e., increase engagement, active learning, etc.)?
- Has the implementation of the technology been mapped to the course schedule to determine if it represents a consistent and persistent change or a situational change?
- Does the technology need to be pilot tested? How can I do a dry run to ensure that the students and I feel comfortable with the course changes?
- Will I need to reconsider the amount of time I spend delivering content in my traditional 50-minute blocks or do something else?
- Will I feel comfortable with my role in the course if it changes how I interact with the class (i.e., more active learning and engagement)?
- Will the students feel comfortable with the technology and their changed role within the classroom?
- Am I prepared to deal with the challenge that comes from change in the classroom, which can include an initial push back from students if the technology does not work as prescribed at the start?
- Have I realistically evaluated my time and priorities so that I can pursue educational innovation, but not at the risk of my promotion and tenure requirements?

Also, there are collateral considerations that come into play. As Gabrielle seeks to answer this why statement, she comes to the conclusion that changes within her course may well affect other courses as well—the interconnectedness within the educational system. She also questions how to best construct learning activities, not as a result of wanting technology, but instead by choosing technologies that can help the learning activity.

The Sixth Why: How Can Learning Experiences Be Organized for Effective Instruction?

Tyler's third question prompts us to consider how educational experiences can be mapped in a manner to provide continuity of application of the technology relevant to the needs of the student and the proposed educational outcomes.

Gabrielle considers how to address this question and reflects upon all of her earlier issues and research. Answering this why statement is, in many ways, the culmination of a number of the points she has been pondering to bring technology to the classroom. So what is Gabrielle to do, and how will she identify the topics to be covered and identify the different instructional methodologies and activities that would go into the delivery of the course?

To consider the example of the mobile learning device, the faculty member could map different activities within the course to different applications of the technology or at different levels of learning. Perhaps the first application of the technology is to identify relevant facts that relate to the discussion taking place (e.g., lower-level Bloom content). The next application of technology is to expand upon the facts to construct an effective argument, which would require a much better understanding and a connection of different constructs to create a coherent point. The culmination is the student using the technology to educate others regarding his or her findings. Historically, teaching, learning, and assessment were linked to a fixed location, albeit a classroom or experiential site, and there was little or no departure from that except for highly structured journeys into the world beyond the classroom. But as technology has advanced, so too has the opportunity to change how we define the fixed learning space.

Gabrielle is faced with an interesting dilemma and tries to understand how to address the blurring between onsite and distance learning that now creates many variations of the educational experience. One alternative Gabrielle considers is the implementation of hybrid or blended courses,[5] which are becoming more popular and represent what could be interpreted as onsite and distance learning combined for course delivery. For example, instead of teaching a three-credit–hour course with the normal amount of seat time—3 hours per week for 15 weeks—the course is delivered partially via an e-learning methodology, and the class only meets 3 hours per week for 7 of the 15 weeks only for discussions and assessments. The seat time is reduced by half, but the course is still the same amount of credits. This methodology would also permit more active learning because the time spent providing the traditional lecture is significantly reduced.

Another consideration Gabrielle explores is the ability to capture educational content either simultaneously with the course delivery or at another time and then make the material available for later use. The example in this case is the digital capture and rendering of audio and possibly video; this is then released after a class for students to reuse as they see fit to help them learn. So in this example, one type of course delivery creates digitized content to support itself or even provide the content platform to change the course either at that time or in the future. To continue this example, Gabrielle could record and digitize a course during one semester. The next time the course is taught, she could use the portions that will not change as online resources and spend the remaining time discussing cases and engaging students in active learning. As with every instance, the key to this approach is ensuring that the appropriate technology is used to facilitate teaching, learning, and assessment so that the outcomes of the program are met and that the students are helped to learn and grow.

Reflective Exercise

Think back on a class you recently taught in which you saw the 1000-yard stare on the face of a student sitting less than 50 feet away. At that particular point in time, the student could have been almost anywhere but in the classroom. How could the use of technology help you engage this learner? Does proximity necessitate student engagement?

_____

_____

_____

_____

The Seventh Why: How Can the Effectiveness of Learning Experiences Be Evaluated?

The answer to this why statement from Tyler's fourth question[1] is the understanding of whether the intended outcomes have been documented through an assessment process. When considering technologic support for assessment, an entire spectrum of technological possibilities and opportunities are available. The remainder of this response is not going to examine assessment practices (see Chapter 4), but it will instead focus on how assessment can be facilitated or enhanced via a technology-mediated process when appropriate.

Let us examine some of the features of assessment that many faculty consider important, and then see if technology could play a role. The first example finds Gabrielle considering how to best get feedback from her students to ensure that material is being understood and that course concepts are being related to one another. Historically, this has occurred by asking students to raise their hands or by calling on students. But does either of these really assess understanding? Possibly, but not necessarily. Now consider the role of technology. The use of audience response systems allows faculty members to pose questions to students who then anonymously click their individual answers. The aggregate answers can be displayed on a projection slide and used to gauge students' understanding and application of the course material. As such, the use of audience response systems provides information for formative and summative assessments.[6] The results are electronically collected and then can be projected in various graphic formats. The results are anonymous, so the faculty member can easily identify whether the content is being understood by the class and if there is a problem without any student feeling singled out. Think of the power provided to the students by allowing them to interact with a faculty member and the course materials in a nonthreatening manner.

> Audience response systems create opportunities for student engagement.

A benefit to the use of audience response systems is their ability to create opportunities for engagement with the students by asking probing or ethical questions to stimulate discussion. Gabrielle was recently talking with a faculty colleague who enjoys using audience response systems in class and, although she thought it would be beneficial to ask multiple-choice questions with one correct answer, she learned that there are many other things she can do with the systems. She learned that asking complex questions with two or more correct answers is possible, fosters discussion, and is an effective engagement strategy.

Audience response systems can also be used to create different gaming opportunities, such as educational *Jeopardy*. Games offer the opportunity for timed responses, and students can respond as a group after playing a game independently in a manner consistent with assessment methodologies that are based on Individual or Team Readiness Assurance Tests (IRAT or TRAT). In essence, anything that could be done to encourage students to get involved can be done through the use of audience response systems.

But what about the why statement of adopting an audience response system? Unless the faculty are appropriately trained on its use and understand its role in teaching, learning, and assessment, adopting this technology will suffer from the fate discussed earlier. Expectations can be raised, but without a satisfactory outcome, the technology will be a disappointment to faculty and students alike. Whatever the chosen technology-mediated assessment vehicle, it must be selected and implemented for the right reasons. Online testing systems via computers and handheld devices can provide students with instant feedback, both in a formative and summative nature. The systems can also allow for the development of extensive test banks of questions, as well as provide in-depth question analytic features. But the more the faculty try to accomplish with technology, the more complicated the process becomes. Online testing as described in this example may also require hardware support and possibly even standardized student technology, which creates expense and a different type of technology support.

The final example for answering this question is through e-folios, which are electronic (digital) portfolios that allow the student to gather and store information, in a structured or unstructured environment, for review by faculty and for personal use at a later time. These e-folios can

E-portfolios can be used for courses, programs, and as a longitudinal means of assessing student growth.

be used for courses, programs, and as a longitudinal means of evaluating student growth. Nearly any artifact of learning that a student produces could be embedded within an e-folio. But why is the information being gathered, and how is it benefiting the student? Answering this question is important in that students should not be asked to compile an evidence-rich portfolio if faculty do not have resources to review, evaluate, and provide effective feedback on the portfolio. The *perception* of the value of e-folios can sometimes overshadow how to use them effectively, and if this occurs, the result is diminished value and use, regardless of the intent.

Online assessment either by a computer or handheld device can be linear (one question after another) or Web-centric (questions build upon each other), as well as summative or formative. Some versions of online assessment software provide instant feedback and allow the student to see his or her mistakes as well as provide feedback. But with this technology comes a challenge. With online assessment the student needs some hardware and the skills to use it. The same is true from the faculty perspective; faculty will require the skills to use the assessment software. Again, just because it involves technology does not mean that it is the best thing to do.

Summary

Gabrielle has a lot to think about as she considers the implementation of technology in her course. She is engaged in a long process of self-reflection and investigation to answer a number of complicated questions—the questions of why to implement technology and how technology can benefit teaching, learning, and assessment. What she thought would be a quick set of questions to ask and answer turned into a much longer journey than she ever expected. Her eyes became open to the fact that the area of technology is ever changing, and her journey to technology integration will extend over a lifetime in academia with many turns, twists, and choices. This journey of Gabrielle's is reflective of those quintessential lines from the Robert Frost poem *The Road Not Taken*—"Two roads diverged in a wood, and I, I took the one less traveled by, and that has made all the difference."[7] Gabrielle's journey to enhance her classroom with technology is borne from the fact that she has chosen the path less traveled and has been an entrepreneur. Will you be willing to do the same when faced with a similar choice?

References

1. Tyler RW. *Basic Principles of Curriculum and Instruction.* Chicago, IL: The University of Chicago Press; 1949.
2. Kvavik RB, Caruso JB. ECAR study of students and information technology 2005: convenience, connection, control, and learning. http://www.educause.edu/ir/library/pdf/ers0506/rs/ERS0506w.pdf. Accessed August 18, 2009.

3. Council for Higher Education Accreditation. *Accreditation and Assuring Quality in Distance Learning: CHEA Monograph Series 2002, Number 1.* Washington, DC: Council for Higher Education Accreditation; 2002.

4. Robinson ET. Survey of technology use at colleges and schools of pharmacy in 2006: an exploratory study. *J Pharm Teach.* 2007;14(2):105–118.

5. Garrison DR, Vaughan ND. *Blended Learning in Higher Education: Framework, Principles, and Guidelines.* San Francisco, CA: John Wiley; 2008.

6. Cain JJ, Robinson ET. A primer on audience response systems: current applications and future considerations. *Am J Pharm Educ.* 2008;72(4):article 77.

7. Frost R. *The Road Not Taken.* http://poetrypages.lemon8.nl/life/roadnottaken/roadnottaken.htm. Accessed August 18, 2009.

CHAPTER 7

What Matters in Facilitation of a Small Group or Seminar?

Zubin Austin, PhD, MBA, MIS, BSPharm

Introduction

Traditional lecture-based, didactic methods of instruction may be suitable in some situations, for example the transmission of content where outcomes are clear and circumstances are unambiguous. Within professional education, there is an increasing recognition of the limitations of didactic instruction when addressing highly contextualized problems in which judgment and contingency planning are required. Professional practice itself is frequently characterized by the need to exercise professional judgment and discretion, by situations where there is no clear, single correct answer, and cases where the least worst alternative must be selected because no best option exists.

In recognition of the unique and context-specific nature of professional practice, small-group teaching and learning strategies are frequently used within professional education. However, small-group teaching and learning is not a one-size-fits-all solution to all educational problems or situations, and no single, uniform definition of small-group teaching and learning exists. Several characteristics of this methodology are uniquely well-suited to professional education, and they will be discussed in this chapter. When applied in an appropriate and context-sensitive manner, small-group teaching can facilitate learning and integration of knowledge, skills, and attitudes. Although the logistical, financial, and resource implications of small-group methods may be significant, so too are the potential dividends of this approach.

> The world of education is filled with broken paradoxes— and with the lifeless results. We separate teaching from learning. Result: teachers who talk but don't listen and students who listen but do not talk.[1]
>
> P. Palmer

In this chapter, an attempt will be made to answer the following questions about small-group teaching and learning:

- What is small-group teaching and learning?
- How is small-group teaching and learning different from other methods? In what situations might it be preferred?
- What can you do to prepare yourself for the role of a small-group facilitator?
- What can you do to help your students prepare themselves for the role of small-group learners?
- How can you apply facilitation and small-group process skills to enhance the success of learners in the small groups you facilitate?

What Is Small-Group Teaching and Learning?

Small-group teaching and learning typically involves the following:

- A fewer number of students than traditional lecture-based formats, usually 6 to15 students, depending on the circumstances
- A facilitator or educator who may or may not be a content or subject-matter expert but one who is able to motivate students, elicit positive performance, and balance content and process issues within the group
- A high degree of interaction among all members of the group
- Shared responsibility for outcomes between learners and the instructor or facilitator
- Emphasis on not only acquisition of knowledge, but also application of skills and demonstration of attitudes
- An environment in which students engage in active learning involving a variety of learning styles, not simply limited to reading and writing

A critical feature of most effective small-group teaching and learning environments is the centrality of group discussion, group work, and group responsibility. Through group discussion and group work, students learn to negotiate meanings, confirm their understanding, share their expertise (not simply what they have read in a textbook, but also their personal experiences), become familiar and comfortable with the language and rhetoric of the field, and perhaps most importantly, acquire greater confidence and competence in self-expression. An ancillary benefit of this method includes greater opportunities for faculty–student interaction, of critical importance in professional socialization and the modeling and mentoring that lies at the heart of professional education.

Small-group teaching and learning is a methodology that has been successfully used in a variety of situations, including the following:

- *Problem-based learning.* Students collectively identify learning objectives within an area and utilize real-world situations to acquire knowledge, skills, and attitudes required for practice.

- *Case-based learning.* Content experts provide real-world cases as a prompt to groups of students to generate interest in and questions about an area of study.
- *Just-in-time learning.* Learners (generally immersed within a clinical or professional context) bring their self-identified knowledge and skills gaps to a facilitated small group and use this personal experience as a starting point for knowledge and skills acquisition.
- *Skills-based learning.* Learning activities are modeled, demonstrated, rehearsed, and evaluated by students to develop new or complex psychomotor skills.
- *Application-based learning.* Previously learned material is applied within a complex or different context to ensure students are able to apply previously acquired knowledge and skills in a flexible, adaptive, confident, and situationally appropriate manner.

What Is My Job? The Role of Facilitator in Small-Group Teaching and Learning

Effective facilitation of small groups is essential for success. Indicators of unsuccessful small-group facilitation include the following:

- A teacher-centered didactic lecture style, rather than a student-centered dialogue.
- A facilitator who talks more frequently and for longer periods of time than students in the group.
- Students who are unwilling or reluctant to speak, share ideas and experiences, ask questions, or engage with one another and the group.
- Students who do not perceive value to adequate preparation before each session.
- Asymmetrical student engagement (i.e., one or a few students dominate all conversation, block others from participating, or appear overly eager to please the facilitator).
- Expectation by students that they will be given correct answers by the facilitator, rather than work collegially to derive the best solutions together.

Effective facilitators recognize that their individual behaviors have a profound influence on how the group functions and the performance norms the group establishes. A facilitator that is disinterested, undemocratic, overly didactic, or overly passive sets the tone for how students expect the group to function. Many facilitators all too quickly fall back upon their content or subject matter expertise and would prefer to exercise their authority as an expert rather than deal with silence, students grappling with difficulties, or confusion among learners. As a facilitator, there are several key elements that you may wish to consider:

- The *physical environment* is critical for successful facilitation. Seemingly small environmental issues—for example, exchanging a rectangular table for a round table—will produce significant differences with respect to verbal and nonverbal communication patterns (including eye contact). A small-group session in which students' seats are arranged auditorium style will discourage interaction and heighten passive learning tendencies. Wherever possible, use round tables, learner circles, or other methods that ensure that all participants can see and interact with one another with minimal obstruction. Avoid configurations in which all students see the facilitator but do not necessarily see one another. Attentiveness to room temperature, lighting conditions, air circulation, comfort of seats and tables, etc., is also necessary to ensure that students can focus on group discussions and are not distracted by environmental conditions.

- *Group size* is a highly contentious topic, with some arguing that small-group facilitation can only truly be undertaken with eight or fewer students, but others demonstrate that it is possible to use effective facilitation skills in groups of several hundred students. As the facilitator, you must determine the optimal group size based on personal comfort and confidence, nature of the learning activity, type of learners involved, environmental conditions, and practical or logistic constraints based on finite resources. In general, small-group facilitation with fewer than 5 students or more than 15 students may become more challenging; at the lower end, very small groups may not have adequate diversity to truly unleash the benefits of small-group methods; and at the upper end, larger groups may not allow sufficient individual face time and participation and may result in the formation of subgroups or cliques. Many educators agree that the optimal small-group size is usually six to nine students. At least one study has indicated that, from a student satisfaction perspective, a group size of 10 to 12 students is optimal.[2]

- The *configuration of a group* to optimize learning is also contentious. Some argue that homogenous groups, formed by clustering students with similar learning styles, educational backgrounds, ethnocultural backgrounds, academic strengths, grade point averages, personal interests, or learning needs, may be more efficient than randomly assembled groups. Others argue that such engineering of groups deprives students of diversity of opinions and experiences, a critical feature of small-group learning. Though no consensus exists regarding how to best configure a group of learners, you need to be aware that *assembly effects* clearly do exist; the other learners in a group do influence how a group develops and performs. Most educators and students perceive great value in mixing students with different academic strengths so that those students who may be stronger in some areas can assist other students. Deliberately engineering groups to avoid mixing students can deprive them of important opportunities to learn tolerance and acceptance of different viewpoints and backgrounds and (more importantly) does not prepare them for the real world in which management of such diversity is a workplace success factor.

- The *structure of a small group* may influence success and outcomes. When a group of students first comes together, there is a natural tendency for them to self-compare and benchmark based on academic abilities, status, influence, or other factors. There may be an equally natural tendency for students to fall into self-prescribed roles within the group; for example, the quiet, studious student does all the library-based research, the confident, charismatic student does all the talking, or the tech-savvy student handles computer-related issues. Such division of labor may be appropriate in some circumstances, but students may require facilitation to push them out of their self-imposed comfort zone to allow them to acquire new competencies. The rotation of roles and responsibilities (starting with more comfortable roles first, then moving to less well-known ones) provides important learning opportunities and ensures that the small-group structure does not produce stagnation. Many successful facilitators outline group process—rather than content or expertise—roles. Such roles include timekeeping, recording, idea generation, reality testing, resource gatekeeping, etc. Structuring groups around these process roles and ensuring a rotation through various responsibilities to avoid stereotyping or stagnation can be a useful method for utilizing structure within small-group teaching and learning. As the facilitator, you must be vigilant to ensure that students do not remain trapped within their own comfort zones and that all students have equal opportunities to learn, develop, perform, and lead.

- As a facilitator, it is helpful for you to work with students to ensure groups are *cohesive and communicate effectively*. Effective communication is the cornerstone of effective small-group work. Attentiveness to students' verbal and nonverbal cues is critical, particularly if there are concerns regarding respect issues. You should neither demonstrate nor condone or ignore comments, gestures, or signals (including rolled eyes, smirks, etc.) that may discourage students from contributing. In-group or cliquey conversations or coded language among some students specifically designed to exclude others should be dealt with quickly and firmly. For effective communication to occur, speaking and listening must both occur. Ground rules to establish a respectful atmosphere for learning are essential. It is important for you to remain attuned to conversations, to ensure that all students contribute to the best of their abilities, that no student is blocked or scorned, and that taking turns is the norm. The cohesiveness of the group provides an important measure of how willing individual students are to coordinate their efforts for the overall benefit of the group. Highly cohesive groups will, for example, meet frequently outside scheduled times, use *we* rather than *I* in discussions, demonstrate a friendly, supportive attitude toward one another, and will likely be more successful as a group and as individuals in advancing learning. Low-cohesion groups may be marked by absenteeism and excuse making, emergence of cliques or factions within the group, and a strong divergence in attainment of outcomes.

- *Fostering a democratic discussion environment* in which all group members feel safe and valued is an important skill for facilitators. Using clear and purposeful group structures and teaching methods can ensure that groups spend more time interacting and less time simply listening to the facilitator talk. As a general rule, infrequent intervention by the facilitator will allow the group to develop its own norms and strategies for ensuring successful outcomes. Although you clearly have a role in establishing group learning outcomes, students themselves must feel invested in the process; learning outcomes cannot be what you impose on the student, but instead what the group (students plus facilitator) jointly identifies as salient, attainable, and important. Similarly, although you may wish to learn in a specific way, you must recognize that individual students and the group as a whole may have different methods and learning styles, and these must be respected. You should not dictate processes for achieving agreed-upon outcomes, but instead remind groups of these outcomes and foster an environment of collective responsibility to ensure all group members achieve these objectives within the available time and resource constraints.

Skills for effective facilitation are many and diverse, and each facilitator brings his or her own interests, strengths, and experiences to a group. The previously outlined core competencies for effective facilitation provide only a starting point in small-group teaching and learning. Effective facilitators must learn to be flexible and adaptive to evolving needs and circumstances and remember that their primary obligation is to foster a group culture and dynamic that reinforces group accountability for processes, outcomes, and learning.

How Do I Get Things Started with Small-Group Teaching and Learning?

First impressions are critical to ensure success in educational settings. Students need to feel both comfortable and confident in their environment to optimize learning. Small-group teaching and learning provides you with opportunities to engage students, but for some facilitators, getting started can be daunting. Although there is no checklist available to ensure the perfect start to a small-group relationship, the following tips and techniques have proven useful to many facilitators. They may be things to consider when you are first starting to work with a small group:

- *Pay attention to the small details.* Room location, configuration, temperature, lighting, etc., may not have much to do with you as a facilitator, but your interest in, and concern about, these environmental attributes signal your interest in and concern about your learners. Even if these things cannot be changed or fixed, simply acknowledging them and respecting the impact they may have on learners is important.

- *Introduce yourself and explain (from your perspective) why you are here.* Students benefit from understanding the life experiences of their instructors. Simply introducing yourself by name and giving them a brief resume is not the same as providing them with a context for understanding how your professional life and personal interests have led you to this role as a small-group facilitator. Such an introduction provides them with more context to understand you and a more personal reason to want to engage with you and the group.

- *Have students introduce themselves and explain (from their perspective) why they are here.* Just as students need a context to understand facilitators, all group members benefit from understanding one another. Do not assume that simply because students may be classmates or have been in the same program for several years that they actually know anything about one another. Structuring time to allow for this networking is useful and can help build group cohesion.

- *Have a sense of humor and try to be relaxed and flexible.* Being a facilitator can be daunting—as daunting as being a student in a small group. Remember that for everyone, getting started can be stressful. Using humor, informal storytelling and anecdote sharing, and other activities as icebreakers are good ways of starting to build the cohesion that characterizes effective groups.

Above all else, remember that *well begun is half done.* The way in which you engage learners in the environment will set the pattern for success in your small group's activities.

What Is Their Job? The Role of Learners in Small-Group Teaching and Learning

Students who enter professional programs have frequently mastered traditional lecture-based, didactic methods of teaching, learning, and assessment. For some of these students, the notion of a learner-centered, small-group process may be intimidating, idealistic, or simply a waste of time. Many learners are not accustomed to this learning model, so they may not be prepared for the different expectations, responsibilities, and rewards associated with collaborative small-group learning. In some cases, students may even resist this method of instruction; because they succeeded in the traditional didactic lecture-based format, they may believe small-group methods may actually adversely affect their personal academic performance.

You can help students embrace small-group methods by illustrating how this instructional format is essential for workplace success. Skills such as listening, presenting ideas, persuasive (yet respectful) articulation of differing ideas, negotiation of conflict, management of diversity, and working as part of a team are as important to professional working life and success as mastery of content and knowledge. Equally important, small-group work in an academic setting gives students the opportunity to develop self-appraisal, self-direction, and independent-reflection skills necessary for lifelong learning.

Learners who are new to small-group sessions may require assistance in understanding what is normal for a group of students. They may observe other small groups and compare those group processes with their own, leading to summary (and perhaps inaccurate) judgments that their own group is dysfunctional or works really well. The reality, of course, is that all groups develop and work differently, and individual students must assume collective responsibility to ensure effective group functioning for everyone's mutual benefit.

You may assist students in their roles by articulating a generic model for team functioning, to reassure students that their experience is not unusual, and to provide them with a road map for team evolution. The stages of group formation include the following[3]:

- *Forming.* In this first stage, group members are introduced to one another for the first time. During this stage, there is a natural (though perhaps unhelpful) tendency for group members to assess one another, establish hierarchies, and jockey for dominance and positional power. More charismatic and confident (though not necessarily more competent) individuals may assume more primary positions, and first impressions may lead to lasting stereotypes. You can assist learners in this phase by providing structured opportunities for individuals to showcase their experiences and strengths rather than relying upon informal social mechanisms to provide advantage to extroverted individuals at the expense of somewhat more introverted ones. Clearly identifying objectives, having clearly structured or unambiguous tasks, and providing opportunities for individuals with different strengths and talents to come to the fore can facilitate forming.

- *Storming.* In the life cycle of most small groups, formation is usually a somewhat formal and polite process in which individuals do not wish to appear too different from one another for fear of social sanction. When a group has formed and actually begins to work together, differences that may have been hidden, overlooked, or simply not apparent may become more conspicuous. This is particularly the case when the activities that the group undertakes become more complex or ambiguous and the responsibility or accountability for outcomes heightens. The second stage of group formation, storming, occurs when these differences lead to outright disagreement and in some cases overt hostilities. This is a natural and inevitable part of group work, and you should alert students to the importance and role of conflict in small-group teaching and learning. Although many learners are conflict-averse or conflict-avoidant, it is important for students to recognize that, without conflict, progress may be suboptimal. It is through the healthy, forceful, and respectful exchange of ideas that learning occurs. During the storming stage, students may expend considerable effort to try to avoid conflict entirely, believing this is the hallmark of an effective group. In fact, the opposite is true; groups that do not storm do not usually function as effectively as possible. The key during this stage is for students to learn how to respectfully but vigorously disagree with one another, how to articulate their perspectives, how to win (and lose) arguments gracefully, all the while remaining engaged with the group and committed to the group's objectives. Failure to storm may actually indicate disengagement and disinterest; it is through storming that the group and its individual members learn, grow, and develop.
- *Norming.* In some unfortunate cases, the storming stage may prove fatal to a group; some small groups have such acute storming stages that they are not able to recover. Fortunately, this is relatively infrequent, and you need to remain vigilant during storming to ensure successful transition to the third stage of group formation—norming. During norming, groups begin to develop their own culture and their own rules for engagement, performance, conflict management, defining success, etc. Groups that successfully navigate the storm frequently cohere in unexpected ways. Signal events in norming include a gradual transition away from *I* statements to *we* statements, an informal and relaxed atmosphere among group members, self-identification as friends rather than fellow workers, and a sense of shared purpose rather than everyone doing their own thing. During norming, the role of the facilitator may gradually diminish as the group works through issues in a more consensual and democratic manner. Whereas during storming you may have to intervene more

frequently to establish ground rules, ensure fair play, and encourage cooperation rather than competition; whereas during norming you may become just another group member. In some circumstances, unfortunately, unacceptable standards may emerge during norming. In some groups, acceptance of academic dishonesty, plagiarism, laziness, or other undesirable activities may become normalized. Despite group acceptance of these norms and this group culture, you must ensure that students recognize and respond appropriately to these less-than-desirable group norms.

- *Performing.* When a small group is able to successfully navigate the perilous waters of forming, storming, and norming, they frequently are able to reach the penultimate stage of performing. During this stage, groups function effectively to the best of their diverse abilities. Performance is generally characterized by common ground among all group members; commitment to a shared vision, outcome, or objective; real engagement and interest in the task and one another; the ability to deal with uncertainty and ambiguity with creativity; and the ability to draw upon the diverse strengths and experiences of individual group members. During this stage, you as the facilitator become relatively unimportant; the group facilitates itself with minimal input and control by the facilitator. To facilitate a performing group is to admire and marvel at how the whole is greater than the sum of the parts.

- *Adjourning.* In the final stage of group formation, small groups must disband and move on after completion of their task. Celebrating the accomplishments and success of the group are important positive reinforcers, but you must also encourage students to recognize that all things come to an end and that there is much to learn and much to accomplish from other groups and other experiences. Facilitators frequently overlook the importance and value of a formal adjournment of a group's efforts. For students who have been immersed in their group's work, there may be a strong psychological need for formal acknowledgment and closure to allow them to gracefully move forward in their academic and personal lives. It is an appropriate and necessary role of the facilitator to provide this acknowledgment and closure in a manner that empowers and enables students to look forward with expectation rather than reflect backward on the good old days.

Students may benefit from understanding these stages of group evolution and in normalizing their own experiences based on this model. Recognizing that much of the learning associated with small-group work is about processes rather than content, understanding the ways in which human beings relate and interact with one another by actually experiencing it through small-group work, and reflecting upon it during and after can be a profoundly important developmental experience.

The roles and responsibilities of students within a small-group environment may be aligned to the stages of group formation previously noted; students will be required to assume different jobs contingent upon the functioning and level of the group itself. This means that an individual student's role will evolve as the group evolves and as that student's skill set advances.

Some facilitators have successfully utilized learning and group-work contracts to alert students to what is expected of them within a small-group environment and what they can expect from their fellow students and facilitator. Care must be taken not to simply impose a pro forma contract on students; rather, it is the process of crafting, discussing, and drafting the contract itself that provides the most learning and opportunity for buy-in. In general, most contracts address (but are not limited to) the following elements:

- Willingness to contribute to the best of one's ability
- Respecting other group members and the facilitator, as evidenced by respectful, active listening; taking turns; and appropriate verbal and nonverbal communication
- Following through on commitments to other group members
- Ensuring that all group members have an equal opportunity to contribute
- Maintaining and upholding academic standards of conduct and behavior
- Engaging in honest self-appraisal and peer assessment
- Flexibility in assuming roles and responsibilities and ensuring equitable distribution of responsibilities and rewards among all group members
- Dealing with disagreement and managing conflict constructively
- Embracing (not simply tolerating or accepting) individual group members' diverse backgrounds, experiences, and perspectives

In some cases, the development and drafting of a group work contract can be a valuable forming activity that allows individuals to get to know one another through cooperative work that is not linked to specific or hierarchical skills, knowledge, or talent. Rather than frame the contract as simply a lofty discussion of ideal behaviors, students should be encouraged to discuss concrete consequences of nonadherence and strategies for the group to monitor, respond to, and correct individuals' behaviors if they deviate from agreed-upon standards.

How Do We Work Together as Facilitators and Learners in Small-Group Collaboration?

Small groups are generally not the most efficient vehicles for simple distribution of information, but they are effective mechanisms of facilitating higher-order understanding of concepts and developing and improving strategies for problem identification and problem solving. To achieve these objectives, students must engage in meaningful communication directed toward specific goals and outcomes.

To do so, Jaques[2] has enumerated a variety of techniques for effective facilitation of small groups:

- Ensure that all group members have an agreed-upon series of ground rules, common expectations, or a learning contract that clearly outlines behavioral norms and consequences for deviation.
- The facilitator must ensure that the task, activity, or learning challenge is appropriate for the students at a developmentally appropriate level for the group. For example, highly contextualized or ambiguous cases should not be given to groups who are just forming or storming because this may further exacerbate individual differences and grievances; instead, such cases are better placed during the performing stage of a group's evolution.
- As a facilitator, learn how to use silence effectively, and do not become uncomfortable or embarrassed by it. For example, when posing a question, do not frame it in such a way that the answer is self-evident. Do not answer it yourself or continuously reformat it to make it simpler or to ensure that students have understood it. Do not misinterpret silence as lack of understanding—students need time to think and formulate a response. After you have posed a question, give the students at least 10 seconds before you say anything else.
- When the 10 seconds you have given the students has passed, give them 10 more seconds. As a general rule, any time you have the urge to make a statement or ask a question, wait 10 seconds to see if one of the students asks that question or makes that statement. Remember, as learners they already know quite a bit—they just need more time than you do to formulate their thoughts and articulate their ideas.
- Observe, listen, and watch in an honest and unflinching way. Do not overlook unflattering nonverbal cues students may be sending you—respond to them instead of ignoring them. The speed with which you accurately respond to the nonverbal cues students send you conveys a powerful message to them about how interested you are in their learning.

Jaques[2] has enumerated seven group structures and strategies for effective small-group facilitation:

1. *The group round.* This strategy is particularly well-placed at the beginning of a session so that everyone is involved and contributing from the start. In this format, each student is given a brief time (less than one minute) to say something—anything—about the session, topic, homework, group process, etc. By hearing from everyone at the beginning, confidence builds that all voices deserve to be heard. An interesting variation on the group round is to avoid a sequential

speaker's format and instead invite the first speaker to nominate the second speaker, who in turn nominates the third speaker, etc. This provides diversity, interest, and lack of routine to the group round.

2. *The buzz group.* As a tool for encouraging less forthcoming students, the buzz group allows those who may be hesitant to speak in front of a whole group the opportunity to test drive their ideas with one other person first. In a buzz group, the facilitator pairs off students to work on a specific task or discuss a specific topic; the pair then shares their discussion with the larger group. This provides a safer route to engage less talkative or more reticent students and allows them to build up their confidence in speaking in front of the whole group.

3. *The snowball group.* This is an extension of the buzz group and is particularly helpful for small groups with 14 or more members. In snowballing, pairs that were created in the buzz group then join together, now as a group of four rather than a pair of two. This incremental approach to speaking in front of progressively larger groups can be effective, but care must be taken to ensure that it does not become redundant. One suggestion is to make the task of the four-member group more sophisticated or different from the task of the two-member pair to ensure that all learners remain engaged.

4. *The fishbowl.* With groups of 10 or more, the fishbowl provides a unique opportunity to learn about learning through observation. In the fishbowl, half of the group serves as discussants and problem solvers, while the other half of the group observes them in action. The roles are then reversed, with the observers now becoming the discussants. In this way, students have the opportunity to observe other students learning, interacting, and problem solving, a powerful trigger for self-reflection and personal development.

5. *The crossover.* In a crossover, subgroups are formed to facilitate greater participation by individual students. After a predetermined time, an activity, or an outcome, subgroups are reconstituted with different members. This reconstitution ensures that all students have the opportunity to work with everyone but in a smaller, more intimate environment than the entire group. The crossover also permits seeding of ideas among subgroups.

6. *Circular questioning.* In this method of facilitation, each student is limited to asking one question (or stating one comment); the next student must build upon that question (or comment) in framing his or her new question or comment, and so on. Circular questioning imposes intellectual discipline and focus on learners by forcing them to prioritize ideas; it also ensures that more vocal individuals do not monopolize air time during discussion and emphasizes the interdependent nature of the group.

7. *The horseshoe.* Also known as the workshop method, the horseshoe involves alternating between small-group activities and traditional, didactic lecture-style theory bursts. By providing no more than 15 to 20 minutes of highly focused and situationally relevant factual content in an efficient and targeted manner, learners are better able to immediately apply knowledge to case discussions or problems. Facilitators who utilize the horseshoe must demonstrate discipline in *not* exceeding the 15- to 20-minute theory burst and allowing sufficient time for small-group discussion. Frequently alternating between theory burst and group work is generally engaging for students, efficient in balancing knowledge transmission with application and skill development, and provides opportunities for both formal and informal learning.

As a facilitator, there are many options available to enhance collaborative learning. As previously outlined, by experimenting with a variety of strategies you will learn how to customize them based on the small group's specific needs and your individual interests.

What Matters in Assessment of Small-Group Learning?

Although many instructors support the notion of small-group learning as effective, there is some question about how to fairly and efficiently assess individual students, particularly in the context of a professional curriculum where individuals are expected to demonstrate individual competencies. Recognizing that the environment for learning may not be the same as the environment for assessment, some facilitators may conclude that small-group learning is somehow unfair if it is not also coupled with small-group assessment, and small-group assessment may not be possible if individual accountability for learning is an expectation.

If you are involved in small-group teaching and learning, it is essential to recognize the importance of assessment both as a measure of learning and as a way of motivating students to want to contribute and learn. The reality for many learners continues to be that assessment and assessment methods drive learning; alignment of teaching, learning, and assessment methods is integral to effective teaching. Thus, the question arises, If I am teaching using small-group methods, how can I possibly test using traditional, individual methods?

The key to understanding this dilemma is to recognize the multiple forms of assessment that are available. Formative assessment is used to provide feedback to learners on their development and progress through an educational program or class. Formative assessment is best when it is continuous and embedded in the teaching and learning directly; when formative assessment is an add-on, it can appear burdensome and problematic to students. Ongoing feedback to students to help them build their confidence and accuracy of self-assessment skills can be woven into facilitation activities by, for example, allocating time in each session for self- and peer reflection or assessment. As a facilitator, you can use formative assessment on a regular basis to understand how students value the educational experience and to help them develop the self-reflection skills necessary for life after school. Asking learners to reflect on their own performance and the performance of their peers, then pushing them to identify specific situations, comments, or events rather than vague generalities, provides both formative assessment and an opportunity to develop important self-assessment skills.

Summative assessment is, of course, an important part of an educational program. Summative assessment allows for more formal testing of knowledge and benchmarking of skills progression. Ideally, learners have received sufficient formative assessment during the course of learning to be able to perform effectively when summative assessments are required. The principle of aligning assessment with teaching and learning is important, but it does not necessarily mean that simply because group learning methods were used that individual assessment methods cannot be applied. The key is transparency, opportunities to learn and develop through feedback, and sufficient and clear notice given to students that they will be assessed individually even if they are learning in a group environment. Such structures encourage both individual and group accountability for learning outcomes.

Recently, there has been interest in the role and value of group-based assessments; for example, group projects, reports, or presentations, and even group-based objective structured clinical examinations (OSCEs). Although such forms of assessment may be psychometrically stable and robust, their value must be balanced against the need within a particular educational program for individual learners to be accountable. Facilitators need to have the flexibility and creativity to allow for a variety of different assessment methods, both formative and summative, that align with teaching and learning objectives. Overreliance on one or two types of assessment and providing insufficient formative assessment to support summative assessment must be avoided if alignment is to occur.

How Do We Put It All Together? Pearls for Educators

For most teachers, the time and effort required to successfully facilitate small-group teaching and learning is significant but is more than compensated by the outcomes, level of student engagement and motivation, and opportunities to get to know students better as learners and as human beings. Small-group teaching and learning may make some facilitators feel vulnerable; without the protective cloak of content expertise or the safety of a large screen and a PowerPoint presentation, facilitators also allow students

> More structure, less intervention.[3]
>
> D. Jaques

> Being a democratic discussion leader involves making the right sort of nudges and interventions. The role can be made a lot less demanding by using more structure and less intervention in the group process.[4]
>
> M. Guela

to get to know them better as human beings. Each facilitator therefore brings his or her own personality, passion, and foibles to this job.

There are no one-size-fits-all solutions or road maps for facilitators who wish to optimize teaching and learning. Every individual is unique. Nonetheless, over many years of small-group teaching and learning in a variety of contexts and settings, a collective wisdom is evolving regarding strategies, tactics, guidelines, ideas, and dos and don'ts of effective facilitation. These pearls are by no means comprehensive, nor are they vetted, approved, or tested in any other objective manner. You should use your judgment and discretion in interpreting these ideas, recognizing that what works for one may not work for another. As a starting point, however, these pearls may provide a bootstrap for those beginning their facilitation career or for those interested in examining ways of improving their practice.

- Have a goal for the session. Simple or refined, a goal provides direction and focus and provides a benchmark for students to track their progress.
- Extract yourself from the interaction. Remember the purpose of small-group work—to assist in acquiring knowledge, skills, and behaviors by facilitating the involvement of learners, not by downloading information.
- Identify both quiet and dominant students. Work with both of them to find a happy medium.
- Use your own concrete and personal experiences to humanize the process. Students respond well to a judiciously placed and salient story from the trenches. Do not overuse this technique, otherwise you will be doing all the talking, but once in awhile it can be very effective.
- Know the difference between open- and closed-ended questions, and generally use open-ended questions more frequently. Open-ended questions have no specified or expected answer, so they do not limit or close down conversation, and they tend to promote more questions, reflection, and thinking. Closed-ended questions usually have a specified desirable answer and are therefore dead-ends in terms of small-group discussions.

> Prepare yourself for facilitating groups.[5]
>
> J. Westberg, J. Hilliard

- Use advanced organizers to prepare students for the next session. Not only will this force you as the facilitator to be organized and plan ahead in a strategic manner, it will also provide students with a clearer understanding of how each session relates to the previous and subsequent sessions.

Before we can facilitate, we need to reflect upon and learn from our own experiences as a learner and a teacher. Westberg and Hilliard[5] have developed a checklist to facilitate self-appraisal. The two core areas they concentrate on are (1) reflection on self-identified characteristics of effective small-group teachers and (2) reflection on the understandings and capabilities of the facilitator. Through a series of questions and probes, the checklist walks you through your own assumptions and biases regarding what constitutes effective small-group facilitation.

> Know what to do, when, and how.[2]
> D. Jaques

Understanding the theory of group formation and dynamics is useful but may be of limited value when confronted with conflict, disagreement, or other threats to a positive group climate that encourages interaction. Consider the following tips:

- *Glance around the group frequently.* Avoid limiting your eye contact to one or a few students, and make sure you rotate your gaze frequently and fairly. This indicates to each student that they matter to you, and you are not favoring one person over another.

- *Do not ignore uncomfortable cues students send you.* Frequently, students will communicate confusion, uncertainty, dislike, or boredom in a nonverbal manner. These cues may be subtle but are definitely observable if you are paying attention—a sharp indrawn breath, a snort of frustration, frequent shifting of position, or a slight frown are all ways for students to let you know what they think. Do not avoid or overlook these signs and then claim that no one told you there was a problem. Frequently, students will not use words to express their true feelings, but these feelings do get expressed. Although it may be easier to pretend we have not noticed what is communicated (but not spoken), in the long run this leads to greater problems in group cohesion and performance.

- *Use your nonverbal skills effectively.* The correct nonverbal cue communicated to a student at the correct time can fundamentally reorient a drifting conversation. Raising your eyebrows, nodding, and smiling are effective, nonverbal methods for inviting students to participate in a conversation. For some students, a verbal invitation may be too daunting or intimidating; the nonverbal invitation provides greater comfort and security and may be more effective than using words in some circumstances. Developing and consistently using your repertoire of nonverbal skills to engage students in conversation, encourage them to stop dominating conversation, or help them to recognize the appropriateness (or lack thereof) of what they have said can be more effective and less threatening than using verbal communication. Such *bringing in* and *shutting out* nonverbal strategies should be considered a core part of your small-group facilitation technique.

- *Reflecting and deflecting questions.* Frequently, students will want to defer to your authority and your expertise and simply want you to tell them the right answer. As discussed previously, it is important to not be trapped in this role, and instead allow students to cooperatively derive solutions to problems and answers to questions. When asked a blunt question (such as What do you think? or What is the right answer?), the effective use of reflecting and deflecting questions can be of assistance. For example, if a student says "I don't understand—what does this mean?" you can say "That's a good question. What does the rest of the group think?" instead of answering it yourself. Students will soon realize that they collectively have significant knowledge and experience to answer most questions and that your role is to facilitate the process, not to simply answer all the questions they may have.

- *Supporting and valuing.* Though it may seem self-evident, it is essential that facilitators do not communicate, verbally or nonverbally, judgment or derision to students. Unfortunately, some facilitators may inadvertently allow a look of surprise or a vague look of disgust to cross his or her face when confronted with a student's comment. Such looks send powerful signals to students that they are not valued, and this will result in not only that individual student shutting down, but a chill could potentially spread across the entire group. Developing strategies that acknowledge a student's contribution while still recognizing that additional work is necessary is important for a facilitator. For example, if a student makes a completely incorrect statement, rather than stating "That was wrong" or communicating this sentiment nonverbally, an affirming "Thank you for that comment. Does anyone else have any other opinions?" is a gentle and effective way of reorienting a discussion without devaluing the student's contribution.

- *Checking in.* Many students feel stress and anxiety in small-group settings. As a result, they may not communicate verbally as clearly as they would like to or as clearly as they could in a less public setting. Effective facilitators use the skill of checking in to confirm they have understood what the student has said and to give the student an additional opportunity to publicly explain him- or herself. For example, a well-placed "I'm not sure I understood what you just said. Did you mean . . ." can provide a face-saving way for a student to clarify an ambiguous statement.

- *Building.* To facilitate cohesion within the group, building is a strategy that should be considered. Building involves explicitly linking students' comments to one another in a way that illustrates how each student is meaningfully contributing to the overall progress of the group. Facilitators should be explicit when using building as a facilitation strategy to encourage everyone to contribute to the group's overall goal.

- *Redirecting.* At times, a student may make an outrageous or completely inappropriate remark. Rarely is it appropriate to publicly rebuke a student in front of the group because this will simply build resentment and fear (although, in some extreme circumstances, a public rebuke may be required if a comment is particularly inflammatory and inappropriate). Redirecting is the facilitation skill used to change topics to avoid further focus on a specific area. Redirection must be done artfully so you do not appear to be ignoring uncomfortable topics. Facilitators need to develop a repertoire of redirection strategies that can be applied in a way that does not appear formulaic. Some strategies that are effective can include taking a break or a time out, then starting the discussion with a new topic or a statement such as "Let's revisit what we discussed about half an hour ago to see where we are now."

> Get the small things right.[6]
> R. Tiberius

Recognizing that small-group interaction is simply another form of human interaction, pay attention to the small details to create an environment that is inclusive, welcoming, and comfortable for students. This means you should do the following:

- Set the stage by ensuring the room you are working in is conducive to learning, discussion, and thinking. Lighting, temperature, air circulation, etc., need to be appropriate. Chairs and tables should be comfortable and arranged in a manner to emphasize collaborative and collegial discussion. Use overhead or PowerPoint projectors and other technologies judiciously because they may serve to distance you from students and reinforce a noncollaborative, teacher-centered learning environment instead of a learner-centered space.
- Introduce yourself and say a few words about your experience, background, interests, and limitations.
- Ensure that the students know one another, or else have them introduce themselves. Use fun (but not overly cloying) icebreaking exercises so students can start to become comfortable with the group.
- Initially, it is appropriate for the facilitator to assume greater prominence and leadership in establishing objectives, group processes, etc. This prominence should wane with time, and the group itself should be making these decisions.
- Be organized! Make sure you have the materials you need so you do not appear to be disorganized, disinterested, or preoccupied. Students deserve to know that, during each session, their learning is your top priority. Wherever possible, ensure that students receive materials in advance of each session. Although not all of them may read it or do what you would like them to do with it, most students will appreciate the effort you have made to get the material to them in advance and will recognize this as your commitment to their learning.
- Use humor, anecdotes, and your own experiences (good and not so good) as a way of building rapport with students. Remember that all of us learn not simply from success, but also from lack of success,

and your willingness to share these stories and experiences with students will make a difference in the way the group functions.

Summary

To unleash the power of small-group teaching and learning is to enable individual students to recognize that they are better able to learn, grow, and develop through interdependent group-based work. This may seem illogical and counterintuitive to some, an idealistic fantasy to others, or simply a time-consuming task with limited evidence of improved outcomes. To those who have worked as small-group facilitators and who have actively engaged in refining their facilitation practice to enhance learning, the advantages of this approach are clear and striking. Although small-group teaching and learning is not necessary or effective in all cases and circumstances, openness to using this approach in appropriate situations is beneficial.

Reflective Exercise

Reflect upon your most positive and your most negative team or group working experience in which you were required to learn and perform with other people. How have these experiences shaped your interest in, willingness to participate in, and opinions about small-group–based collaborative learning? What biases and assumptions do you have about this model of learning based on your previous experiences?

_____

_____

_____

_____

Reflective Exercise

Reflect upon your most recent experience with facilitating a small group. What were the accomplishments and challenges you faced? To what extent were these accomplishments and challenges a function of the individuals (and their personalities) that were in the group versus the nature and structure of the small group itself?

_____

_____

_____

_____

Reflective Exercise

Within small-group collaborative settings there is frequently a tension between group-based learning and individual performance and assessment. As you reflect upon your own experiences as a facilitator or a small-group learner, what has been most successful in helping to negotiate this tension?

_____

_____

_____

_____

_____

_____

Reflective Exercise

Reflect on your own teaching and learning style. How does your style influence your role as a facilitator? Does it serve as a barrier or an enabler to small-group collaborative learning?

_____

_____

_____

_____

_____

_____

References

1. Palmer PJ. _The Courage to Teach: Exploring the Inner Landscape of a Teacher's Life_. San Francisco, CA: John Wiley and Sons; 1998:68.
2. Jaques D. ABCs of learning and teaching in medicine: teaching small groups. _BMJ_. 2003;326:492–494.
3. Jaques D. _Learning in Groups_. 3rd ed. London, England: Kogan-Page; 2000.
4. Guela M. Clinical discussion sessions and small groups. _Surg Neurol_. 1997; 47:399–402.
5. Westberg J, Hilliard J. _Fostering Learning in Small Groups: A Practical Guide_. New York, NY: Springer Publishing Company; 1996.
6. Tiberius R. _Small-Group Teaching: A Trouble-Shooting Guide_. London, England: Kogan-Page; 1999.

What Matters in Laboratory Learning and Teaching?

Jennifer Kirwin, PharmD, BCPS
Jenny A. Van Amburgh, BSPharm, PharmD, CDE

Introduction: Why a Chapter About Laboratory Teaching?

The laboratory is an environment in which pharmacy students can apply knowledge, develop and practice skills, and demonstrate professional attitudes and values. Entry-level pharmacists need to master skills in drug information, dispensing, therapeutic drug monitoring, patient counseling, and extemporaneous compounding, and they increasingly need to be able to assess patients through the use of interviews and physical assessment techniques. Collaborative practice, medication therapy management, and other advanced pharmacy practice activities are now more readily available to practitioners. Students can practice all of these skills in a laboratory. The notable advantage of the laboratory environment is that the instructor can both control the content of the activities and assess the student's knowledge, skills, or values at the individual level. Achieving these goals is challenging and often impossible in a large lecture-style classroom (where instructors rarely have the time to individually observe each student) or in introductory or advanced pharmacy practice experiences (where preceptors are unable to control the situations to which students are exposed).

The educational potential of pharmacy laboratories is great, but resources to guide pharmacy educators on laboratory coordination and instruction are relatively sparse. A search of published print and online sources yielded limited descriptive evidence on pharmacy laboratory course placement, pharmacy laboratory design, and links between laboratory courses and broader curricular planning and programmatic assessment. In many instances,

In the laboratory environment, the instructor can both control the content of the activities and assess the students' knowledge, skills, or values at the individual level.

recommendations on pharmacy laboratory design and assessment have been adapted from guides written for use in the basic science laboratory. In this chapter, we will attempt to provide a road map connecting the overall design of a pharmacy laboratory to specific teaching activities and assessment strategies. First, we will present general concepts with specific applications to pharmacy practice laboratories, and then we will conclude the chapter with examples from pharmaceutical sciences courses.

Throughout our chapter, we ask you to participate by considering several questions about your laboratory course. After answering each set of questions, you can review the information presented and then return to the initial questions—hopefully with new ideas. This model embraces the active learning and reflective loop that is a key part of learning in the laboratory setting.

After reading this chapter, you should be able to answer the following questions:

- What is the rationale for laboratory-based teaching?
- What are the key elements of laboratory learning?
- What factors should be considered in the development of assessments that measure targeted knowledge, skills, attitudes, and values?
- What are the day-to-day considerations for effectively coordinating a laboratory as they relate to the use of space and personnel and to safety issues?
- How do I use the results of laboratory assessments and student and peer feedback to improve my laboratory course?

Why Include a Laboratory Course?

Since pharmaceutical care was first highlighted by Hepler and Strand in their seminal paper, the patient care laboratory has become a mainstay of pharmacy education, though the course may go by any one of several names, including pharmaceutical-care laboratory, skills laboratory, or integrated practice skills laboratory.[1] The 2007 ACPE Accreditation Standards include laboratory teaching as one of the desired (as opposed to required) components of a doctor of pharmacy program.[2] Usual laboratory activities currently go beyond prescription processing and ask students to address a wide variety of professional situations. As a laboratory coordinator or instructor, you should carefully consider the purpose of your laboratory course within the context of your specific academic program. In their book *A Handbook for Teachers in Universities and Colleges*, Newble and Cannon describe the two main purposes for laboratory-based teaching: (1) learning skills and techniques and (2) learning the process of scientific inquiry.[3] In our experience, the practice laboratory offers an environment where you can teach and assess the former while allowing

What is the purpose of your laboratory course? What skills and techniques will students be expected to master following completion of the course?

students the opportunity to apply previously learned concepts to simulated practice situations. Students generally complete organized activities that allow them to develop skills (e.g., drug dispensing, physical assessment, patient counseling, and manipulation of sterile products), attitudes (e.g., approachability and professional presentation of oneself), and values (e.g., respect for others, honesty, care, and compassion) that are characteristic of the profession of pharmacy.[4,5]

What Matters About Learning in the Laboratory?

Laboratory-based education is said to have originated with the work of Kurt Lewin, a German-born teacher and researcher. Lewin is credited with developing the foundation for modern laboratory teaching when he first organized "basic skills training groups" (later T-groups) where participants worked in small groups to alternately respond to complex situations and then critically analyze the experience.[6] These experiences allowed participants to process situations from a variety of perspectives to facilitate understanding and improve acceptance of alternative ideas. Lewin initially used these methods in research about intergroup prejudice, but they were later applied to address a wide variety of social inequities.[7]

Several key elements from Lewin's T-group method are applicable to laboratory training in the health professions. Inclusion of these key elements in the laboratory experience will ensure that students get the most out of the activity[7]:

- *The use of cognitive organizers or maps.* Evidence-based aids should be used to add to participants' preexisting knowledge or explore alternative views.
- *The right climate.* A laboratory environment should be nonjudgmental and trusting to allow participants to challenge and perhaps change their behavior or convictions.
- *A chance for the presentation of self.* The laboratory experience should provide an opportunity for participants to disclose information about their preexisting knowledge, attitudes, and beliefs.
- *Experimentation, practice, and application.* Opportunities should be provided where participants can try out new thoughts, behaviors, or techniques before taking them out into the real world.
- *Appropriate feedback.* Timely criticism, based on direct observation, should be provided to help participants understand the impact of their actions.

Laboratory courses are commonly included in health profession education, and most educators agree that there has to be a safe place for students to practice skills and techniques before they work with patients. However, the idea that laboratory teaching is indispensible should ideally be supported by broad-based studies providing evidence that this teaching environment is more effective than others in the achievement of specific skills. Unfortunately, such supportive findings are not readily available in pharmacy or other health professions literature. Several recently published articles highlight the need for laboratory instructors in medical training to document the unique contributions of laboratory-based education to the curriculum.[8,9] Pharmacy laboratory instructors should be prepared to do the same. Laboratory courses are expensive to run and require talented, well-trained personnel to design, conduct, and manage them. Good documentation that laboratory teaching achieves unique educational end points may eventually be necessary to support the continuing need for space, staff, and supplies. To that end, this chapter offers suggestions on how to build assessment of educational outcomes into the *design* of your pharmacy practice laboratory course. As such, at the start of your laboratory course, you will have a system in place to assess the course's educational impact on student learning.

What Matters in the Design of a Laboratory Course? The Foundational Principles of Laboratory Experiences

---

Reflective Exercise

Consider what you want the students to be able to do by the last day of the laboratory class that they cannot do at the start of your class. Using the systems approach (Chapter 3), think about the students you will teach (the input). Where are they in terms of their stage of development? With what knowledge, skills, and attitudes do you except them to begin the laboratory? Take a minute to record your thoughts in column A of **Table 8–1**. Now, think about the students who have already completed your course. What makes them different from the first group (the output)? Detail these characteristics in column B. How does your course help students get from A to B (the process)?[10]

Table 8–1 Planning the Laboratory: Reflection on Students

	Before Your Course (Column A)	After Your Course (Column B)	What the Students Need to Learn (The Difference Between A and B)
Knowledge			
Skills			
Attitudes			
Values			

The characteristics that you want your students to develop as a result of your laboratory become the overarching purpose(s) of the course. They provide the foundation for the rest of your course design and assessment plans.

Course Mapping

After identifying the overarching purpose(s) of the laboratory course, your next step is to prepare detailed objectives that the learner should be able to achieve at the conclusion of the course. As with other instructional objectives, these objectives should be specific and measurable, and they should tie into the more global outcome statements used by the academic program. **Table 8–2** describes some of the objectives we use in our laboratory course. In the following sections, we will then map, in the style of Newble and Cannon,[3] the laboratory activities and assessment methods to these objectives. You are encouraged to use a similar format to outline the objectives for your laboratory course. Please refer to Appendix 8–1 where you can start your course map. In the first column of the table in Appendix 8–1, list the objectives for your laboratory course.

Planning Activities

As described in Chapter 1, the teacher's primary goal should be student learning. In the laboratory, special attention must be paid to the organization of, and rationale for, each activity. Mapping laboratory activities to the list of laboratory course objectives can ensure that each objective is addressed by an activity in the laboratory and, conversely, that each activity encourages the student to develop professional attributes that are important to the overall goals of the program.

You already know how fast pharmacy practice is changing. Students are going into a wide variety of practice environments, and the list of skills they will need to enable them to deliver effective, patient-centered care is getting progressively longer and more complex. As such, it is the responsibility of each pharmacy program to make sure that every student graduates with a generalist set of skills to be used and applied to any practice setting.

Table 8–2 Example of Learning Objectives

Objectives

Given a case, counsel a patient on adherence, proper medication use, adverse effects, self-monitoring, need for follow-up, and relevant lifestyle changes as indicated for a particular medical condition.

Given filled medication orders, stock containers, and written prescriptions, evaluate the orders in preparation for dispensing to the patient, and, when indicated, suggest corrections to be made.

Demonstrate correct technique for administration of medications via the following routes: subcutaneous injection, intramuscular injection, inhalation, and instillation into the eye.

A review of the pharmacy literature revealed several publications that describe the content taught in practice laboratory courses. In a 2005 paper, Chereson and colleagues described the survey results of pharmacy practitioners and their opinions of the skills necessary for patient-centered pharmacy practice.[5] The authors surveyed community pharmacists (including those in chain and independent pharmacies) and hospital pharmacists who participated as experiential preceptors for a college of pharmacy. The researchers reported that the 10 most important skills or abilities for students to learn were the following:

1. Communication with other healthcare professionals
2. Documentation of interventions
3. Drug administration techniques
4. Drug information skills
5. Interpretation and verification of prescriptions
6. Monitoring of drug therapy
7. Nonprescription recommendations and counseling
8. Patient counseling
9. Prescription processing (entering and preparation for dispensing)
10. Profile review for drug-therapy problems

Table 8–3 provides an expanded list of skills and abilities commonly taught in pharmacy practice laboratories according to the literature reviewed for this chapter.[5,11–16]

A 2007 article by Spray and Parnapy describes the results of a survey of colleges and schools of pharmacy to determine the patient assessment skills currently being taught.[17] Based on this survey, the top 12 patient clinical assessment skills being taught are the following:

1. Abdominal exam
2. Cardiovascular exam
3. Gastrointestinal–hepatic assessment
4. Head, eyes, ears, nose, and throat exam
5. Laboratory values
6. Mental status assessment
7. Musculoskeletal exam
8. Neurological exam
9. Pain assessment
10. Principles of patient encounters
11. Pulmonary exam
12. Vital signs

The authors stated that several of the respondents wrote in additional assessments that were taught at their institutions, including skin, hair, and nails; peripheral vascular; and diabetic foot exams. Additional details about

Table 8–3 Topics Commonly Included in Patient-Care Laboratories

Administer immunizations

Apply drug information skills

Communicate drug administration techniques

Communicate with healthcare providers

Counsel and teach patients how to use home diagnostic devices

Determine appropriateness of medication

Document assessments (SOAP, QuEST/SCHOLAR)

Document interventions

Incorporate health promotion and disease prevention activities

Interpret laboratory values

Interpret prescription and verify completeness and accuracy

Interview patients

Monitor drug therapy

Obtain information from, and document actions and recommendations in, a patient chart

Perform extemporaneous compounding

Perform patient counseling

Practice physical assessments skills

Prepare parenteral products

Process prescriptions (i.e., enter prescription into computer and onto patient profile and prepare prescription for dispensing)

Provide disease state management

Provide nonprescription recommendations and counseling

Review patient profiles for drug therapy problems

Select drug and dosage forms

Select drug supply

Use simulations and standardized patients for physical assessment skills and counseling

equipment and personnel needs were provided in the article to facilitate implementation of these topics in other laboratory courses.

These lists are not comprehensive but rather offer a sampling of what is currently taught in many pharmacy practice laboratory courses. You need to decide which activities are best-suited for your laboratory course based on when the course is taught in the curriculum, what previous experiences your students have had, and the specific objectives of your laboratory course. Activities can be created in which students practice these skills and abilities on simulated patients with a variety of medical conditions. These activities should allow for concurrent or subsequent reinforcement of learned material from courses in pharmacology, patho-physiology, and pharmacotherapeutics. The laboratory setting might also reinforce or compliment introductory pharmacy practice experiences by asking students to create a patient scenario based on something they have experienced or by reflecting on a past activity in light of new information learned. Also, activities and discussions might be used to improve students' awareness of professionalism, the role of the pharmacist in health promotion and disease prevention, and interdisciplinary team practice.[11,14] Laboratory courses can be the bridge between didactic course work and practice experiences.

Reflective Exercise

Return to Appendix 8–1. In the column on the right, list the learning activities that students will be asked to perform that relate to the learning objectives listed in the left column. As an example, see **Table 8–4**, which provides our course map with inclusion of the learning objectives and related activities.

Table 8–4 Example Activities Matched to Course Objectives

Objectives	Teaching and Learning Activities
• Given a case, counsel a patient on adherence, proper medication use, adverse effects, self-monitoring, need for follow-up, and relevant lifestyle changes as indicated for a particular medical problem.	• View examples of communications techniques (online, in class) • Have students watch videos and critique in class or as homework • In-class discussion about patient counseling • Videotape student counseling of simulated or standardized patients in lab; self-assess video tapes
• Given filled medication orders, stock bottles and written prescriptions, evaluate the orders in preparation for dispensing to the patient, and, when indicated, suggest corrections to be made.	• In-lab discussion of checking strategies and review of sample orders • Create timed mock final check exercises for students to complete in lab
• Demonstrate the correct technique for administration of medications via the following routes: subcutaneous injection, intramuscular injection, inhalation, and instillation into the eye.	• Complete lab work sheets with partner to learn SC injection, IM injection, respiratory medication administration, and proper administration of ocular medications • Counsel patients when indicated in videotaped consultations

Planning Assessments

When you have determined what will be taught, it is time to consider how you will verify that the students have learned the material. This is course assessment, and it can document several things: (1) whether or not the student has attained a given level of competence, (2) how effectively the activities led to learning of a particular topic, and (3) where you might consider making changes to your course the next time around. We refer you to the assessment chapter (Chapter 4) to acquire a foundational knowledge of assessment and a working knowledge of key tools in your assessment toolbox.

For each laboratory activity that you listed in your course map, you now need to decide what to evaluate and then find or create an assessment tool that can measure those key components. For example, in a patient counseling session, you might be assessing the student's knowledge of what information needs to be provided to the patient (i.e., level of knowledge in the cognitive domain) as well as how effectively the student delivered the information to the patient (i.e., level of communication skill in the psychomotor domain). You might also consider evaluating the student's professionalism as part of the activity (i.e., attitudes in the affective domain). Therefore, your assessment tools need to be able to measure knowledge, skills, and attitudes.

Two assessment techniques commonly used in the laboratory are performance assessments and rubrics. As described in Chapter 4, performance assessments are used to evaluate the actual process of doing. Examples of performance assessments used in the laboratory setting are the *objective structured clinical examination* (OSCE), which can be quite complicated to administer; and the *practical examination*, which is less complicated to administer. These can be designed to be reliable and valid performance assessments that can be used to assess the student's knowledge as well as communication, physical assessment skills, and level of professionalism.

When developing OSCEs, you should consider the following[18,19]:

- *What is to be assessed?* OSCEs are commonly used to evaluate the mastery of practical skills, problem solving and clinical reasoning skills, and laboratory data interpretation. Often these examinations are high stakes or used as progression requirements in a pharmacy program.
- *How many OSCE stations should you have?* The number of stations will depend on how many students need to be assessed, how long a student will need to spend at a station, and how many hours the students have to complete the examination.
- *How much time should be spent at each station?* Five minutes per station is probably most frequently used, but times can range from 4 to 15 minutes.
- *How will the students be assessed at each station?* You will need to create assessment tools that can be *reliably* used in each OSCE station.

Have you evaluated the climate in the laboratory? What is the flow of activities, and is it conducive to teaching, learning, and assessment?

Depending on the activity, you could create a checklist that the evaluator uses to determine whether the students can or cannot perform various steps in an activity, or it may be best to create a rubric or rating scale for the assessment.

- *What resources will be needed—how much space, how many evaluators, how much time?* As you design your OSCE blueprint, you must consider your work space (this will impact the number of OSCE stations), the number of students that need to complete the OSCE, the number of people needed to assist in the setup and evaluation of the students, and how much time you will need to conduct the examination. It is helpful to create a checklist of all the resources needed prior to designing the OSCE.

- *How will the stations be organized?* You need to consider the blueprint of the OSCE stations. How will the students move from one station to the next? Will you include rest stations in between stations? You want to make sure that you have evenly distributed the different activities so that you do not have several high-order or complex stations in a row. When the design of the stations has been created, consider sharing this with the students so they know what to expect for the layout. Keep in mind that developing the blueprint is usually the most protracted stage of the OSCE process.

- *How will the students be notified that it is time to move to the next OSCE station?* Will each evaluator notify the students when time is up, or will a stopwatch or timer be used to alert students to move to the next station? This will depend on the layout of the examination—whether it is held all in one room or spread out among several rooms.

- *How will you determine the threshold for passing the OSCE?* Several methods may be used, but in general, methods for setting the passing standard are either item-centered (known as fixed or absolute) or person-centered (relative). Fixed standards are determined using a group of subject matter experts who individually evaluate each item to determine what percentage of minimally competent test takers will correctly answer the question. This is then used to determine an overall cutoff score for the exam. Relative standards are determined by the subject matter experts by considering the relationship between the test scores and important factors such as skills, education, and experience. In this case, the cutoff score is the score that best differentiates those test takers characterized as passing and those as failing.[20]

Would a performance assessment—an objective structured clinical exam (OSCE) or practical exam—be an appropriate summative assessment technique in your laboratory course?

Rubrics are another common assessment tool used in laboratory courses to evaluate all components—a student's knowledge, skills, and attitudes.[21–24]

The four basic elements in the development of a rubric are described in Chapter 4.

The laboratory environment supports the use of a wide variety of assessment methods. Regardless of the particular assessment tool used, you need to be able to document that each individual student and the class as a whole have met a reasonable expectation of proficiency on each specific objective. In other words, successful completion of an activity must be directly linked to a course objective as measured by a valid assessment. By designing your assessment tools as you are developing your laboratory course objectives and activities, you are more likely to ensure that the three components (objectives, learning activities, and assessment) remain connected.

You might also consider how you will establish interrater reliability if your assessment instruments will be used by more than one evaluator. Also, will the tools be used by the students as part of peer or self-assessments? Will the assessments occur in real time? Will activities be recorded using audiovisual equipment to be evaluated at a later time? Thinking about these components in advance can help you set clear expectations and give students ample time to prepare to meet your standards.

Reflective Exercise

Let us finish up the course map. Please return to Appendix 8–1. You should be able to plot your assessments in the third column to clearly demonstrate how each activity is linked to a course objective. See **Table 8–5** for an example of a completed map of laboratory objectives and activities.

As the Laboratory Coordinator, What Operational Issues Need to Be Considered?

Along with the course design, the laboratory coordinator needs to also consider the day-to-day operations of the laboratory. Who can access the space? How is the laboratory kept supplied and safe for student use? What are the laboratory rules?

Use of Space

We encourage you to consider how to best accommodate the learner in the laboratory space provided. In several published abstracts, authors have described the physical and curricular redesigns of pharmacy practice laboratories to allow for the simulation of a variety of practices. Laboratory space has been redesigned to allow for more contemporary practice in prescription dispensing, patient counseling, and physical assessment.[25,26]

Table 8–5 Example of Completed Map with Objectives, Activities, and Assessments

Objectives	Teaching and Learning Activities	Assessments
• Given a case, counsel a patient on adherence, proper medication use, adverse effects, self-monitoring, need for follow-up, and relevant lifestyle changes as indicated for a particular medical problem.	• View examples of communications techniques (online, in class) • Have students watch videos and critique in class or as homework • In-class discussion about patient counseling • Videotape student counseling of simulated or standardized patients in lab; self-assess videotapes	• View another videotaped encounter at beginning of the exam and write a critique of the session • Grade student critiques of video-taped counseling sessions • Questions on written exam • Evaluation of counseling session with standardized patient by lab instructor • Student reflection on counseling strengths and limitations
• Given filled medication orders, stock bottles, and written prescriptions, evaluate the orders in preparation for dispensing to the patient, and when indicated, suggest corrections to be made.	• In-lab discussion of checking strategies and review of sample orders • Create timed mock final check exercises for students to complete in lab	• Score on final check exercises
• Demonstrate correct technique for administration of medications via the following routes: subcutaneous injection, intramuscular injection, inhalation, and instillation into the eye.	• Complete lab work sheets with partner to learn SC injection, IM injection, respiratory medication administration, and proper administration of ocular medications • Counsel patients when indicated in videotaped consultations	• Performance on lab work sheets • Performance on patient consultations • Questions on written exam

When there is to be more than one activity per laboratory section, have you thought about work flow and whether or not everyone has enough room to work safely? Attention paid to the flow of laboratory activities will minimize confusion and increase the likelihood that students can focus their energy and attention on the learning activities, rather than navigating a crowded, noisy, disorganized laboratory space.

Who Will Maintain and Service Laboratory Supplies and Equipment?

Depending on the nature of the laboratory, there may be a need for someone to oversee the use of supplies, order equipment, and maintain sensitive technology. This may be especially important when laboratory devices and supplies are also used by the school for other purposes (e.g., the laboratory might loan out blood pressure cuffs or point-of-care testing devices to conduct a health screening day). Schools have a variety of systems for laboratory maintenance, and instructors should be sure to familiarize themselves with the available resources. If you are serving as the laboratory course coordinator, be sure to seek the advice of your school administrator to discuss your budget needs for startup as well as ongoing maintenance and upkeep of the laboratory.

Who Will Be Involved in Running the Laboratory?

Laboratory instructors are routinely referred to as managers because they are responsible for more than teaching content; they must also effectively coordinate many small groups of students and facilitate the activities of a variety of adjunct laboratory instructors.[27] Often many people assist with the delivery of a laboratory, and the course coordinator must ensure that these individuals fulfill their individual roles while working together effectively. You may be working with one or all of the following individuals in your laboratory:

- *Course coordinator.* This person is responsible for academic decisions related to course administration. This person may or may not be responsible for maintaining the physical laboratory space that the course uses. A course coordinator may oversee many sections of the laboratory course or may coordinate more than one course at a time.

- *Laboratory instructors.* There may be additional qualified personnel hired to act as laboratory instructors. They generally work under the direction of the course coordinator to implement the course activities. In the case of pharmacy skills laboratories, licensed practitioners from the local area often participate as instructors on an adjunct basis. They may be responsible for evaluations and/or assist students with laboratory activities. Often pharmacy residents or new graduates participate as laboratory instructors. This can be a very rewarding way to stay connected to your school or college of pharmacy.

- *Teaching assistants (TAs).* Teaching assistants are an invaluable resource in the science laboratory. In many basic science laboratories, TAs may serve as laboratory instructors and may have varying levels of responsibility for administering the laboratory. Many higher education institutions have compiled guidebooks and training manuals for use by teaching assistants and graduate students as they learn how to teach. Excellent compilations have been assembled by the University of Medicine and Dentistry of New Jersey (http://cte.umdnj.edu/traditional_teaching/traditional_laboratory.cfm) and the Michigan State University Teaching Assistant Program (http://www.tap.msu.edu/handbook/docs/2009-2010_handbook.pdf).

- *Lay people or actors.* Last, you may choose to use additional people in your laboratory to play the role of patients in student activities. These people usually follow some sort of predetermined script and may be referred to as *simulated* patients (where someone plays the role of the patient but may not necessarily present an identical character to each student) or *standardized* patients (simulated patients who are also standardized, meaning they respond to each student the same way to ensure a uniform experience). The use of standardized patients allows for a uniform assessment of skills, but it also requires more training and coordination on the part of the course coordinator. Patient actors may or may not be paid. Instructors might also consider connecting with local theater groups to recruit local actors to play the role of patients.[12,13,15,28]

Regardless of the number or type of participants serving as staff in your laboratory, you will need to consider how each participant will be recruited, what remuneration will be provided (if any), and who will be responsible for the training of these individuals on course policies and activities.

How Will You Control for Multiple Evaluators or Multiple Laboratory Sections?

When planning activities, it is important to consider the ramifications of multiple laboratory sections and multiple evaluators. Every effort should be made to maintain the integrity of student work by discouraging students from communicating the twists and turns within a particular laboratory case with their colleagues in other sections. Individual, Internet-ready workstations allow students to resolve drug-related problems with a variety of resources, but unfortunately they also allow quick and easy transmission of material to peers via e-mail and Internet chat. Likewise, when multiple laboratory sections are facilitated by multiple laboratory personnel, it is even more important to use valid and reliable assessment tools whenever possible to ensure interrater reliability of the assessments. Similar assessment rubrics should be used across all activities of a similar kind in the semester or in the curriculum. Though challenging to develop, using assessment tools that have demonstrated interrater reliability can strengthen the activity and reduce student frustration with the use of multiple evaluators.[29]

Have You Adequately Considered the Safety Needs of Students and Staff in the Laboratory?

This is one of the most critical topics in this chapter. The exact nature of safety procedures will depend on the type of laboratory being offered. Safety rules in a chemistry laboratory will likely differ from rules for a pharmacy practice skills laboratory. At a minimum, you should consider policies that address the following questions:

- Can students bring food or drink into the laboratory?
- What are your expectations about clothing or footwear? Is it safe to allow open-toed shoes or loose hair or jewelry?

- Do laboratory staff and students know the proper ways to handle injuries or accidents? Do you have protective materials available (e.g., gloves) to respond to accidents?
- How will you dispose of medically or chemically hazardous materials? Do you need to arrange for services to remove filled disposal containers from the laboratory when they are full?
- Are you modeling safe, appropriate procedures while demonstrating laboratory activities?

Information about laboratory safety can be found in a variety of locations, including teaching assistant training manuals (online or in your institution) and the U.S. Occupational Safety and Health Administration (www.osha.gov).

What Matters with Applications to Pharmaceutical Science Laboratories?

Instructors planning laboratories for the pharmaceutical sciences have to consider many of the same foundational components as found in pharmacy practice laboratories: Why is this laboratory needed? What are the knowledge, skills, and attitudinal objectives of the laboratory? Given the students' prior preparation, what is the content and presentation of the learning exercises so that students achieve the objectives? And what assessments will you use to document that the objectives have been achieved? Two types of pharmaceutical science laboratories illustrate unique issues in this field: simulation laboratories and compounding laboratories.

Simulation

Simulations are replacing wet laboratories. Several examples follow. In anatomy, physiology, and pathophysiology, computer simulations such as A.D.A.M. (www.adameducation.com) create virtual patients that, during guided laboratory sessions, let students navigate through the body and visualize the pathogenesis of diseases and their progression. In biopharmaceutics and pharmacokinetics, laboratory sessions can be organized around a cluster of interactive computer simulations. Developed by faculty in the Department of Clinical Pharmacology at Christchurch Medical School, New Zealand, 16 simulations are provided so that students can explore the impact of modifying variables in such concepts as metabolism and clearance, protein-binding, pharmacodynamics, and pharmacogenetics (www.icp.org.nz). Computer simulations also can be used in laboratory sessions to challenge students in the application of course principles to the calculation of dosing and determination of plasma drug concentrations under varied patient profiles. A catalog of pharmacokinetic software compiled by David Bourne, PhD, of the University of Oklahoma is available at http://www.boomer.org/pkin/soft.html. Last, due to high cost, expensive laboratory equipment may not be available for pharmaceutical analysis laboratories. Arrangements such as the one between the pharmaceutical sciences faculty at the University of British Columbia (UBC) and researchers at Western Washington University (WWU) may be a solution. Using Internet-based technologies, the WWU Integrated Laboratory Network provided remote access to its gas chromatography-mass spectrometry so that students at UBC's pharmacy program could "actively engage with chromatographic and mass spectral theory and data for qualitative and quantitative analyses."[30] In these four examples, the infrastructure of the computer laboratory and its physical and technologic upkeep are considerations.

Although literature describing laboratories for the pharmaceutical sciences is sparse, reports of educational innovations in the related fields of science, technology, engineering, and math (STEM) are available. Through its Division of Undergraduate Education (DUE) and its Transforming Undergraduate Education in Science, Technology, Engineering and Mathematics (TUES) program, the National Science Foundation funds "efforts to create, adapt, and disseminate new learning materials and teaching strategies to reflect advances both in STEM disciplines and in what is known about teaching and learning."[31] For example, the University of Wisconsin–River Falls's four-year project Developing Computer Simulations Integrating Biomedical Research Techniques with Bioinformatics Tools for Case-Based Learning in Introductory Biology Courses[32] may provide simulations, and the evaluation of their effectiveness, that will be valuable in planning the content for pharmacy laboratories.

Compounding

Compounding continues as a function of pharmacy practice. Two major bodies related to pharmacy education implicitly and explicitly call for it; the American Association of Colleges of Pharmacy's 2004 CAPE Educational Outcomes calls for patient-specific care[33] (that could involve personalized medication solutions and individualized formulations), and knowledge of extemporaneous preparations and sterile products are included in the 2010 North American Pharmacist Licensure Examination (NAPLEX) Blueprint.[34]

With the growth of niche compounding markets, such as pediatrics, geriatrics, veterinary medicine, total parenteral nutrition, and home healthcare, as well as the continuing need for alternative dosing formulations, compounding remains a part of contemporary practice. Eighty-seven percent of independent pharmacists in four Midwestern states offered compounding in their pharmacies, and 84 percent of respondents said that compounding should be a part of the PharmD curriculum.[35]

But what is the breadth and depth of the content? The literature is extremely sparse on these topics. A 2005 survey revealed that although all responding schools of pharmacy indicated that they included "some instruction on compounded sterile products," "only 13% of schools felt that their students had adequate training in compounding sterile preparations before graduation."[36] And when capsule compounding was taught in a first-year pharmaceutical-care laboratory, 87 percent of students successfully completed the task; however, when retested in the second year, only 17 percent retained the skill.[37]

Lacking national guidelines or recommendations for the elements that should be covered in a compounding laboratory, faculty are left with developing their own institutional-specific efforts. Objectives can be developed with input from internal and external constituents, the laboratory sessions can be designed within the time and space limits of the curriculum and the facility, and students can be assessed (and potentially reassessed) to determine if the skills have been developed and retained. Those who are teaching, or planning to teach or modify, pharmaceutical sciences laboratory should complete the table in Appendix 8–1 to help organize the objectives (input), teaching and learning activities (processes), and assessments (outcomes) of their laboratory sessions.

What Matters About Continuous Quality Improvements and Feedback?

When the laboratory has run for a period of time and the dust has settled, it is time to objectively assess how it went. Some institutions have an established process that encourages instructors to review their course after each cycle. However, even if this is not an expectation at your institution, an annual reflection can help measure the success of your course and allow you to make meaningful, achievable plans for improvement the next time around. Consider how you might measure success. For example, some instructors may look at the percentage of students who successfully achieved each course objective or the percentage of students who passed a final practical exam. Others might use measures of student satisfaction or a composite of all of the above.

Commonly, instructors solicit feedback about courses from students using standardized course or instructor evaluations. Peer feedback (from faculty in the school or from other laboratory instructors) may also provide valuable data about your course. Self-reflection is a critical component of course evaluation. Integration of these three components—student evaluation, peer evaluation, and self-reflection—provides the most complete picture of the course and should be the foundation for annual assessment. Periodically, you might consider soliciting feedback from external sources— from accreditation bodies or from real-world practitioners. These outside perspectives can validate the content being offered and help ensure that the activities are realistic and applicable to practice. **Figure 8–1** provides a depiction of the contributors to comprehensive course evaluation.

How will your students evaluate the laboratory experience? What features of the laboratory course are most important to assess?

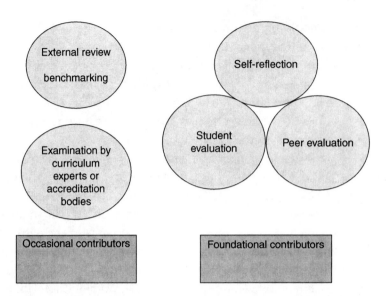

Figure 8–1 Contributors to Comprehensive Course Evaluation

As you make improvements to your course, we encourage you to share your ideas, successes, and challenges. Use this process as an opportunity to identify potential scholarship in the area of teaching and learning methods. (See Chapter 14 for more information on how to connect your teaching with scholarship.) Applying research principles to your course can help strengthen the course modifications being made, assess the effectiveness of the change, and help the larger academy of pharmacy instructors move forward.

What Will Matter in the Future?

It is beyond the scope of our chapter to include an exhaustive description of all available instructional resources for laboratory courses, and there is no doubt that such a list would quickly become out of date. In our research for this chapter, a number of databases and search strategies were found to be most helpful. As you develop and refine your own laboratory course, consider using the resources described in **Table 8–6.**

Summary

Laboratory teaching provides students with the opportunity to experience learning situations found in the real world, but in the laboratory they are associated with less risk and more feedback. As a laboratory instructor, you can have a substantial role in the students' development of knowledge, skills, attitudes, and values that are important to the pharmacy profession.

Table 8-6 Recommended Resources on Laboratory Course

Resource Name and Access Information	Keywords to Consider
Medline (www.pubmed.com)	Assessment
ERIC (www.eric.ed.gov)	Communications
American Association of Colleges of Pharmacy (www.AACP.org) and *American Journal of Pharmaceutical Education* (www.ajpe.org)	Laboratory Laboratory instruction OSCEs
Internet search of laboratory instruction and TA prep materials	Patient assessment
Currents in Pharmacy Teaching and Learning	Patient counseling
National Science Foundation (www.nsf.gov) Course, Curriculum, and Laboratory Improvement Program STEM (Science, Technology, Engineering, and Math) Program	Pharmaceutical care Physical assessment Practice laboratory Simulated patients Simulations Standardized patients Teaching laboratory

With careful course planning and assessment, laboratory courses can offer high-quality learning experiences with valid assessments and provide reliable documentation of educational achievements.

Acknowledgment

The authors thank Mansoor Amiji, PhD, for his valuable input in developing the content of the pharmaceutical sciences laboratory section.

References

1. Hepler CD, Strand LM. Opportunities and responsibilities in pharmaceutical care. *Am J Hosp Pharm.* 1990;47:533–543.
2. Accreditation Council for Pharmacy Education. *Accreditation Standards and Guidelines for the Professional Program in Pharmacy Leading to the Doctor of Pharmacy Degree.* Chicago, IL: Accreditation Council for Pharmacy Education; 2006.
3. Newble D, Cannon R. *A Handbook for Teachers in Universities and Colleges.* 3rd ed. London, England: Kogan Page Limited; 1995.
4. Roth MT, Zlatic TD. Development of student professionalism. *Pharmacotherapy.* 2009;29(6):749–756.
5. Chereson RS, Bilger R, Mohr S, Wuller C. Design of a pharmaceutical care laboratory: a survey of practitioners. *Am J Pharm Educ.* 2005;69(1):article 3.
6. Smith MK. Kurt Lewin: groups, experiential learning and action research. http://www.infed.org/thinkers/et-lewin.htm. Updated June 18, 2009. Accessed August 15, 2009.

7. Adams M, Bell LA, Griffin P. *Teaching for Diversity and Social Justice: A Sourcebook*. New York, NY: Routledge; 1997.

8. Lynagh M, Burton R, Sanson-Fisher R. A systematic review of medical skills laboratory training: where to from here? *Med Educ.* 2007;41:879–887.

9. Hofstein A, Lunetta VN. The laboratory in science education: foundations for the twenty-first century. *Sci Ed.* 2004;88:28–54.

10. Streichler R. Graduate teaching assistant handbook. http://ctd.ucsd.edu/resources/tahandbook.pdf. Accessed June 5, 2009.

11. Fernandez R, Parker D, Kalus JS, Miller D, Compton S. Using a human patient simulation mannequin to teach interdisciplinary team skills to pharmacy students. *Am J Pharm Educ.* 2007;71(3):article 51.

12. Rickles NM, Tieu P, Myers L, Galal S, Chung V. The impact of a standardized patient program on student learning of communication skills. *Am J Pharm Educ.* 2009;73(1):article 4.

13. Schultz KK, Marks A. Community-based collaboration with high school theater students as standardized patients. *Am J Pharm Educ.* 2007;71(2):article 29.

14. Crawford SY. Pharmacists' roles in health promotion and disease prevention. *Am J Pharm Educ.* 2005;69(4):article 73.

15. Glasser D, Ahrens R, Caffee A, Johnson M. Standardized patient assessment in disease state management model. *Am J Pharm Educ.* 2002;66:72–78.

16. Darbishire PL, Plake KS, Nash CL. Active-learning laboratory session to teach the four M's of diabetes care. *Am J Pharm Educ.* 2009;73(2):article 22.

17. Spray JW, Parnapy SA. Teaching patient assessment skills to doctor of pharmacy students: the TOPAS study. *Am J Pharm Educ.* 2007;71(4):article 4.

18. Harden RM. Twelve tips for organizing objectively structured clinical examination (OSCE). *Med Teach.* 1990;12:259–264.

19. Austin Z, O'Byrne C, Pugsley J, Quero Munoz L. Development and validation processes for an objective structured clinical examination (OSCE) for entry-to-practice certification in pharmacy: the Canadian experience. *Am J Pharm Educ.* 2003;67(30):article 76.

20. Fielding DW, Page GG, Rogers WT, O'Byrne CC, Schulzer M, Moody KG. Standard setting for a test of pharmacy practice knowledge: applications in high-stakes testing. *Am J Pharm Educ.* 1996;60:20–29.

21. Brown MC, Conway J, Sorenson TD. Development and implementation of a scoring rubric for aseptic technique. *Am J Pharm Educ.* 2006;70(6):article 133.

22. Brown MC. Internet-based medical chart for documentation and evaluation of simulated patient care activities. *Am J Pharm Educ.* 2005;69(2):article 30.

23. Mackellar A, Ashcroft DM, Bell D, Higman JD, Marriot J. Identifying criteria for the assessment of pharmacy students' communication skills with patients. *Am J Pharm Educ.* 2007;71(3):article 50.

24. Kimberlin CL. Communicating with patients: skills assessment in US colleges of pharmacy. *Am J Pharm Educ.* 2006;70(3):article 67.

25. Brown TA. Renovation of a dispensing laboratory into a multi-functional teaching area. *Am J Pharm Educ.* 1999;63:87S.

26. Deloatch KH, Brock TP, Pittman AW. Design and renovation of a pharmaceutical care teaching space. *Am J Pharm Educ.* 1998;62:129S.

27. Michigan State University. Teaching labs more effectively. http://www.msu.edu/unit/taprog/thoughts/tt11.doc. Accessed August 10, 2009.

28. Austin Z, Tabak D. Design of a new professional practice laboratory course using standardized patients. *Am J Pharm Educ.* 1998;62:271–279.

29. Rickles N, Kirwin J, Brown TA. Development and integration of a communication skills evaluation form for use across the pharmacy curriculum. *Am J Pharm Educ.* 2009;73(4):article 57.

30. Albon SP, Cancilla DA, Hubball H. Using remote access to scientific instrumentation to create authentic learning activities in pharmaceutical analysis. *Am J Pharm Educ.* 2006;70(5):article 121.

31. National Science Foundation. Transforming undergraduate education in science, technology, engineering and mathematics (TUES). http://nsf.gov/funding/pgm_summ.jsp?pims_id=5741&org=DUE&from=home. Accessed December 27, 2009.

32. National Science Foundation. Award Abstract #0717577, developing computer simulations integrating biomedical research techniques with bioinformatics tools for case-based learning in introductory biology courses. http://www.nsf.gov/awardsearch/showAward.do?AwardNumber=0717577. Accessed December 27, 2009.

33. American Association of Colleges of Pharmacy. Educational outcomes 2004. http://www.aacp.org/resources/education/Documents/CAPE2004.pdf. Accessed December 28, 2009.

34. National Boards of Pharmacy. NAPLEX Blueprint. 2009. http://www.nabp.net/ftpfiles/bulletins/NB042010.pdf. Accessed December 28, 2009.

35. Martin KS, McPherson TB, Fontane PE, Berry T, Chereson R, Bilger R. Independent community pharmacists' perspective on compounding in contemporary pharmacy education. *Am J Pharm Ed.* 2009;73(3):article 54.

36. Helluma M, Alverson SP, Monk-Tutor MR. Instruction on compounded sterile preparations at US schools of pharmacy [abstract]. *Am J Health Syst Pharm.* 2007;64:2267–2274.

37. Eley JG, Birnie C. Retention of compounding skills among pharmacy students. *Am J Pharm Ed.* 2006;70(6):article 132.

Appendix 8–1
Your Course Mapping Process

Objectives	Teaching and Learning Activities	Assessments

CHAPTER 9

What Matters in Experiential Education?

Lynne M. Sylvia, PharmD

Introduction

Approximately 30 percent of a four-year professional pharmacy curriculum must be devoted to experiential education. Introductory pharmacy practice experiences (IPPEs) must comprise at least 5 percent of the curriculum, and at least 25 percent of the curriculum must be allocated to advanced pharmacy practice experiences (APPEs).[1] Based on these figures, the average pharmacy student is engaged in at least 300 hours of IPPEs and 36 weeks of APPEs to meet the requirement for completion of the PharmD degree.

Meeting the experiential educational needs of all pharmacy students is a daunting task for schools of pharmacy. To achieve this end, schools are increasingly relying on part-time or volunteer faculty to serve as experiential preceptors. Given the number of students currently enrolled in PharmD programs, it is not uncommon for a practice site and its practitioner preceptors to be affiliated with more than one school of pharmacy as a provider of experiential education. The current demand for quality experiential sites and qualified preceptors has raised a number of reasonable concerns within the academy of pharmacy. Primary concerns are whether practitioner preceptors are being adequately prepared and trained to provide experiential education and whether experiences are being standardized based on predetermined outcomes.[2,3] The adage "see one, do one, teach one" that has conveyed a rather simplistic approach to clinical teaching is no longer applicable.[4] To facilitate the growth and development of contemporary pharmacy practitioners, experiential preceptors

> Introductory pharmacy practice experiences (IPPEs) are practice experiences offered in various practice settings during the early sequencing of the curriculum for purposes of providing transitional experiential activities and directed exposure to pharmaceutical care.
>
> Beck DE, Thomas SG, Janer AL. Introductory practice experiences: a conceptual framework. *Am J Pharm Educ.* Summer 1996; 60:122–131

Advanced pharmacy practice experiences (APPEs) are a series of required and elective experiences offered in the final year of the PharmD program that are of sufficient intensity, duration, and breadth (in terms of patients and disease states that pharmacists are likely to encounter when providing care) to enable achievement of stated competencies.[1]

> Accreditation Council for Pharmacy Education

must appreciate the multidimensional aspects of clinical teaching, particularly how their teaching strategies and their design of clinical experiences can influence learning.

What Is Experiential Education?

In the broadest sense, experiential education involves *learning* through *experience* in an *immediate* and *relevant* setting. As an IPPE or APPE preceptor, what type of learning experience are you currently offering your students? Is the experience relevant and reflective of contemporary practice? Are your students directly involved in the day-to-day activities of the pharmacy? As you will learn in this chapter, experiential education should actively engage the student in activities that have real consequences.[5,6] To maximize the potential for learning in experiential education, all of the learner's senses should be engaged.

Providing a quality experience that engages all of the student's senses is challenging, and this needs to be recognized up front. For learning to happen, each IPPE and APPE must be a well-designed, facilitated experience that allows students the opportunity to increase their knowledge, develop skills, and become professionally socialized. Providing such an experience requires that you, the preceptor, have a fundamental understanding of the three domains of learning: cognitive, psychomotor, and affective (see Chapters 2 and 4). You must also appreciate that your teaching or precepting style may need to vary on an hourly basis. You will need to identify when it is best to instruct, model, coach, or facilitate learning through mentoring. The setting of learning will also present unique challenges to you and your students. Compared to the didactic teaching environment (e.g., lecture hall or classroom), a relevant practice setting is uncontrolled and fraught with unanticipated interruptions. These frequent interruptions in your teaching may be viewed as a hindrance; however, they are a realistic component of contemporary pharmacy practice, and their presence reflects that your experiential setting is dynamic. As an IPPE or APPE preceptor, you must learn how to maximize a teaching moment in the face of such distractions and to teach students how to adapt to interruptions in pharmacy work flow. And in this dynamic environment, you still need to apply systems thinking (see Chapter 3) to identify and organize the inputs in your experiential setting as well as processes to maximize the learning experience. Each of these challenges needs to be recognized and embraced to facilitate quality experiential education.

In this chapter, you will be asked to reflect on your current role as an experiential preceptor (i.e., IPPE, APPE, or residency preceptor) and to map the experience that you are currently offering your students or residents in your practice setting. Mapping will involve a close examination of your experiential rotation, and it will most likely expose areas of both excellence and needed change in your program. Newly appointed practice faculty members, volunteer faculty, and residency preceptors can also use the mapping exercise to design new experiential rotations. Overall, this chapter will address the unique challenges of experiential education by providing answers to the following questions:

- What are the basic tenets of experiential education?
- Which teaching strategies have been shown to be most effective in the experiential setting in terms of facilitating the development of professional competence?
- How does the preceptor adapt his or her teaching role to maximize the opportunity for experiential learning?
- Which tools and techniques are best-suited for the assessment of clinical knowledge, skills, and attitudes acquired through experiential learning?

What Matters in Learning in Experiential Education?

Experiential learning involves "a direct encounter with the phenomena being studied rather than merely thinking about the encounter, or only considering the possibility of doing something about it."[7] Not all experiences result in student learning. Before designing an IPPE or APPE, you should be familiar with the basic principles or tenets of experiential education. These tenets are revealed through a historic review of experiential education.

Learning through experience, or experiential education, is the oldest form of education. More than 2,500 years ago, Confucius conveyed his philosophy of learning by the words, "Tell me and I will forget, show me and I may remember, *involve me* and I will understand"[8] (emphasis added). These words have become a motto for experiential education. A basic tenet of learning through experience, conveyed in the words of Confucius, is that students learn best by *doing*. Observation of experienced practitioners or seeing practice has a place in experiential education, particularly during introductory experiences. However, the bulk of the experience, whether an IPPE or APPE, should extend beyond observation or exposure to include direct engagement.

In the 1930s, John Dewey described two other basic principles of experiential education, *interaction* and *continuity*.[9,10] Dewey, an American philosopher and educator, criticized traditional education, describing it as unnecessarily long and restrictive.[11] He believed that learning could best be achieved through involving students in real-life tasks. For example, math and fractions could be learned by applying these concepts to cooking or by figuring out how long it would take someone on horseback to get from one place to another.[11] These real-life experiences could not only enhance learning but also enable the student to connect with his or her society and develop a social conscience. Dewey encouraged fellow educators to study the nature of human experience before attempting to engage students in experiential learning. He argued against generalizing experiences. No one experience would be rewarding for all students. Dewey's theory on experiential education is based on the premise that "one's present experience is a function of the *interaction* between one's past experiences and the present situation" (emphasis added).[9] As such, Dewey believed in constructivism, that students create knowledge by relating their unique set of past experiences to the current situation. Based on Dewey's theory, there is not only an interaction between experiences but also *continuity*. What a student learns from one experience, whether positive or negative, will influence all of that student's future experiences. Dewey's philosophy on experiential education offers us a number of insights about our roles as IPPE or APPE preceptors. In particular, we are reminded that experiential education consists of a series of experiences, with each event influencing the next. Moreover, there is an individualized or subjective element to learning through experience; what one student takes away from an experience may be largely different from that of another student.

Kolb, who describes himself as a contemporary advocate of experiential education, built on the work of others, including John Dewey, Kurt Lewin, and Jean Piaget, to create an experiential learning model.[12] According to Kolb, experiential education offers the student the opportunity to test information learned in the classroom against real-life experiences. The interaction between concrete experiences and prior knowledge leads to new knowledge.[12] Kolb describes the process of experiential learning as a four-phase cycle.[12] The first phase is a *concrete experience* (e.g., a patient encounter, the receipt of a medication order, or a question presented on rounds by a physician). Following this experience, the student should be asked to examine it from many different perspectives based on all of the senses. This second phase is known as *reflective observation*. What did he or she see, hear, or observe during the encounter? What actually transpired? What were the roles of all the parties involved? Was a task completed? If so, what was the quality of the end product? What were the behaviors or expectations of the patient or fellow healthcare providers? Reflection offers the student the opportunity to identify the actions that took place during the encounter and the result of these actions. The third phase is *abstract conceptualization*. During this phase, the student is asked to dig deeper and attempt to identify the general principles that underlie the experience. Questions that should be asked include the following: What could explain the observations? How will these observations influence future attempts to perform this task? Was I, the student, prepared for the situation? If not, how will I become better prepared for a similar situation in the future? The last step is *active exper-imentation* in which the student applies these general principles and theories to future encounters. The following example illustrates the Kolb experiential learning cycle:

Phase 1, concrete experience. A student is asked to interview a patient to obtain a drug allergy history.

Phase 2, reflective observation. The task is achieved. The student identi-fies that it took 20 minutes to complete the interview. The patient was able to clarify the type of allergic reaction that he had to penicillin, and he also reported that he tolerated a number of cephalosporins in the past. The student observed that the nature of the patient's allergy to penicillin and ability to tolerate cephalosporins were not listed in the patient's medical record.

Phase 3, abstract conceptualization. The student makes an association between the time it took to conduct the interview and the haphazard nature of his questioning of the patient. To better prepare for future encounters of this type, the student will need to develop a structured interview process and determine the best order of questioning. Two general principles or theories are identified by the student: (1) a struc-tured interview process may allow for time-efficiency in allergy history taking, and (2) asking patients if they can tolerate structurally similar drugs (e.g., cephalosporins) should be a standard component when assessing history of penicillin allergy.

Phase 4, active experimentation. The student uses a self-developed, struc-tured allergy interview process and documentation form for future encounters. The student also compares and contrasts allergy information documented in the medical record versus that obtained through the direct patient interview. He tests his hypothesis regarding the frequency with which charted penicillin allergy histories include documentation of tolerance to cross-reactive or structurally similar compounds.

Kolb's model reminds us of two additional tenets of experiential edu-cation: *reflection* and *independent learning*. These elements apply not only to the student in the experiential model, but also to the preceptor. Before any future experiences are undertaken, both the teacher and the student should reflect on the current experience. Both the teacher and the student should also have the opportunity for independent learning. As a precep-tor, the application of Kolb's model prompts you to reflect on your role as a teacher. What have you learned about your teaching from the con-crete experience? What did you observe about yourself in the role of a teacher? What theories have you identified about your teaching methods, and how will you experiment in the future to test these theories? For those of you who may find Kolb's model too abstract, consider a more simplified three-stage experiential learning cycle. The three stages are *do* (go forth and have an experience), *review* (assess what happened and identify what can be learned from the experience), and *plan* (plan a way to approach the next experience based on what was learned from the current experience).[11]

Reflective Exercise

Table 9–1 lists the basic tenets or principles of experiential education discussed in this section. The table also provides areas for your comments and reflections. If you are currently offering an APPE or IPPE at your practice site, how are you applying each of these principles to your program? As a new preceptor, how will you ensure that these principles are applied to the design of your IPPE, APPE, or residency program?

Table 9–1 Tenets of Experiential Education

Basic Tenet	Reflection and Planning
Active Student Engagement To what extent does your IPPE or APPE consist of observation or exposure? What patient-care activities are students directly involved in? Are they realistic and immediate?	
Interaction and Continuity How do you account for students' past experiences? Do you review student portfolios? How do you or will you introduce students to your practice?	
Reflection Do you encourage reflective exercises? Are you and your students engaged in reflective activities? When and how are these activities employed?	
Independent Learning To what extent are students engaged in independent learning activities? Do they develop individualized goals and courses of action to achieve these goals?	
Planning To what extent do you review each experience? How do you apply the reflections and observations of both students and preceptors to the planning of future experiences?	

What Matters in the Design of Experiential Education?

A quality experience has been defined as "a well-planned, outcomes-focused training experience with adequate supervision and assessment by a qualified preceptor within a learning-rich practice environment."[6] Of the many features of experiential education packed into this definition, *well-planned* is the most essential. You are more likely to offer an experience that meets current quality standards if you prepare and plan for the IPPE or APPE well in advance of student placement. During the planning stage, each of the following questions should be asked and answered.

> Quality experiential education is "a well-planned, outcomes-focused training experience with adequate supervision and assessment by a qualified preceptor within a learning-rich practice environment."[6]
>
> American College of Clinical Pharmacy

What Is the Ultimate Goal of the Experiential Program (IPPE, APPE, Residency) with Which I Am Affiliated?

The goals of an experiential program are typically described in the IPPE and APPE preceptor manuals provided by your affiliated college or school of pharmacy. The goal of experiential education, in general, has also been described by the Accreditation Council for Pharmacy Education (ACPE)[1] and in an American College of Clinical Pharmacy (ACCP) white paper on quality experiential education.[6] Goals for residency training are provided by a number of organizations, including the American Society of Health-System Pharmacists. The statements provided by each of these organizations convey a consistent message. The ultimate goal of experiential learning in pharmacy is the development of professional competence. Having the knowledge, skills, and attitudes necessary for the provision of patient-focused and population-based care constitutes professional competence. Nimmo and Holland have defined professional competence in the form of an equation[13]:

$$\text{Professional Competence} = \text{Skills} + \text{Professional Socialization} + \text{Judgment}$$

Skills reflected in this equation include problem solving, critical thinking, communication, and psychomotor action (e.g., drug-order entry, IV admixture preparation, physical assessment, administration of immunizations). Displaying the attitudes, behaviors, and values of a professional, or being professionally socialized, is another component of competence, as is the ability to apply sound clinical judgment. The latter skill is acquired through practice with feedback and reflection. Keeping our goal in mind, how will you design a clinical experience that allows for the development and assessment of each of these components? As in the systems approach, the starting point of your planning process is the recognition of the end point (the aim or goal) of experiential learning—professional competence.

Is There a Learning-Rich Practice Environment?

A learning-rich environment is one that provides the student with an opportunity to meet the expectations of the specific learning experience, whether introductory or advanced. It can be defined on the basis of both qualitative and quantitative measures. One learning environment may be better-suited or more learning-rich for an IPPE, whereas another may offer a better setting for an APPE. To make this determination, you need to be familiar with the fundamental differences between the IPPE and the APPE (see **Table 9–2**).

Whether you are designing an IPPE or an APPE, a learning-rich environment is one that offers ample opportunity for direct patient contact. As noted by Parsell and Bligh, "Patients play a crucial part in the development of clinical reasoning, communication skills and professional attitudes, and their relevance to real life provides essential motivation for learners."[4] During an IPPE, students should have the opportunity to develop empathy and an understanding of illness through direct patient exposure. During successive IPPEs and APPEs, students can then come to know the patient through continued interaction. As described by Hepler and Strand, knowing the patient is the first step in the provision of pharmaceutical care.[14] A learning-rich environment provides this opportunity. As part of your planning, what extent of exposure to patients can you offer the student in the IPPE or APPE? Be creative. In an IPPE, could students attend your diabetes education classes and interview patients about their knowledge of their disease? Could they obtain medication histories from patients or assist

Table 9–2 Characteristics of IPPEs and APPEs

Characteristic	IPPE	APPE
Competencies to be achieved from the experience	Process and dispense new and refill medication orders.	Practice as a member of an interdisciplinary team.
	Conduct patient interviews to obtain patient information.	Identify, evaluate, and communicate to patients and healthcare providers the appropriateness of patient-specific drug therapy.
	Create patient profiles.	
	Interact with other healthcare professionals.	Consult with patients regarding self-care products.
	Assess patient care literacy and compliance.	Recommend drug therapy.
	Interact with pharmacy technicians in the delivery of pharmacy services.	Provide patient education to a diverse patient population.
	Bill third parties for pharmacy services.	Manage the drug regimen through monitoring and assessment of patients.
Placement in curriculum	IPPEs start in first professional year.	APPEs take place in the fourth professional year.
Student's level of interaction	The student's interaction ranges from shadowing and observation to direct involvement in patient care.	The majority of the student's experience involves direct patient care.
Primary roles of preceptor	The preceptor primarily instructs and models.	The preceptor primarily models, coaches, and facilitates.

patients in selecting OTC medications in a community pharmacy setting? As you plan for patient exposure, remember the need to obtain clearance for student contact with patients. What immunizations must the students have to be in contact with patients at your practice site? Do the students need to undergo training regarding the Health Insurance Portability and Accountability Act (HIPAA), and when can this be achieved?

Learning-rich also means resource-rich and preceptor-rich. Identify the inputs that you will need to maximize the learning experience. In terms of resources, how will the students access patient-specific information at your site? What drug information systems will the students be able to use? Is there adequate physical work space for the students and an adequate number of computers for the students' use? An additional resource that will need to be considered is you, the preceptor. How much time per day or week will you be able to devote to the precepting of students? Will you be the sole preceptor at your site, or will other preceptors be engaged in the program? Good precepting takes time—time to prepare the experience, coach the students, supervise them as they attempt to assume professional responsibility for patient care, and time to provide quality feedback.

A team-based approach to precepting at your site may allow for more contact time between students and the preceptor and for students to be integrated within the entire pharmacy department or practice setting. If multiple preceptors will be involved at your site, a substantial amount of planning will need to be done to orchestrate and execute an outcomes-based experience. At least six months prior to student placement, your team should begin a series of meetings to share learning styles, teaching philosophies, and teaching strategies. The affiliated college's preceptor manual will need to be reviewed by the team to ensure standardization and consistency in assessment. Through collaboration and planning, you will be able to identify which preceptors have the time and expertise to model and coach drug distribution skills, problem-solving skills, direct patient care skills at the bedside or in the clinic, and literature evaluation skills through coordination of a journal club. If you are coordinating a team-based approach to precepting at your site, a number of resources are at your disposal to help develop effective preceptors. Each of the following resources provides valuable guidance for the development of a preceptor-rich program:

- *Education Scholar (www.educationscholar.org)*. This Web-based program was developed by the Western University of Health Sciences and the American Association of Colleges of Pharmacy (AACP). It provides educational modules to assist faculty in adopting learner-centered teaching methods; see the module on experiential education.
- *ACCP Academy Teaching and Learning Certificate Program* (www. accp.com/academy/teachingAndLearning.aspx). The American College

of Clinical Pharmacy (ACCP) designed this program to assist in the recruitment, motivation, and preparation of clinical educators.

- *AACP Professional Experience Program (PEP) Library of Resources* (http://www.peplibrary.vcu.edu/index.html). This online library of resources on experiential education is sponsored by Virginia Commonwealth University.
- "Teaching Rounds," *British Medical Journal.* A series of articles called "Teaching Rounds" in *BMJ* showcases a variety of topics related to clinical teaching.[15–20]

How Do I Design an Experience That Is Outcomes-Focused?

The design of an IPPE or APPE should be based on the outcome statements specific to that experience. These statements are provided in your IPPE or APPE preceptor manual from your affiliated college or school of pharmacy. Outcomes are measurable statements of performance that reflect the acquisition and application of knowledge, skills, and behaviors (see Chapter 4 for a discussion of outcome statements). Applying them to the design of your IPPE or APPE allows for consistency or standardization in experiential education. Sample outcomes for an IPPE and an APPE are provided in **Table 9–3**.

Note the differences and similarities between the outcomes of the introductory and advanced practice experiences. What concrete experiences can you offer students that will allow them to achieve these specific outcomes? What activities routinely performed by you or other pharmacists in your practice setting demonstrate patient-focused care and population-focused care? Could these activities or components be learned and subsequently performed by IPPE or APPE students at their specific stage of development? Do the activities have real consequences? Answering

---

Table 9–3 Sample Outcome Statements for an IPPE and an APPE

IPPE in First Professional Year	APPE in Acute Patient Care
Develop a covenantal relationship with the patient as the first step in the provision of pharmaceutical care.	Identify population-based drug therapy and monitoring requirements.
Assist in the preparation, compounding, and dispensing of patient-specific drug therapy.	Communicate effectively with patients, preceptors, and other members of the healthcare team.
Apply principles of pharmacy management to the provision of pharmaceutical care.	Recommend patient-specific therapeutic plans based on the unique clinical, psychosocial, cultural, and educational needs of each patient.
Demonstrate professionalism and leadership by carrying out duties in a professional manner, including the use of time-management, organizational, and ethical skills.	Demonstrate professionalism and leadership by carrying out duties in a professional manner, including the use of time-management, organizational, and ethical skills.

these questions will result in the generation of a list of potential activities relating to each of the outcome statements of the specific experiences. Activities for the sample IPPE may include participation on rounds or in a clinic to observe the patient–pharmacist relationship, assistance in IV drug preparation and compounding, and involvement in management projects involving procurement and appropriate storage of drugs. Activities for the sample APPE may include participation in patient discharge counseling, medication reconciliation, and target drug programs, including renal dosing of medications, IV to PO drug conversion, and antimicrobial stewardship. Most important, the activities that you engage students in should reflect contemporary practice, be measurable, and be specific to the desired outcomes of the IPPE or APPE.

How Do I Identify and Set Realistic Expectations for My Students?

Scenario: You are a newly appointed preceptor, and you are currently precepting your first APPE student. It is the end of week 1 of the APPE. Two days ago, you assigned a 12-minute oral case presentation to your student. He was asked to summarize a patient case in the medically accepted format and to SOAP out the patient's primary medical problem. You also asked the student to investigate a specific drug-related problem involving this patient and to provide an evidence-based plan for the resolution of this drug problem. Today, when listening to the student's presentation, you note that it deviates from the medically accepted format, and it lacks sufficient detail. The student uses many unacceptable medical abbreviations, and his knowledge of the drug-related problem appears rudimentary. He refers to evidence-based guidelines as the source of his decision making; however, he recites the content of these guidelines rather than applying them to the unique patient situation. Based on the assessment tool provided by the college, you calculate a failing grade for the oral presentation. The student is devastated by the failing grade, and you are questioning your abilities as a preceptor. You think your expectations were realistic, but were they?

Throughout the literature on experiential education, preceptors are advised to set realistic expectations for their students, but how do you gauge whether your expectations are realistic? Setting realistic expectations requires that you have knowledge of the pharmacy curriculum in total, knowledge of the individual student as a learner, and general knowledge of the levels of cognitive, psychomotor, and affective learning. Setting realistic expectations does not mean lowering your standards. Instead, *realistic* refers to attainable expectations based on where your student is in his or her journey to professional competence.

The learner's existing knowledge and clinical capabilities must be taken into account.[4]

G. Parsell, J. Bligh

To set realistic expectations, you need to plan ahead and identify those inputs, just like you did in Chapter 3. Start by reviewing the pharmacy curriculum. What courses has the student completed prior to undertaking your IPPE or APPE? What courses has the student yet to complete? Second, learn about your learner. What types of IPPEs or APPEs did he or she previously complete, and what was the nature of the learner's prior work experience? What types of patient care or population-based care activities were previously undertaken by the student? By asking questions of the student and by doing your homework regarding the college's curriculum, you will be more apt to set realistic expectations for the IPPE or APPE that are consistent with the college's outcome statements.

To set realistic expectations, you also need to be familiar with the levels of cognitive learning. In the 1950s, Bloom described a taxonomy of cognitive learning in which recall of information is considered to be the lowest level of learning.[21] In increasing order, higher levels of learning are comprehension, application, analysis, synthesis, and evaluation (see Chapter 2 for further discussion of Bloom's Taxonomy). Typically, entry-level APPE students have a lot of knowledge, and they can recall lists of adverse effects of drugs, basic mechanisms of drug action, and the stepwise approaches to the treatment of common diseases as per evidence-based guidelines. But what is the depth of their knowledge and comprehension? Have they questioned the evidence-based guidelines, their derivation, and the extent to which they can be extrapolated to the care of a specific patient? To what extent have they analyzed patient-specific information over a longitudinal period? Although APPE students have had some opportunity to apply data and synthesize treatment plans in their didactic education, these skills have not yet been mastered at the time of entry into APPEs. Expecting mastery of these skills at the start of APPEs or during IPPEs is unrealistic. To set realistic expectations for experiential education, you need to gauge your student's level of learning at the start of the IPPE or APPE.

Gauging a student's learning is interpreted by some as measuring the extent of the student's knowledge upon entry into the IPPE or APPE. Keep in mind that administering a pretest written exam can help you identify the extent of the student's retention of knowledge or recall of information; however, this tool is less effective at measuring higher levels of learning, such as analysis and synthesis. Moreover, a written exam cannot effectively measure a student's psychomotor skills or level of professionalism. An entry-level objective structured clinical examination (OSCE) would be an effective assessment technique in this setting in that it would allow for the assessment of knowledge, skills, and attitudes. As discussed in Chapter 8, an OSCE takes time to plan, requires numerous resources, and may be cost prohibitive. In lieu of an OSCE, how could you gauge the extent of the student's knowledge, skills, and professional attitudes at the start of the clinical experience?

Consider the development of a number of orientation-based activities in your IPPE or APPE. During the first week of the experience, engage the students in nongraded role-playing exercises, interactive cases, and disease state management discussions. Ask them to share their understanding of therapeutic concepts or disease states, and ask them to use Bloom's Taxonomy to identify their levels of learning of the topics. Through discussion, students can gain self-awareness of the need to dig deeper into learning and to work toward comprehension and analysis rather than relying solely on information recall. Early in the experience, you can also identify the students' current perceptions of health, wellness, and illness and their attitudes toward healthcare providers and patients. Ask students to observe the interpersonal relationships between patients and physicians, nurses and pharmacists, and pharmacists and patients. Engage students in discussions to determine the extent to which they are professionally socialized. By employing discussion-based and skill-based activities in the early stages of the IPPE or APPE, you will be better able to customize the experience to the individual learner and set realistic benchmarks and expectations for the entire experience.

Getting back to our scenario, were the preceptor's expectations unrealistic? This question cannot be answered based on the information provided. Was this the student's first APPE? Was the case study format modeled for the student? Was the student clear as to the expectations of the exercise? What were the student's prior experiences, and what feedback had he or she received about prior case presentations? What did the student's portfolio reveal? Answers to all of these questions need to be obtained during an orientation period to set realistic expectations for the experience.

Reflective Exercise

Please refer to the mapping exercise in Appendix 9–1. In column 1, list the primary outcomes of the IPPE or APPE that you are currently precepting or planning to precept. In column 2, list the activities that your students are currently engaged in or will be engaged in that will demonstrate the achievement of these outcomes.

What Matters in the Role of the Preceptor?

If you accept that the experiential learner advances along a continuum from a dependent to an independent learner, then you must also accept that your role as teacher must be adaptable to the learner's needs. As an experiential educator, you will serve as an instructor, model, coach, and facilitator of learning. Your challenge is to identify which teaching role

> Learners move from being dependent on their teachers to becoming collaborators, and finally toward being independent, self-directed learners and practitioners.[22]
> F.T. Stritter, R.M. Baker, E.J. Shahady

best serves the learner at the given time and at his or her stage of development. The following scenario will be used to illustrate the varied roles of the experiential educator.

> *Scenario*: At your practice site, students are involved in the assessment of patients with suspicion of heparin-induced thrombocytopenia (HIT). The students receive a daily printout of all patients who were ordered an enzyme-linked immunosorbent assay (ELISA) for determination of a platelet factor 4 antibody. Students are then responsible for reviewing the patient's medical records, laboratory values, and clinical status to calculate a 4T's score. This score, ranging from 0 to 8, is used to estimate the probability of HIT. Depending on the score and the results of the ELISA, an intervention in the care of the patient may be warranted.

Before the student can engage in this clinical program, you must ensure that he or she has adequate knowledge of the mechanism by which heparin causes thrombocytopenia, the sensitivity and specificity of the assay technique, alternative causes of thrombocytopenia, and the calculation and interpretation of the 4T's score. This stage of learning will typically require instruction. The term *instructor* conjures up visions of a classroom and a lecturer and the process of transmitting knowledge. In the experiential setting, instruction should take on another vision, one in which there is active discussion between the teacher and the learner. Before adding to the student's knowledge in the area of HIT, you should engage the student in a discussion to identify what he or she already understands about the topic. Experiential education should build on what was previously learned in the didactic portion of the pharmacy program, and there is rarely the need for standard lecturing. Start your instructional session by asking the student what he or she currently understands about the pathophysiology of HIT, about the assay techniques, and about the 4T's score. Prior to the discussion, provide the student with a key reading on the topic, or have the student conduct an independent literature search to identify a key reading. During the ensuing discussion, fill in the gaps of the student's knowledge of the topic, and focus on measuring the student's comprehension of the topic. Using this approach, you are instructing and transmitting needed knowledge, but the student is not a passive participant in the learning process. You are also offering the student the ability to construct new knowledge from his or her existing knowledge of the topic.

Having the foundational knowledge of HIT and the 4T's scoring system is not enough. For the student to participate in the clinical program, he or she needs to know how to apply this knowledge to the care of patients. This type of learning will require modeling on the part of the preceptor. Modeling involves walking the student through the problem-solving process in both the literal and figurative senses. In this scenario, you would physically walk the student to the patient care area, physically show the student where medical records are stored or how this information is accessed via the computer system, walk the student to the lab to discuss the specificity and sensitivity of the assay results, and walk the student to the nursing station and the patient's bedside to visually examine the patient for signs of HIT. As you physically walk the student through the process, you also walk him or her through your mental process of solving the clinical problem. Talk aloud and share your strategy of thinking. How do you determine the extent of decline in the platelet count? If there are missing pieces of information, how do you account for them in your assessment? How do you weigh each patient finding and put the pieces together to calculate the 4T's score? Which interdisciplinary team members help you in providing this service, and how do you interact and work with these individuals in a collaborative manner? You need to model not only the process of thinking, but also the professional demeanor and interpersonal skills that are necessary to provide this patient care service.

After observing, reflecting, and conceptualizing the process, it is now time for the student to actively experiment and engage in the program. As the preceptor, your job is not done. As the student attempts to calculate the 4T's score on his or her own, the student may get stuck in the process and need your assistance. At this stage of learning, you will serve as a coach. A good coach sets the ground rules for the game but allows the student to carry the ball. As a coach, you will listen and observe. You will work with the student to solve a patient problem, but the student will take the lead. When the student is veering off the mark, you will set him or her back on course. Instead of instructing, you will ask the student questions to identify what he or she is thinking and why he or she is taking or planning to take a particular course of action. You will help the student develop the ability to self-police or self-regulate his or her actions. You will provide positive feedback and reinforcement, and you will also correct mistakes. Most important, you will loosen the reins of control so that the student can develop the confidence and competence to eventually perform the task in your absence.

Facilitation is the stage of learning in which the student is independently providing the patient care service. At this stage, you have determined that the student is ready to assume responsibility for the task or some part of the task. Keep in mind that facilitation is not always achieved in experiential education, and the coaching stage is typically protracted. The student may become proficient enough to assume responsibility for a part or parts of the problem-solving process, but not the entire process. In the previous scenario, the student may develop the psychomotor and cognitive abilities to obtain the information needed to calculate the 4T's score;

however, the student may still require your assistance to put all of the pieces together to provide a final assessment of the patient. In this regard, you may be able to serve as a facilitator for part of the process but continue to coach the student through the more sophisticated and multidimensional assessment and plan.

Reflective Exercise

Identify one clinical activity that your students perform that is listed in your experiential course map. How do you currently teach the students so that they can eventually assume responsibility for this activity? Outline the process in **Table 9–4**. How are you providing instruction? Modeling? Coaching? Are you serving as a facilitator of learning and allowing the student to function independently? If you are a new preceptor and are planning a student-based activity, outline the process you will use to teach this skill.

What Matters in Teaching Strategies That Promote Learning in Experiential Education?

Choose those strategies that challenge the student, encourage self-directed learning, and provide ongoing constructive criticism.[6]
American College of Clinical Pharmacy

In the previous section, you were reminded of the varied roles of an experiential preceptor. You will instruct, model, coach, and facilitate. But how will you master these roles in your fast-paced, uncontrolled, contemporary pharmacy practice setting? Being a coach, model, and facilitator takes time. How do you maximize your time for teaching so you serve as an effective preceptor? The following teaching strategies are recommended to do just that.

The Socratic Method of Teaching

Socrates' philosophy on learning and teaching was deeply rooted in the belief that truth (knowledge) can best be achieved through questioning. The Socratic method of teaching stems from this philosophy. Using this method, the teacher reduces a concept into a series of small questions. Systematic questioning of the student encourages critical thinking, and

---

Table 9–4 Outline Your Educational Plan

Activity: _____

Instruction:

Modeling:

Coaching:

Facilitation:

finding answers to these questions allows the student to distill the truth on his or her own. The following example illustrates the Socratic method:

Non-Socratic approach:
Student: I don't understand how beta-blockers work in heart failure.
Preceptor: They block the beta-receptor that was downregulated due to chronic stimulation by norepinephrine. Beta-blockade leads to upregulation of the receptor, thereby increasing cardiac output.
Student: Oh.

Socratic method:
Student: I don't understand how beta-blockers work in heart failure.
Preceptor: In heart failure, how does the body compensate for a reduction in cardiac output?
Student: By increasing the heart rate and releasing renin to eventually increase preload.
Preceptor: How does the body increase the heart rate and release of renin?
Student: It seems like norepinephrine would be involved, but I'm not sure. Is this correct?
Preceptor: Yes. Why don't you review the pathophysiology of heart failure with a focus on the role of compensatory mediators, specifically norepinephrine? We can continue the discussion after you sort this piece out.

In this example, the Socratic teacher used questions to identify the student's level of understanding of the topic versus telling or transmitting the answer to the student. Using this method, the teacher was able to identify where the student had a gap in his or her understanding and what assumptions were being made. The Socratic method offers the student the opportunity to share his or her thoughts aloud and to trace out the implications of what he or she is saying. Most important, the student is held responsible for his or her own learning, and the seeds are sown for self-directed learning. Whenever possible and feasible, the Socratic method is advised as the preferred strategy for clinical teaching. To facilitate learning through the Socratic process, see **Table 9–5** for examples of the types of questions used in clinical coaching.

The One-Minute Preceptor Technique

Described in 1992, the One-Minute Preceptor technique largely involves clinical questioning with feedback, and it extends from the Socratic teaching model.[23] This method allows you to initially diagnose the learner then teach through discussion in a timely manner. The One-Minute Preceptor technique, originally designed for use in ambulatory clinics and medical offices, is based on the premise that the duration of a clinical teaching encounter averages 10 minutes. The initial six minutes of the encounter are typically devoted to presentation of the clinical problem by the learner.

Table 9–5 Coaching Questions and Their Purpose

Purpose of Question	Example
To measure knowledge or recall	What is the goal blood pressure in a patient with diabetes?
To clarify or aid the student in organizing his or her thoughts (comprehension)	What was your understanding about the physician's choice of a thiazide for this patient?
To extend the discussion and examine whether the student can take the situation further (application, analysis)	Why did you choose an ACE inhibitor as the drug of choice for the patient?
	What if this patient has heart failure? Diabetes?
	If the patient was also receiving ciprofloxacin, how would this influence your decision?
To prompt the student to consider additional pertinent factors; to offer the student some support or aid in providing a more acceptable response	Have you considered the fact that the patient has a family history of depression?
	How might the patient's social history influence your choice of drug therapy?
For justification; to identify if the student can support his or her position with evidence	What evidence from the case led you to that conclusion?
	Could you explain your reasoning?

Source: Adapted from Kleffner JH, Hendrickson WD. Effective clinical teaching. http://www.utexas.edu/pharmacy/general/experiential/practitioner/exercises.pdf. Accessed September 1, 2009.

The next three minutes are expended on an attempt by the teacher to clarify the problem. For example, the teacher may ask questions to identify whether a patient's fever has escalated or whether any new medications have been added to the patient's drug regimen. This leaves 1 minute out of 10 for discussion or teaching. How will you use this minute? The One-Minute Preceptor approach offers you a teaching strategy that maximizes the limited time that you have for clinical teaching. With continued use, this method helps you restructure a 10-minute teaching encounter to make the best use of that time. The One-Minute Preceptor method[23] is illustrated in the following clinical teaching scenario.

Scenario: After having your student go on rounds with you on the cardiology team for the past two weeks, you feel that he is ready to go on rounds without you today while you work in another area of the pharmacy. During rounds today, your student sees a patient who was admitted from the cardiology clinic due to a diffuse skin rash. There is suspicion that the rash is drug-induced, and your student was asked to investigate all potential drug causes. Following rounds, your student presents this case to you. He shares that the patient is awaiting orthotopic heart transplantation and is on home milrinone therapy. During rounds, the patient stated that he thought the rash was just a sunburn from being exposed to the sun while mowing his lawn. He uses a riding lawn mower, and he does his lawn over the course of a few days in sections at a time. The rash is only on the sun-exposed areas of his skin, and there is some bluish discoloration to the skin on the distal extremities. As your student is presenting this case, you realize that you are very familiar with this patient. You recall that his diuretic therapy was recently changed from furosemide, which he has taken for years, to torsemide. He was started on amiodarone four months ago. Immediately, you suspect amiodarone-induced photosensitivity as the cause of this admission. How do you best proceed as a clinical teacher?

In this scenario, the preceptor is faced with a common dilemma. Should she tell the student what she suspects is the cause of the skin rash? How long will it take the student to put the pieces together on his own? Because the preceptor has already loosened the reins and allowed the student to go on rounds without her, the student is most likely in the coaching and facilitating stages of learning. The preceptor wants the student to have the opportunity to find the knowledge on his own, but she is pressed for time. She decides to try the One-Minute Preceptor method.[23] It involves five steps or microskills that should be followed in order. The microskills are as follows:

1. *Get a commitment.* As the preceptor, instead of sharing your opinion of the case or where you think the student should look for additional information, ask the student for his thoughts on the clinical situation. What does the student think is going on with this patient? How does he intend to proceed with solving this problem? As the preceptor, do not take over the situation, and do not provide your solution to the problem. Avoid saying, "This is obviously a case of . . ." Asking the student to commit to a position on the case allows you to assess his reasoning skills. Moreover, it places responsibility for the care of the patient in the hands of the student. In this scenario, assume that the student commits to the position that torsemide-induced photosensitivity is the most likely explanation for the patient's drug rash.

2. *Probe for supporting evidence.* After the student has made a commitment, ask probing questions to identify the evidence that supports his position. In this scenario, questions could include the following: What patient-specific findings led to your position that the rash is most likely photosensitivity? What other potential causes for the rash did you consider but found to be irrelevant? Why do you feel it is important to consider torsemide as a potential cause of the rash? The goal here is not to lead the student down your path to your solution but to identify whether the student can substantiate his own claim based on evidence from the case. Was this a lucky guess on the part of the student, or did he truly build

an evidence-based argument? The goal with this step is to help the student perfect his reasoning skills. This is also a good place to identify misconceptions. For example, the student may be committed to the position that only drugs started within the past few weeks should be considered as a cause of the patient's rash. This misconception can be corrected later.

3. *Reinforce what was done well.* For the student to develop sound clinical judgment and reasoning skills, he needs to receive feedback. Start by providing positive feedback specific to the student's actions and behaviors. For example, "Your presentation of the case was well organized and detailed. In particular, you were attentive to the timeline, and this is crucial in the assessment of a drug-induced rash." Avoid general comments such as "good job"; the student will not be sure what was good about it.

4. *Give guidance about errors and omissions.* In short, you need to correct mistakes. Constructive comments should be as specific as possible. An omission in this case may have been the lack of attention to the bluish discoloration of the skin. Offer guidance by directing the student's attention to this finding by asking questions such as, How do you account for the skin discoloration? Is this a consistent finding in drug-induced photosensitivity? In some cases, the student may have committed an error in judgment; or his behavior toward you, the patient, or another healthcare provider may be in need of correction. Keep in mind that unnoted mistakes are apt to be repeated.

5. *Teach a general principle.* Almost every case illustrates a general principle or concept that can be applied or extrapolated to future cases. In this step, ask yourself, What one teaching point do I want the student to get from this case? If the student is confronted with another drug-induced dilemma in the future, what strategic step is he most likely to forget to apply? As an example, in this case the student may not have understood the difference between phototoxicity and photoallergy. He may have been focusing his investigation on drugs that cause skin reactions via an immunologic response (i.e., photoallergy), not drugs that cause chemically mediated direct toxic effects to the skin (i.e., phototoxicity). Take a minute to teach this concept. When the student sees another patient with suspected photosensitivity in the future, he may readily apply this general concept and be able to move on to higher levels of inquiry or problem solving.

When you use the One-Minute Preceptor technique, each encounter needs to be concluded within a reasonable amount of time. Time management is crucial in clinical teaching. To conclude an encounter, offer the student guidance on resolution of the problem. What are your expectations of the student? How much additional time can be expended on this problem? In this case, a sample conclusion offered by the preceptor could be, "I think we need to resolve this problem within the hour. Please make this a priority activity. When you have investigated the issues that we discussed, please get back to me and we will review the data together to devise a course of action."

The One-Minute Preceptor technique has been widely adopted by faculty involved in medical residency and fellowship training. Its utility has been assessed by both faculty members and students.[24–27] In one randomized controlled trial, medical students exposed to this teaching method were found to have increased motivation to do outside reading, and they reported more frequent feedback from teachers and more involvement in clinical decision making as compared to a control group of their peers.[25] This teaching technique offers the opportunity for reflective observation and conceptualization based on a concrete experience. In this regard, it addresses the core components of Kolb's experiential learning model.

What Matters in Assessment?

> ### Reflective Exercise
>
> Fill out column 3 of the mapping exercise in Appendix 9–1. How do you currently assess performance and achievement of the outcomes in your APPE or IPPE? *What* assessment tools are you employing? *When* are assessments performed? *How many* assessments are being performed relative to each outcome measure?

Evaluating performance is a key component of quality experiential education. Assessments should be provided in a thoughtful and purposeful manner. The methods and instruments that you use to assess performance are largely determined by your affiliated school or college of pharmacy or residency program. Before assuming the role of preceptor, these methods should be carefully reviewed with a focus on the following.

Assessment Tools and Instruments

To demonstrate achievement of each experiential outcome, the student will typically perform a number of different activities at different times and at different frequencies throughout the experience. These activities often need to be assessed using different instruments or assessment techniques. As such, the assessment process used in experiential education is triangulated and involves a variety of qualitative and quantitative measures (see Chapter 4 for a discussion of triangulation). For each APPE or IPPE outcome, what types of assessments are being used to measure competence? Are both quantitative and qualitative measures being used? As an example, are both the number and quality of pharmacy interventions being considered in the assessment of clinical problem-solving skills? How many observations are being made to assess acquisition of a skill? For example, is achievement of oral communication skills based on your observation of one oral presentation, two oral presentations, or a variety of activities performed throughout the APPE? Before engaging in assessment, take a global look at the current APPE or IPPE assessment plan. What is being assessed, how is each outcome being assessed, and how often are the assessments being performed?

A variety of assessment methods are used in experiential education, ranging from checklists to portfolios, and the utility of each method needs to be appreciated.[28] A checklist approach can be used to identify whether students can or cannot perform specific tasks. This method offers the evaluator only two scoring choices: can perform (yes) or cannot perform (no).[29] The quality of the performance is not addressed, thus a checklist approach should not be used when the quality of the performance matters. The merits of rubric-based assessments were described in Chapter 4. Rubrics provide detailed descriptions of performance at different levels. These criteria-based assessment tools can be used to assess the acquisition and application of knowledge, skills, and professional behaviors. Rubrics are associated with a high degree of interrater reliability; students can use them to self-assess their level of performance prior to and during the experience, and the use of rubrics minimizes subjectivity in the assessment process.[28,29] Compared to scale-based assessments (i.e., 1 = poor and 5 = excellent), rubrics identify what constitutes a stellar performance in addition to what specific features of a performance need to be improved.

As mentioned in Chapter 4, the reflective portfolio provides a purposeful collection of the student's work that was gathered over time, thereby offering a longitudinal depiction of the student's journey to professional competence. The portfolio should provide evidence of competence relative to specific outcomes (e.g., samples of care plans developed by the student, written pharmacy consults, written drug evaluations or guidelines) and evidence of reflection or introspection performed at various stages of the student's professional development. A review of the student's portfolio prior to and following the IPPE or APPE can offer insight about the student's achievements and areas that need to be developed in addition to his or her current attitudes and healthcare beliefs. Guideline 15.1 of the current ACPE Accreditation Standards is specific to the use of portfolios to document student learning and the attainment of desired competencies.[1] As noted by Plaza and others, the use of a student portfolio as an assessment technique presents a number of challenges to the experiential preceptor.[30] Before engaging in the assessment of portfolios, you will need to identify the purpose of the assessment (formative or summative), whether it will be performed electronically or via a paper process, and whether the assessment will be qualitative or both quantitative and qualitative.

The assessment of portfolios should be standardized and rubric-based to minimize interrater variability in the evaluation.

Reflective writing, whether included in a portfolio or as a journal, is a vital component of experiential learning. Reflections have been shown to give meaning to the clinical experience and to help students develop into mindful practitioners. Reflective writing should not be conducted as a knee-jerk reaction to a clinical encounter. Instead, reflective writing needs to be taught, for it to be thoughtful and purposeful. Wald and colleagues recently described the use of field notes with structured questions or prompts to facilitate reflective writing.[31] Following a clinical encounter, medical students were asked to complete a field note in response to structured questions that focused on specific aspects of the encounter. The use of these prompts or questions was effective in helping the students organize their thoughts and express their ideas. Wald and colleagues also had physicians and psychologists provide one-on-one guided feedback to the students about their reflections.[31] As noted by these investigators, "quality feedback affects willingness and ability to reflect and should promote critical thinking."[31] As such, before employing reflective writing in an IPPE or APPE, attention should be given to the reflective writing process in addition to the type and frequency of feedback to be provided to the student.

Timing of the Assessments

At the very least, assessment of the student's performance in all outcome areas should be performed at the midpoint and upon completion of the experience. A midpoint evaluation is a formative assessment; the intent is to offer feedback on areas of deficiency so that performance can be improved. This assessment should also provide feedback on positive aspects of performance and identify performance areas that have not yet been addressed during the IPPE or APPE. Keep in mind that the intent of a formative assessment is to share observations and information about the student's performance with the goal of "narrowing the gap between actual and desired performance."[19] The summative assessment is performed at the completion of the experience, thereby providing a final evaluation, judgment, or grade of the student's performance. If a comprehensive formative assessment is provided at the midpoint of the experience, and constructive feedback is offered throughout the experience, then there should be no surprises during the summative evaluation.

Self-Assessments

Students should have an opportunity to assess their own performance during the experience. Lifelong learners are reflective practitioners who respond to internal feedback. Opportunities for self-assessment build self-awareness, the foundation for lifelong learning. During formative assessments, students

> Good clinical teaching = asking questions.

> To assess the learner's level of knowledge quickly, the teacher needs only two tools: good questions and the ability to listen and observe.[16]
>
> D.M. Irby,
> L. Wilkerson

should be offered the opportunity to self-assess using the same evaluation instrument(s) that you use to provide external feedback.

Preceptor Evaluations

How will *your* performance be evaluated? Will students have the opportunity to assess your level of professionalism and your ability to serve as an instructor, coach, and facilitator? Prior to the IPPE or APPE, review the preceptor evaluation process provided by your institution's experiential office. Are there additional aspects of your performance that you would like to receive feedback on? How and when will you be able to access the evaluative comments provided by your students? Will they be provided in a timely manner so you can make necessary changes in upcoming IPPEs or APPEs?

Assessment as Quality Improvement

What information can you gain from the final assessment of the students, and how can you use this information in a feedback loop to modify any of the inputs or processes to improve the IPPE or APPE?

What Matters in Providing Feedback?

> *Scenario*: A student has been late for rounds two days in a row. His absences are noticeable to everyone on the team. Do you take the student aside now, during rounds, to discuss his tardiness? Is it best to talk to him after rounds? He is an otherwise stellar student. Do you let this behavior go for now and instead assume it is because of his long commute to the hospital and the early hour?

> Feedback has the purpose of raising the trainee's self-awareness about their performance and leaves them to choose their future actions.[32]
>
> E.A. Hesketh, J.M. Laidlaw

Providing effective feedback is an essential component of the teaching–learning–assessment process. Constructive feedback should be offered to meet three ends: reinforce good practice, correct mistakes, and modify behavior. The problem with feedback is that it is often not provided. Preceptors are known to avoid offering feedback because they are uncomfortable with calling attention to negative behavior. Many also fear that feedback will adversely affect a student's self-esteem or the teacher–student relationship. The truth about feedback is that it is not synonymous with an evaluation. Feedback should offer information based on observation of the student, thereby being formative rather than summative. Feedback should also be conversational and not confrontational. There is no doubt that providing effective feedback is challenging, but it needs to occur. Lack of it may give the student the impression that all is well when, in fact, all is not well. Equally important, positive feedback is needed to reinforce good practice and encourage the student to take additional risks for continued growth. Some general recommendations and two specific approaches to providing effective, constructive feedback are provided in **Table 9–6**. These recommendations should be applied to provide effective, nonjudgmental feedback in the clinical setting.

Table 9–6 Providing Effective Feedback

General Recommendations*†‡

Inform the students at the start of the IPPE or APPE to expect feedback on a routine basis. They should view this as an expected component of their experience.

Chose a relaxed, private atmosphere for your conversation.

Engage in a two-way conversation with the student.

Be descriptive and nonevaluative. What did you observe about the student's performance that requires feedback? (For example, "I noticed that you have been late for rounds for the past two days," not "Your tardiness is unacceptable and will not be tolerated.")

Be behaviorally anchored. Focus on a behavior that can be changed rather than on any personal traits of the individual.

Observe an activity more than once before offering feedback.

Be specific to the behavior that requires a change rather than commenting on general performance. (For example, "The expectation for rounds is that you are on the medical floor at 8:00 a.m.," not "Your lack of professionalism has really become an issue.")

Time your feedback appropriately. Offer feedback soon after an event has taken place or while an observation is being made. In addition, get in the habit of providing feedback at the end of every day or at the end of each week.

Limit the feedback to only one or two items. Avoid pointing out all negative behaviors or all positive behaviors in a single session.

Balance the feedback session by asking the student to offer his or her own perceptions and plans for improved performance.

Approaches to Providing Feedback

Feedback Sandwich*

Offer two reinforcing statements as the bread and one corrective comment as the jelly.

This method is also referred to as the C–R–C approach, where C = commendation and R = recommendation for improvement.

Provide a reinforcing statement to start the conversation, then provide the corrective comment. An example is as follows:

- *Reinforcing statement*: "You are well-prepared for rounds. By prerounding, you are able to contribute to the team-based discussions because you have accurate medication lists and last night's lab results."
- *Corrective comment*: "I've noticed that you've been late for team rounds for the past two days."
- *Reinforcing statement*: "You contribute well to the team by appropriately forecasting what will be discussed and bringing evidence to support your positions on patient care."

Pendleton Four-Step Model‡

Step 1: The learner is asked to state what is good about his or her performance.

Step 2: The teacher states areas of agreement and elaborates on good performance.

Step 3: The learner states what area of performance could be improved.

Step 4: The teacher states what he or she has observed that could be improved.

---

*Source: Adapted from Cantillon P, Sargeant J. Teaching rounds: giving feedback in clinical settings. *BMJ*. 2008;337:1292–1294.

†Source: Adapted from Ende J. Feedback in clinical medical education. *JAMA*. 1983;250(6):777–781.

‡Source: Adapted from Pendleton D, Schofield T, Tate P, Havelock P. *The Consultation: An Approach to Learning and Teaching*. New York, NY: Oxford University Press; 2003.

Summary

Providing quality experiential education is challenging. In this chapter, you had the opportunity to reflect on how you are currently teaching experiential students and assessing their performance. As a final step in your mapping exercise, please refer to the last column of the table in Appendix 9–1. What are your observations, thoughts, or reflections on the IPPE or APPE that you currently offer? What aspects of the experience could be improved? Which aspects of the experience are working well and should be continued? In the last column, outline the steps that you will need to take to ensure that your IPPE or APPE meets the definition of a quality clinical experience.

References

1. Accreditation Council for Pharmacy Education. Accreditation standards and guidelines: professional degree program. http://www.acpe-accredit.org/standards. Adopted January 15, 2006. Accessed June 15, 2009.
2. Flynn AA, MacKinnon GE. Assessing the capacity of hospitals to partner with academic programs for experiential education. *Am J Pharm Educ*. 2008; 72(5):article 116.
3. Reynolds JR, Briceland LL, Carter JT et al. Experiential education delivery—ensuring success through support and development of the faculty and administrative team: report of the 2004–2005 Professional Affairs Committee. *AJPE*. 2005;69(5):article S9.
4. Parsell G, Bligh J. Recent perspectives on clinical teaching. *Med Educ*. 2001; 35:409–414.
5. Neill J. What is experiential learning? http://wilderdom.com/experiential/ExperientialLearningWhatIs.html. Accessed November 13, 2008.
6. American College of Clinical Pharmacy. Quality experiential education. *Pharmacotherapy*. 2008;28(10):219e–227e.
7. Borzak L, ed. *Field Study. A Sourcebook for Experiential Learning*. Beverly Hills, CA: Sage Publications; 1981.
8. Pickles T. Experiential learning . . . on the Web. http://reviewing.co.uk/research/experiential.learning.htm. Accessed June 9, 2009.
9. Neill J. John Dewey: philosophy of education. http://www.wilderdom.com/experiential/Summary/JohnDeweyExperienceEducation.html. Accessed June 9, 2009.
10. Dewey J. *Experience and Education*. New York, NY: Kappa Delta Pi; 1938.
11. Neill J. John Dewey: philosophy of education. http://wilderdom.com/experiential/JohnDeweyPhilosophyEducation.html. Accessed November 13, 2008.
12. Kolb DA. *Experiential Learning: Experience as the Source of Learning and Development*. Englewood Cliffs, NJ: Prentice Hall Inc; 1984.
13. Nimmo CM, Holland RW. Transitions in pharmacy practice, part 2: who does what and why. *Am J Health Syst Pharm*. 1999;56:1981–1987.
14. Hepler CD, Strand LM. Opportunities and responsibilities in pharmaceutical care. *Am J Hosp Pharm*. 1990;47:533–543.
15. Steinert Y. Teaching rounds: the problem "junior": whose problem is it? *BMJ*. 2008;336:150–153.

16. Irby DM, Wilkerson L. Teaching rounds: teaching when time is limited. *BMJ.* 2008;336:384–387.

17. Cruess SR, Cruess RL, Steinert Y. Teaching rounds: role modeling—making the most of a powerful teaching strategy. *BMJ.* 2008;336:718–721.

18. Driessen E, van Tartwijk J, Dornan T. Teaching rounds: the self-critical doctor: helping students become more reflective. *BMJ.* 2008;336:827–830.

19. Cantillon P, Sargeant J. Teaching rounds: giving feedback in clinical settings. *BMJ.* 2008;337:1292–1294.

20. Ker J, Cantillon P, Ambrose L. Teaching rounds: teaching on a ward round. *BMJ.* 2009;338:770–772.

21. Bloom BS. *Taxonomy of Educational Objectives, Handbook I: The Cognitive Domain.* New York, NY: David McKay Co Inc; 1956.

22. Stritter FT, Baker RM, Shahady EJ. Clinical instruction. In: McGaghie CD, Frey JJ, eds. *Handbook for the Academic Physician.* New York, NY: Springer-Verlag; 1988.

23. Neher JO, Gordon KC, Myer B, Stevens N. A five-step microskills model of clinical teaching. *J Am Board Fam Pract.* 1992;5:419–424.

24. Aagaard E, Teherani A, Irby D. Effectiveness of the one-minute preceptor model for diagnosing the patient and the learner: proof of a concept. *Acad Med.* 2004;79:42–49.

25. Furney SL, Orsini AN, Orsetti KE, Stern DT, Gruppen JD, Irby DM. Teaching the one-minute preceptor: a randomized controlled trial. *J Gen Intern Med.* 2001;16:620–624.

26. Irby DM, Aagard E, Teherani A. Teaching points identified by preceptors observing one-minute preceptor and traditional preceptor encounters. *Acad Med.* 2004;7:50–55.

27. Teherani A, O'Sullivan P, Aagaard E, Morrison E, Irby D. Student perceptions of the one-minute preceptor and traditional preceptor models. *Med Educ.* 2007;29:323–327.

28. Boyce EG. Finding and using readily available sources of assessment data. *Am J Pharm Educ.* 2008;72(5):article 102.

29. Medina MS. Assessing student performance during experiential rotations. *Am J Health Syst Pharm.* 2008;65:1502,1504–1506.

30. Plaza CM, Draugalis JR, Slack MK, Skrepnek GH, Sauer KA. Use of reflective portfolios in health sciences education. *Am J Pharm Educ.* 2007;71(2):article 34.

31. Wald HS, Davis SW, Reis SP et al. Reflecting on reflections: enhancement of medical education curriculum with structured field notes and guided feedback. *Acad Med.* 2009;84:830–837.

32. Hesketh EA, Laidlaw JM. Developing the teaching instinct: 1: feedback. *Med Teach.* 2002;24:245–248.

Appendix 9–1
Mapping Exercise

Desired Outcomes	Teaching and Learning Activities	Assessments (Type, Frequency, Timing)	Reflection

What Matters in Dealing with Students?

CHAPTER 10

What Matters in Developing Professionals and Professionalism?

Dana P. Hammer, RPh, MS, PhD

Introduction

A number of years ago, it may have seemed odd to see a chapter about professionalism in a pharmacy education text. After all, pharmacy is a profession, right? And those who are members of this profession have already passed a number of tests of professional competence, such as admittance to and successful completion of pharmacy school, as well as a national licensing examination. Thus, professionalism is assumed to be a part of who we are and what we do in education and practice, and we should not have to worry about it—it takes care of itself. So why has so much attention been devoted to this topic in pharmacy and other health-care profession education in the last few years?

There are three primary reasons that the topic is important to discuss and pay attention to—one is the importance of professionalism in providing patient care; the second is that pharmacy continues to struggle with its professional status; the third is that professionalism of our members and would-be members is perceived to be in need of improvement. This chapter addresses each of these areas, with a focus on the latter and how we can help to develop students' professionalism in pharmacy education. In this chapter, an attempt will be made to answer the following questions:

- Why does professionalism matter?
- How is professionalism defined?

- What strategies have been shown to be effective in promoting student (and faculty!) professionalism throughout the PharmD degree program and beyond?
- What works with regard to assessing the professionalism of students?

Why Professionalism Matters

The cornerstone of any profession is providing ethical, individual, unselfish service to those in need of our knowledge and skills. To provide the best care we can to those whom we serve, it is important for us to embody a character of service, willingness, cooperation, and excellence. We must have a sense of caring for others as our primary responsibility. It is likely that the more we are willing to use our knowledge and skills in providing patient care, the better the care will be. Improving how well we provide care to patients should also help us be better perceived by our health professions' colleagues. We would like for them to see us as partners and team members in the patient care process. It is also important to establish our professionalism with decision makers and society as a whole so that others recognize our value and help us to ensure a future for our profession.

Related to these ideas is pharmacy's status as a profession. Numerous authors enumerate the characteristics of professions[1-3]; those most pertinent to this conversation are autonomy, altruism, and a covenantal relationship with clients. Pharmacy has been considered a quasi-profession among some because we do not shoulder the ultimate responsibility for patient care[3-6]; most of us take orders from prescribers, who do have the ultimate responsibility for a patient's care. And although it would not be appropriate to advocate that we should take full responsibility for patient care, we certainly should heed the arguments for greater and shared responsibilities through the provision of pharmaceutical care and medication therapy management.

Pharmacy has also struggled with its business orientation—pharmacy is the only healthcare profession where, for the most part, members of the profession are not paid for their cognitive services. Free and easy access to pharmacists and their information is an important cornerstone in our profession, but it has also been a burden to professional recognition in that the primary method by which we are reimbursed for our service is through the provision of products. This orientation can be somewhat stifling to a sense of altruism and serving the greater good through our knowledge and skills. This orientation makes it difficult for us to establish relationships with patients even though we know enough about them and their history to really make a difference in their care. The foundation of any profession is a trusted, ethical, confidential relationship with each individual whom we serve. These relationships allow the professional to use his or her knowledge and skills to help these individuals to the best of our abilities. It is difficult to establish and maintain such relationships if we merely provide products to people and nothing else.

The last reason that professionalism is important to discuss (and most pertinent to this text) is a perceived need of improvement of individuals' professionalism. Almost everyday in our current culture, a public role model, celebrity, or professional is chastised for poor behavior. The pharmacy profession is not immune to this scrutiny—a number of publicized events in the past speak to unethical behaviors of some of our members.[7–10] And it certainly does not help increase the public's perception of our professionalism when the vast majority of us do not have individual relationships with our patients—they do not know us, and we do not know them. These phenomena have trickled down to the school level, where many faculty complain that students are less professional these days—more cheating, disruptive behaviors in class, less willingness to accept responsibility, a sense of entitlement, etc. Our class sizes are large, which makes it difficult for us to get to know our students as individuals and help them be positively socialized into our profession.

Reflective Exercise

How do you define professionalism? What examples of student and faculty professionalism, or lack thereof, have you observed in students or instructors?

_____

_____

_____

_____

What Is Professionalism?

Ask 100 people for their definition of professionalism and you are likely to get 100 different answers. Professionalism is a broad concept that means many things. Although professionalism was first discussed by sociologists who were exploring differences between professions and occupations,[11–13] more recent literature describes the foundation of professionalism as putting others' needs above your own.[14,15] It is "demonstrated through a foundation of clinical competence, communication skills, and ethical and legal understanding, upon which is built the aspiration to and wise application of the principles of professionalism: excellence, humanism, accountability, and altruism."[16] The American Board of Internal Medicine (ABIM) describe it as "the basis of medicine's contract with society. It demands placing the interests of patients above those of the physician, setting and maintaining standards of competence and integrity, and providing expert advice to society on matters of health."[17]

> Attributes of professionalism can be considered in several categories—structural, attitudinal, behavioral, and value-based.

The American College of Clinical Pharmacy (ACCP) emphasizes the covenantal or "fiducial" relationship between the patient and the pharmacist as the essence of professionalism—a relationship between the patient and the pharmacist built on trust.[18] The Oath of a Pharmacist and the Code of Ethics for Pharmacists describe professional values such as "considering the welfare of humanity and relief of suffering my primary concerns" and "promoting the good of every patient in a caring, compassionate, and confidential manner."[19,20] Chalmers described professionalism as

> displayed in the way pharmacists conduct themselves in professional situations. This definition implies a demeanor that is created through a combination of behaviors, including courtesy and politeness when dealing with patients, peers, and other health care professionals. Pharmacists should consistently display respect for others and maintain appropriate boundaries of privacy and discretion. Whether dealing with patients or interacting with others on a health care team, it is important to possess—and display—an empathetic manner.[21]

Attributes of professionalism can be considered in several categories: structural, attitudinal, behavioral, and value-based. Structural attributes of professionalism distinguish professions from occupations, as seen in the sociological definitions. Professions are characterized by structural attributes such as the following:

- Specialized knowledge and skills
- Self-imposed and enforced values, behaviors, and codes of ethics
- Professional associations and identity
- Prestige
- Socially vital function
- Specialized client relationship
- Recognition through licensure

Sociologist Richard Hall studied the extent to which members of occupations and professions held certain attitudes to determine how professional they were. He defined professional attitudes as the following:

- The use of the professional organization as a major reference
- A belief in public service
- A belief in self-regulation
- A sense of calling to the field
- Autonomy[22]

The concept of behavioral professionalism was developed to establish the relationship between professional behaviors and the structural and attitudinal attributes of professionalism. It is defined as "behaving in a manner to potentially achieve optimal outcomes in professional tasks and interactions" and includes attributes such as reliability and dependability, confidence, active learning, communicating respectfully and articulately, accepting and applying constructive criticism, behaving ethically, demonstrating a desire to exceed expectations, and putting others' needs above one's own.[23] Value-based attributes are often found in codes of ethics, the oaths of healthcare professions, and other similar documents. Academic medicine most often describes professionalism as a set of values that are demonstrated, which is seen in the aforementioned definitions by Stern[16] and the ABIM.[17] Thus, upon review of the literature, we can determine that professionalism is a complex composite of structural, attitudinal, behavioral, and value-based attributes. No wonder the concept is so broadly used and widely interpreted by professionals, members of occupations, and consumers in any given society. The core of professionalism, however, emphasizes service, altruism, and putting others' needs above your own.

Professionalism Versus Civility

Professionalism can be thought of as the highest form of civility—civility must be present to develop professionalism. Civility could be considered a basic set of accepted behaviors for a society or culture upon which professional behaviors are rooted, such as the demonstration of respect toward one another. We would expect most members of a given culture or society to exhibit at least civil behaviors, but more professional members of that society or culture would be expected to consistently exhibit civil behaviors as well as professional behaviors. For example, communicating articulately, relating empathetically, practicing ethically, exceeding expectations, and putting others' needs above one's own might be considered professional behaviors; they go beyond what we might consider civil behaviors or basic expectations for people in a given society. Many faculty talk about a lack of student professionalism when they are really describing a lack of civil behavior, such as disrespect in the classroom.

> What is the difference between professionalism and civility?

How Does Professionalism Relate to Teaching, Learning, and Assessment?

Some scholars think that the development of student professionalism should be the primary goal of a PharmD degree:

> Schools of pharmacy exist to develop professionally mature pharmacy practitioners who can render pharmaceutical care. As such, our schools' primary reason for being is to develop students into practitioners who can serve patients and their drug therapy needs . . . to do as much as possible to ensure that patients' drug therapy is necessary and appropriate for them and their conditions, and does no unnecessary harm. That is our first obligation. Preparation to accomplish this requires *both* the acquisition of a great deal of knowledge by our students and the development of the

necessary professional attitudes and behaviors. Do schools of pharmacy foster those attitudes and behaviors that protect patients and promote patient care? Have we made technical competence our mission? . . . If all we are interested in is technical competence, then we have become a trade school.[15]

In seven different accreditation standards, the Accreditation Council for Pharmacy Education notes that professionalism is an important component for students, faculty, staff, preceptors, and others who are affiliated with PharmD students.[24] At a minimum, therefore, it is required for schools of pharmacy to address this area. Our responsibility as educators who play a significant role in professionally socializing students is to do so purposefully. Zlatic talks about a fiduciary responsibility that pharmacists have to patients. He describes the same responsibility of faculty to students—teaching is a profession.[25]

Can Professionalism Be Taught?

Some question whether professionalism can be taught. Certainly we can teach students about the concept of professionalism—its various definitions and meanings—similar to what has already been described. But to *develop* professionalism is quite a different matter. Some scholars describe a psychological, developmental, and maturation approach to professionalism. Hilton and Slotnick purport that the essence of professionalism is practical wisdom, which is "acquired only after a prolonged period of experience (and reflection on experience) occurring in concert with the professional's evolving knowledge and skills base."[26] Similarly, Duncan-Hewitt purports that a student's level of cognitive and moral development helps to determine that student's capacity to engage in truly professional behaviors.[27] She also describes the development of student behaviors as a function of mentoring, and there is literature to suggest that some faculty mentors are not functioning at a professional level of cognitive and moral development themselves. Nimmo and Holland apply Krathwohl's Taxonomy of the Affective Domain to the process of changing pharmacists' attitudes and values to practice pharmaceutical care.[28] Krathwohl proposed five stages that are "ordered according to the principle of internalization. Internalization refers to the process whereby a person's affect toward an object passes from a general awareness level to a point where the affect is 'internalized' and consistently guides or controls the person's behavior."[29] Brown and Ferrill describe a similar approach to developing patient advocacy and professionalism in pharmacy students via movement through Bloom's Taxonomy.[30]

Sociological studies note that the most influential factors on the professional socialization process are role models (consider preceptors, faculty, and upperclassmen), the environments in which students are learning (e.g., is the practice site chaotic and disorganized or orderly and calm, and does the school culture promote excellence and service?), and the intrinsic values that students already possess (i.e., what is the character of those we let into our programs?).[31–33] To promote a culture of professionalism within the learning environment, we need to examine what we teach and how we teach it, how students learn (or do not learn) what we are trying to teach, how these efforts relate to students' natural development and maturation, and how our efforts are assessed, if at all.

Reflective Exercise

When you were a student, resident or instructor, did you receive explicit training on professionalism? If you did, what was the nature of this training? If not, how were you professionally socialized?

_____

_____

_____

_____

What Works with Regard to Developing Professionalism in Students?

As one might imagine, there is a paucity of evidence that suggests proven methods to develop student professionalism. The construct itself is so complex, and the development and maturation process are impacted by so many factors, that the development of professionalism is nearly impossible to measure comprehensively in a robust manner such as with a randomized, double-blind, placebo-controlled trial. What we do know, as described in the introductory section, is that some factors seem to have prominent influence on one's professional development. We also know of strategies that seem to enhance certain aspects of professionalism, such as reflection on one's professional behaviors during a medical school clerkship.[34] This section will provide examples of strategies that have been suggested to help develop student (and faculty role model) professionalism across the pharmacy education continuum. Four comprehensive references provide useful strategies and examples that can be used to develop professionalism programs:

- American Pharmacists Association, Academy of Student Pharmacists; Pharmacy Professionalism Toolkit for Students and Faculty, provided by the APhA-ASP/AACP Committee on Student Professionalism[35]

- American Association of Colleges of Pharmacy; 2004 annual meeting school poster abstracts in which schools showcased their efforts toward developing professionalism[36]
- "Student Professionalism," a comprehensive article with many ideas and an extensive bibliography[37]
- *Promoting Civility in Pharmacy Education*, a collection of articles describing how to promote civility in various aspects of pharmacy education, such as large versus small classrooms, experiential education, graduate education, and other topics[38]

School Missions and Program Outcomes

It is paramount, first and foremost, that schools and colleges of pharmacy publicly demonstrate their commitment to the development of professionalism. This may denote a shift in the culture of the school. One school described a school-wide culture change, involving students and faculty, in both curricular and extracurricular programs and activities and how those changes impacted the development of professional socialization and professionalism.[39]

The leadership of schools and colleges of pharmacy must be committed to the development of professionalism. There should be language in schools' mission and vision statements, as well as programmatic and graduation outcomes, related to the development of student professionalism. If professionalism is an outcome that all students must demonstrate to a certain extent prior to graduation, then this requirement should promote professional development and measurement throughout the curriculum. For professionalism to be developed throughout a curriculum, a faculty must first define for itself what professionalism means, as well as articulate its various attributes. When this is done, strategies to develop and measure certain behaviors can be implemented. A white coat ceremony, for example, can help to build pride in and respect for the profession of pharmacy—at least momentarily.[40] Incorporating service learning and volunteer opportunities should help to develop altruism and a service ethic, for example.[41] Extracurricular involvement in professional pharmacy organizations can help to develop leadership and advocacy. Schools also need to hold their faculty and preceptors accountable for demonstrating professionalism and serving as role models for students. At least one school has published its process for threading professionalism throughout its program.[42]

Recruitment

How is pharmacy portrayed in your college's recruitment materials and tools?

Who are the students who are applying to schools of pharmacy? What are their values related to the profession and what the profession aspires to be? What images of pharmacy and pharmacists are portrayed in schools' recruiting tools? What impact do prepharmacy organizations have on the recruitment of students into pharmacy school and these students' professional socialization? Schools and colleges of pharmacy should implement recruitment strategies that attract students who already demonstrate professionalism in their daily lives (e.g., service, compassion, accountability, and commitment). Conversations with counselors from feeder programs should emphasize this orientation, as should all promotional materials and activities. Consider advertisements used by the military to attract new recruits—images of strong, committed, determined, courageous people are shown as members. What can pharmacy school recruiters learn from this? It stands to reason that the more professional someone is upon entry to a pharmacy program, the more professional he or she will be upon graduation, as long as the curricular process does not negatively socialize the person! Recall from the sociological studies that the values and character of a person entering a program strongly predict that person's practice behaviors as professionals.

Admissions Processes

Do schools' admissions processes actively select students with professional traits, or is the greatest concern the candidate's grade point average in prerequisite classes and his or her Pharmacy College Admission Test (PCAT) scores? An interview process seems to be a strategy whereby faculty and other interviewers can get to know a candidate beyond what paper or online applications can provide. Numerous studies have been done to demonstrate the value of interviews in admissions processes and student success.[43-47]

> Reflect on the admission process at your college or school of pharmacy. Is an attempt made to assess the candidate's willingness and readiness for professional socialization?

Other admissions processes used to assess applicant behavior include group interactions and written, impromptu essays. Some investigators have experimented with OSCE-type admissions interviews. Objective structured clinical examinations (OSCEs) are often used in medical education as a means to assess medical students' ability to exhibit certain behaviors and perform skills using standardized patients. This methodology has been adapted for use in the interview process. Interviewees progressed through several "stations, in which they were presented with scenarios that required them to discuss a health-related issue (e.g., the use of placebos) with an interviewer, interact with a standardized confederate while an examiner observed the interpersonal skills displayed, or answer traditional interview questions."[48] This process has been shown to predict medical students' clerkship and licensing exam scores.[49] One also has to consider how much each component of the admissions process weighs in the final decision making. If there is a desire to emphasize professional traits beyond traditional academic performance measures, then measures of those traits should be given significant weight in the selection process.

Didactic Course Work

Helping students develop professionalism can happen throughout the entire continuum of didactic education, usually during the first three years of a traditional four-year PharmD program. Activities and conversations

> A course on professionalism will likely not have much impact. We have already established that development of professionalism occurs through the professional socialization *process*, not just learning about content.

can begin during incoming students' orientation programs—consider professionalism pledge writing; interactions with model practitioners, faculty, local pharmacists, and student pharmacist leaders; exposure to professional organizations; and white coat ceremonies. In the regular curriculum, care should be taken to thread the development and assessment of professionalism throughout various courses and across the academic years, similar to other outcome abilities that the school is trying to develop, such as communication and problem-solving skills. It should be noted that a course on professionalism will likely not have much impact. We have already established that development of professionalism occurs through the professional socialization *process*, not just learning about content.

One must also consider the hidden curriculum, which can be different from the explicit curriculum. Hidden curricula are the underlying messages, attitudes, and values demonstrated by faculty and preceptors. They are often just as powerful, if not more, in shaping student learning. Examples might be faculty who do not enforce or abide by school policy and preceptors who may tell students that what they learn in the real world is the only thing that counts. There could also be examples of inconsistent socialization, that is, what students learn in the classroom is very different from what they experience in pharmacy practice environments.[50] Additionally, some schools have established committees of faculty, administrators, students, or practitioners to help devise strategies for the development of professionalism throughout an entire program. One outcome of such an endeavor might be the development of common classroom expectations that are consistent in all syllabi across the curriculum, thereby sending a consistent message of behavioral expectations for students.

Large Classes

> Where are my shushers?

One challenge that seems to plague faculty is how to improve student behavior in large lecture courses. It seems that the larger the class, the more disruptive or nonengaged students can be. It is easy for them to hide and be anonymous, not to mention that a mob mentality kicks in, where people are more likely to behave disrespectfully in groups than one on one. However, there is literature to support that faculty behavior can also be to blame for poor student behavior; if faculty seem unprepared, aloof, disrespectful toward students, do not start and end class on time, etc., they are more likely to encounter incivilities from students.[51] The good news is that there are successful strategies for reducing these classroom incivilities, such as providing clear behavioral expectations up front, engaging students in active learning, treating students with respect and as individuals, getting to know them beyond being seat warmers (like learning their names), and periodically asking for their feedback about how class is going.[38]

Some faculty have engaged students in the classroom to help minimize disruptions. For example, one faculty member asks for volunteer shushers during each lecture. It is the responsibility of the shushers to shush the rest of the class if ambient conversation becomes too distracting. Sometimes the faculty member will humorously prompt the shushers if the need arises: "Where are my shushers?" (K. DeLoatch, e-mail communication, April 2010).

Newer faculty members seem to have more difficulty with classroom management than more experienced faculty because often new faculty are close in age to the students they are teaching. This proximity in age and experience can create a conflict in itself. Newer faculty often want to befriend students, they may not be as confident in their teaching skills and content expertise, and they want students to think positively of them so they can be more flexible with regard to making exceptions. All of these qualities can lead to greater incivility and a lack of respect by the students toward the faculty member.[38]

It is important to work on demonstrating confidence and control, even if you do not feel you are confident or in control. Some faculty may go overboard on this, however. To cover up insecurities about teaching, the faculty member may come across as overconfident, as if he or she is trying to overtly establish who is in control here and who is the expert. This sort of behavior can also lead to student frustration and incivility. To overcome some of the mistakes new faculty make in the classroom, engage a mentor—likely a senior faculty member—who is willing to observe your teaching and offer constructive feedback on how to improve. He or she might observe subtle behaviors that you may not be aware of, such as confidence level, tone of voice, and others. **Table 10–1** offers additional strategies for the promotion of civility in a large classroom environment.

Keep in mind that classroom behavior is just one subset of the larger domain of professionalism attributes. Enhancing civility in the classroom, although important, is not the only strategy that should be used to develop student professionalism. Depending on the nature of the course, students could also be assigned certain activities to help develop other attributes, such as empathy. The author has assigned students to attend a support group meeting as part of a social–behavioral pharmacy course and then write a reflective paper about the experience.[52] Also, as part of a general pharmacy practice course in the first professional year, students interviewed a person with diabetes and wrote a summary on the experience.

Small-Group Classes

There are more opportunities to enhance student professionalism in small classes because it is easier to get to know students and have individual contact. It is easier to monitor student behavior and provide feedback. It is also easier to engage students in peer and self-assessment of expected classroom behaviors, as well as hold them accountable (such as making their performance of professional behaviors part of their grade). Classrooms where active learning is the norm, such as skills laboratories, are

> It is easier to monitor student behavior and provide feedback in small-group classes.

Table 10–1 Select Strategies to Promote Civility in the Classroom

Syllabus	Clearly explain your behavioral expectations (no cell phones, laptop use for class only, come to class prepared and ready to learn and engage, etc.). Be sure to explain your expectations in terms of minimizing distractions and maximizing student learning. Consider incorporating language from the school's student handbook, making policy consistent among all faculty, and including students' suggestions about what the expectations should be (such as with an online survey prior to the beginning of the class). Students can also share their opinions about their expectations of instructors, which could be included in the syllabus.
Statement of understanding	Have students sign a sheet that demonstrates they will abide by the expectations set forth in the class. This can be done after a discussion of the expectations with the students.
Grade	Incorporate meeting, exceeding, and not meeting these expectations as part of the course grade. This implies that the instructor has some sort of system by which he or she can validly measure these behaviors.
Active learning strategies	Have students watch a podcast of the lecture prior to class, then use the lecture time to answer questions, go over cases, etc.
	Use enhanced lectures—lecture for 10–15 minutes, then have students work on a case for 5 minutes, then discuss it for 5 minutes, then lecture for another 10 minutes, etc.
	Use audience response systems for questions and answers about the lecture material.
	For additional strategies, see the following resources:
	• Angelo TA, Cross KP. *Classroom Assessment Techniques*. San Francisco, CA: Jossey-Bass; 1993.
	• Bonwell CC, Eison JA. *Active Learning: Creating Excitement in the Classroom*. Washington, DC: The George Washington University, School of Education and Human Development; 1991. ASHE-ERIC Higher Education Report No. 1.
Get to know students' names	Have the students say their names when they ask questions in class, study class composites, hold office hours, arrive a little before class and stay after class for a few minutes to mingle and answer questions, and call on students by name.
Act like you care about the students and their learning	Start class with some small talk, such as asking when the next big exam is in another course, etc. You can also ask what questions remain from the last lecture, the homework assignment, etc.
Collect midterm feedback	Convene a representative focus group, conduct a minisurvey, bring in a member of the university's teaching–learning center, or devise other ways to ask students the following questions:
	• What about the course helped you to meet the learning objectives?
	• What could be changed to better help you meet the learning objectives?

ideal settings for the development of certain professionalism attributes. An example of a professionalism emphasis in a skills-based course series has been described elsewhere.[53] Similar to the discussion about large classrooms, professionalism-related assignments could also be part of a smaller course.

Extracurricular Activities

Technically speaking, extracurricular activities (ECAs) are any experiences that occur outside of the formal curriculum of classes and experiential education.

Most commonly, however, ECAs refer to student involvement in professional student pharmacist organizations. Most, if not all, national pharmacy associations have student chapters. There are also pharmacy-based fraternal organizations and honoraries. These organizations provide invaluable opportunities for students' professional development through a variety of activities, such as leadership, responsibility, participation in health fairs, and the political process. These organizations are often advised by faculty members or practitioners who serve as role models for the student members. One school described how it revamped its ECAs to engage more students in more meaningful ways.[54] Another described strategies to involve students on a satellite campus.[55] Some schools have student professionalism committees[56]—the one at the University of Washington School of Pharmacy offers an annual peer- and faculty-nominated student award. Although it seems that the majority of activities promoted by student pharmacist organizations are professional and service-oriented in nature, attention should also be paid to the organizations' social activities so they do not erode the professionalism being developed among the student members.

Experiential Programs

Experiential training is ideal for the development of student professionalism. It is in these environments where students observe role models in action as well as cut their teeth with regard to practice skills, attitudes, and behaviors. They are no longer warming a seat in a large lecture hall; they are responsible for certain activities meant to develop proficiency in patient care and other professional activities. Several strategies have been proposed to enhance professionalism in these environments. Different strategies address different aspects of professionalism. For example, similar to the discussion of classroom strategies, certain practices are meant to improve student behavior during experiential learning[57]:

> Service learning opportunities also provide environments for students to explore their altruism and compassion, which are the core of professionalism.

- State explicit expectations up front (they should be aligned with the school's expectations and incorporate student suggestions).
- Set high, yet achievable standards.
- Hold students accountable for meeting expectations (i.e., assess their professional behavior!).
- Treat students respectfully and as future colleagues.
- Provide specific, timely feedback early and often, and provide it in a constructive manner.
- Seek student feedback on your performance as a preceptor.
- Be the best role model you can be.

Table 10–2 provides specific examples of activities that can help engage students in experiential learning, which should help improve their practice of professionalism.

Table 10–2 Experiential Learning Activities to Help Improve Student Clinical Skills and Professionalism

Dispensing:

- Talk to students as you carry out this activity. Discuss medications and disease states.
- Have students tell you what they know.
- Discuss other treatment options.
- Have students look for medication changes to recommend to physicians.
- Ask students to discuss their rationale or evidence for any changes.
- Have students calculate pediatric doses.
- Have students do antibiotic callback programs.
- Have students master two key OTC drugs per week.
- Have students talk to patients about OTC drugs.

Adverse drug reporting:

- Stress the importance of preventing errors and learning from errors.
- Have students practice completing a form such as MedWatch.

Patient discussions:

- Give students typical, yet complex, patients to research (two per week).
- Have students assess the patients, determine the patients' needs, develop care plans, and implement the plans.
- Have students follow-up with the patients as needed.

Patient counseling:

- Set aside time for students to counsel patients.
- Choose patients with a range of needs (who are likely to appreciate the interaction).

Community education seminars and talks:

- Students benefit from public speaking.
- Look for opportunities to use students to educate your constituents (community service groups, schools, church groups, nursing homes and assisted living complexes, etc.).

Pharmacy management:

- Talk regularly with students about management tasks and issues, such as sales and profit, staff management, scheduling, pricing of clinical services, laws and regulations, etc.

Toxicology sleuthing:

- Identify a mystery that involves drug product interactions for the student to solve and report on.
- Example: S Milosovich died from a heart attack. Milosovich was being treated for heart disease; however, it appears that he or she was taking another stealth medication.
- Put students on the case of a drug–drug interaction that is possible in patients who take many agents.
- Have students provide a detailed explanation of what is going on.
- Work with the students to see how common these interactions are.

Compounding:

- Talk to students about the process and how compounded products differ from commercial products.
- Involve students by having them perform calculations and compounding at your side.

OTC formulary:

- Have students build and maintain a reference tool to assist in making appropriate OTC medication.
- Add one product per week.
- Require students to present that product to the staff.

Patient counseling:

- Ensure balance in counseling patients about prescription and OTC products.
- New mothers are often an appreciative audience.

Empathy assignment:

- Have students live as a patient with a chronic condition (follow the medication and lifestyle routine for several days).
- Have students use common durable medical equipment (oxygen tank, wheelchair or scooter chair, crutches).

Journal club:

- Help students see the literature as valuable.
- Have students lead a review and analysis of a relevant article (every other week).
- Push articles at students continuously.

Source: Adapted from Thomas RA. Preceptor development: integrating students into your pharmacy practice. Presented at: 2006 Iowa Pharmacist Expo; January 28, 2006; Des Moines, IA.

Source: Adapted from Hobson E, Roth M, Harris I. Active learning to achieve abilities. Presented at: The American College of Clinical Pharmacy Annual Meeting; October 22, 2005; San Francisco, CA.

Other aspects of professionalism can be developed during experiential education. Some schools have employed a patient-centered approach to their programs. As part of introductory practice experiences, one school assigned teams of pharmacy students to patients in the community. Teams consisted of a student from each of the P1, P2, and P3 years; teams were facilitated by two faculty members. Each team of students followed a patient throughout the students' didactic career, meeting weekly to discuss all kinds of issues related to the care of this patient.[39] Other helpful examples are described in the AACP's Professional Experience Program (PEP) library, which can be searched with keywords like professionalism.[58] Service learning opportunities also provide environments for students to explore their altruism and compassion, which are at the core of professionalism. An entire issue of the *American Journal of Pharmaceutical Education* was devoted to this topic and describes multiple strategies.[59]

Role of Staff, Faculty, and Preceptors

The importance of role modeling and mentoring for faculty and preceptors has been mentioned thus far. Schools should also consider the role of staff and other personnel (e.g., graduate students, residents) in their interactions with PharmD students. Ideally, all of these individuals demonstrate high levels of professionalism in everything they do; this, however, is unrealistic. Schools should employ strategies to motivate their employees and others with whom the PharmD students interact to demonstrate positive behaviors, and hold them accountable when they do not. Schools might also consider professionalism-development programs for its employees that are consistent with the strategies for student development. This could be part of a faculty–staff development program. Two pages of the "Student Professionalism" article[37(pp22–23)] are devoted to strategies to develop role models and mentors for students. The bottom line is that faculty, preceptors, and staff should demonstrate professionalism at all times—they should also share their wisdom and passion for the profession of pharmacy in ways that mentor and positively socialize student pharmacists.

Role of Technology

There is an emerging literature of e-professionalism issues. Students in the Millennial generation and beyond communicate primarily through the use of technology. (For more information about generation-related issues in teaching and learning, see Chapter 2.) Many of our schools are high-tech and require individual laptop use in most, if not all, courses. Some campuses deliver the vast majority of their PharmD program via distance learning. Each of these issues can be discussed in the context of professionalism. Chretien and colleagues reported that 60 percent of responding medical schools identified online postings of unprofessional conduct by their students.

Responding schools who did not have a policy in place regarding these behaviors were actively developing a policy.[60] Another commentary discusses ethical concerns with clinicians' social networking and provides guidelines to negotiate these forums responsibly and professionally.[61] Cain and colleagues have explored e-professionalism with pharmacy students.[62–64] One of their strategies to help prevent unprofessional behavior in cyberspace is conducting workshops to help students consider the image they project of themselves as a person and a professional in their online social networks, as well as the potential ramifications of that behavior.[62]

Faculty who teach in classrooms where student use of technology is the norm often describe students using their laptops for purposes other than focusing on class material. Other students choose to use their cell phones frequently in class either for verbal or text-message conversations. All of these behaviors can be distracting to other students and to the faculty member in charge. These behaviors can be prevented by providing clear expectations up front about the acceptable use of technology in the classroom. It is also helpful to reward those who meet or exceed expectations, as well as penalize those who do not. Use of technology in the classroom by the responsible faculty member can help to reduce unprofessional behavior when the technology is being used to engage students in their learning; consider the use of audience response systems, for example, in posing and discussing questions about your lecture material.

There is concern about the potential lack of professional socialization with those degree programs that rely heavily on distance learning and the Internet, without regular face-to-face interaction with faculty, preceptors, other students, and professional organizations. More research in this area is needed to determine if a positive professional socialization process is lacking in these environments.

What Works with Regard to Assessing Professionalism?

Reflective Exercise

In your experience as a student, resident, employee, or instructor, how has your professionalism been assessed (e.g., performance appraisal, clerkship or residency evaluations, etc.)? Was it helpful in improving your professionalism? Why or why not?

_____

_____

_____

_____

Although it is extremely important to implement strategies to develop student professionalism, how will we know if those efforts are working? How will students track their progress as developing professionals? The difficulty of gathering robust evidence for proven strategies to develop professionalism has already been discussed. This does not mean, however, that professional behavior cannot be measured—we just may not be able to exactly pinpoint why certain behaviors do or do not occur. *Measuring Medical Professionalism* is a textbook devoted to doing just that.[16] Attitudes toward professionalism can certainly be measured, and numerous tools exist for that purpose.[65–68] Another self-report instrument helps to identify ethical judgment.[69] There are also a few tools that can be used to document the absence or presence of certain professional behaviors or to evaluate their quality.[23,70–72] This section describes general and specific strategies for the assessment of professionalism and its various attributes.

General Strategies

If student professionalism is listed as an outcome of a PharmD program, then it is incumbent on that program to develop, assess, and provide feedback to individual students about their development of this ability, similar to what happens with other student outcomes (e.g., patient care, problem solving). Ideally, assessment of an ability occurs in relation to where it is explicitly being developed. For example, if the learning objectives of a course or learning experience include performing certain behaviors (e.g., coming to class or another site and turning in assignments on time, engaging in proactive versus disruptive or apathetic behavior, demonstrating respect toward self, peers, and instructors), then these behaviors need to be assessed periodically throughout the course or practice experience. Performance of these behaviors should also be included as part of the grade or contribute toward the pass–fail threshold. One school has gone so far as to say that if a student does not meet professionalism expectations set forth for advanced practice experiences, then that student fails the experience.[71]

> Consider the idea of a 360-degree assessment.

Consider the idea of a 360-degree assessment in which students are assessed by their peers, instructors, and others with whom they come into contact, such as patients and other healthcare providers.[73,74] Although determining an individual's attitudes toward, and self-perception of, his or her professionalism can be valuable, incorporating others' observations of the individual's behaviors is critical for a valid assessment of professionalism. This is especially true for individuals who do not see themselves as others see them.

If students maintain portfolios, then documentation of their professional development and assessments of professionalism could be maintained in the portfolio. Perhaps, similar to other portfolio components, students could reflect on this aspect of their portfolios. Assessment itself implies evaluation *and* feedback—when it comes to professionalism, the power of this feedback cannot be underestimated. If faculty, preceptors, and other mentors can periodically have open and frank conversations with a student about his or her professional development, it could go a long way in helping that student achieve higher levels of professionalism. Also consider the idea of a professionalism award—what criteria would be used to identify the recipient(s)?

How to Assess Student Professionalism

As previously mentioned, it is important to first describe and define how students demonstrate professionalism, part of which probably mirrors expectations you might have of them for classroom and practice site behavior. For the classroom and clinic, it might be helpful in this process to describe the A students—what is it that they do to earn top grades? Decisions then need to be made about the whos, whats, wheres, hows, and whys:

- *Who is being assessed?* Students? Residents? Others?
- *Who will do the assessing?* Self? Peer? Faculty? Preceptor? Patient? Staff?
- *What will be assessed?* Observed behavior? Attitudes?
- *What instrument will be used?* One of those already referenced or one that you might create? More than one?
- *Where will they be assessed?* In class? In clinic? Outside of class or clinic?
- *How often will they be assessed?* Regularly? Only when unprofessional behavior occurs?
- *How will they be provided feedback on the assessment?* Via live conversation? Portfolio? Written communication?
- *Why will they be assessed?* As part of the grade? As part of documentation toward meeting outcomes? So they know how they are developing?

These questions should be answered prior to engaging in some sort of assessment.

For published classroom and clerkship examples, review the work of Hammer and Paulsen[53] and Boyle et al.[71]

What Should You Do When Unprofessional Behavior Occurs?

The answer is easy: it depends. It depends on who is involved, what happened, when it happened, where it happened, and why it happened. This section explores strategies for managing these challenging situations as they arise.

First and foremost, be familiar with school policy. Most schools have conduct or honor codes published in student handbooks. There is likely a process for faculty and preceptors to follow if students demonstrate certain forms of unprofessional behavior, especially those that are more egregious like plagiarism, theft, physical threats, and others. What can be more difficult, however, is when students act unprofessionally in the classroom or practice site, but the behavior may not have been severe enough to initiate a formal review process as described in the student handbook. These situations might involve moderately disruptive students in class, apathetic students at your practice site, and students who make inappropriate comments to faculty, preceptors, patients, fellow students, and others. The following tips can help faculty and preceptors when they are confronted with unprofessional students[75,76]:

- *Respond; do not react.* Make sure to listen, keep calm, and do not become emotional or angry. Some mild behaviors may even be addressed by peers (such as the shusher example previously described) or by you in a lighthearted or humorous way.
- *Address the situation immediately.* Point out that whatever is happening should not be happening, then meet with the student(s) involved outside of class; if you are in a practice setting, meet in a more private area. Meeting personally with the student(s) involved may depend on the severity of the behavior—for example, if someone answered a cell phone in class once and their classmates and you addressed it with that person during class, then you may not feel the need to talk privately about it with the student unless it happens again.
- *When you meet with the student(s) involved, make sure you are not alone.* This is important for your own safety, as well as to prevent any he said, she said situations that might follow.
- *Document what happened.* This is especially important if additional incidents occur. You can also discuss the situation with your assistant or associate dean of students. If a behavioral problem happens in a course or practice setting where professional behavior evaluations occur regularly, then maintaining documentation of this sort and having conversations about behavior with students becomes much easier—it is part of the normal routine of the course or practice experience.

When students demonstrate unprofessional behaviors, do *not* handle them as follows:

- Ignore incivilities, hoping they will go away. *They won't!*
- Laugh off inappropriate comments or behavior.
- Walk away from offensive behavior. Silence = Sanction.
- Argue, become defensive or take it personally.
- Press for an immediate or public explanation of the offensive behavior.

- Make exceptions about assignments or uncivil and unprofessional behavior.
- Go it alone and refrain from talking with colleagues about these issues.

Summary

Professionalism is much more than acting respectfully in the classroom and practice site. It is truly caring about and for patients and others in an altruistic and unselfish manner. It is being a member of a profession, which requires achieving and maintaining a certain competence and expertise and practicing ethically. It is founded upon maintaining individual, trusting relationships with those whom we serve. There are multiple ways to help students develop certain aspects of professionalism as they progress through a professional program. It is also important to consider your own behavior as a role model for students. What spoken and unspoken values and behaviors are they observing in you? Pharmacy schools need to make the development of student professionalism their primary focus because it is the essence of how we serve society.

References

1. Greenwood E. Attributes of a profession. *Soc Work.* July 1957;2:44–55.
2. Vollmer HM, Mills DL, eds. *Professionalization.* Englewood Cliffs, NJ: Prentice Hall, Inc; 1966.
3. Smith MC. Implications of "professionalization" for pharmacy education. *Am J Pharm Educ.* 1970;34(1):16–32.
4. Denzin NK, Mettlin CJ. Incomplete professionalization: the case of pharmacy. *Soc Forces.* 1968;46:375–382.
5. Montague JB Jr. Pharmacy and the concept of professionalism. *J Am Pharm Assoc.* 1968;NS8(5):228–230.
6. Shuval JT, Gilbert L. Attempts at professionalization of pharmacy: an Israel case study. *Soc Sci Med.* 1978;12:19–25.
7. Rankin K. Feds sweep down on unethical pharmacists. *Drug Store News.* July 27, 1992;14(14):4.
8. Pharmacist accused of diluting drugs. *Chain Drug Review.* September, 2001; 23(16):RX26, RX28.
9. Big Spring, Texas pharmacist convicted of drug diversion [press release]. Dallas, TX: US Department of Veterans Affairs, Office of Inspector General, Office of Investigations, South Central Field Office; February 9, 2005.
10. Medicare's Most Wanted. Pharmacies, employees indicted in $2.3 million NJ Medicaid scheme. http://medicaresmostwanted.blogspot.com/2009/11/pharmacies-employees-indicted-in-23.html. Accessed December 4, 2009.
11. Parsons T. *The Social System.* Glencoe, IL: The Free Press; 1951.
12. Strauss G. Professionalism and occupational associations. *Ind Rel.* 1963;2 (3):7–31.
13. Vollmer HM, Mills DL, eds. *Professionalization.* Englewood Cliffs, NJ: Prentice Hall, Inc; 1966.
14. Beardsley RS. Chair report of the APhA-ASP/AACP-COD task force on professionalization: enhancing professionalism in pharmacy education and practice. *Am J Pharm Educ.* 1996;60(suppl):26S–28S.

15. Hammer DP, Berger BA, Beardsley RS, Easton MR. Student professionalism. *Am J Pharm Educ.* 2003;67(3):article 96.

16. Stern DT, ed. *Measuring Medical Professionalism.* New York, NY: Oxford University Press; 2006.

17. American Board of Internal Medicine. Medical Professionalism Project. Medical professionalism in the new millennium: a physician's charter. *Ann Intern Med.* 2002;136(3):244.

18. Roth MT, Zlatic TD. Development of student professionalism. *Pharmacotherapy.* 2009;29(6):749–756.

19. American Pharmacists Association. Oath of a pharmacist. http://www.pharmacist.com/AM/Template.cfm?Section=Oath_of_a_Pharmacist&Template=/CM/HTMLDisplay.cfm&ContentID=18306. Accessed November 28, 2009.

20. American Pharmacists Association. Code of ethics for pharmacists. http://www.pharmacist.com/AM/Template.cfm?Section=Search1&template=/CM/HTMLDisplay.cfm&ContentID=2903. Accessed November 28, 2009.

21. Chalmers RK. Contemporary issues: professionalism in pharmacy. *Tomorrow Pharm.* March 1997:10.

22. Hall RH. Professionalization and bureaucratization. *Am Soc Rev.* February 1968;33:92–104.

23. Purkerson Hammer D, Mason HL, Chalmers RK, Popovich NG, Rupp MT. Development and testing of an instrument to assess behavioral professionalism of pharmacy students. *Am J Pharm Educ.* 2000;64:141–151.

24. Accreditation Council for Pharmacy Education. *Accreditation Standards and Guidelines for the Professional Program in Pharmacy Leading to the Doctor of Pharmacy Degree.* Chicago, IL: Accreditation Council for Pharmacy Education; 2007.

25. Zlatic, T. *Re-Envisioning Professional Education.* Kansas City, MO: American College of Clinical Pharmacy; 2005.

26. Hilton SR, Slotnick HB. Proto-professionalism: how professionalisation occurs across the continuum of medical education. *Med Educ.* 2005;39(1):58.

27. Duncan-Hewitt W. The development of a professional: reinterpretation of the professionalization problem from the perspective of cognitive/moral development. *Am J Pharm Educ.* 2005;69(1):article 6.

28. Nimmo CM, Holland RW. Transitions in pharmacy practice, part 5: walking the tightrope of change. *Am J Health Syst Pharm.* 2000;57(1):64–72.

29. Seels B, Glasgow Z. *Exercises in Instructional Design.* Columbus, OH: Merrill Publishing Company; 1990:28.

30. Brown D, Ferrill MJ. The taxonomy of professionalism: reframing the academic pursuit of professional development. *Am J Pharm Educ.* 2009;73(4):article 68.

31. Merton RK, Reader GG, Kendall PL. *The Student–Physician: Introductory Studies in the Sociology of Medical Education.* Cambridge, MA: Harvard University Press; 1957.

32. Sherlock BJ, Morris RT. The evolution of a professional: a paradigm. *Soc Inq.* 1967;37:27–46.

33. Simpson IH. Patterns of socialization into professions: the case of student nurses. *Soc Inq.* 1967;37:47–54.

34. Baernstein A, Fryer-Edwards K. Promoting reflection on professionalism: a comparison trial of educational interventions for medical students. *Acad Med.* 2003;78(7):742–747.

35. American Pharmacists Association, Academy of Student Pharmacists. Pharmacy professionalism toolkit for students and faculty provided by the APhA-ASP/AACP Committee on Student Professionalism. http://www.pharmacist.com/AM/Template.cfm?Section=Professionalism_Toolkit_for_Students_and_Faculty&Template=/CM/HTMLDisplay.cfm&ContentID=5415. Accessed November 29, 2009.

36. American Association of Colleges of Pharmacy. Meeting abstracts, 105th annual meeting; July 10–14, 2004; Salt Lake City, UT. *Am J Pharm Educ.* 2004;68(2):54–64. http://www.ajpe.org/aj6802/aj680254/aj680254.pdf. Accessed November 29, 2009.

37. Hammer DP, Berger BA, Beardsley RS, Easton MR. Student professionalism. *Am J Pharm Educ.* 2003;67(3): article 96.

38. Berger BA, ed. *Promoting Civility in Pharmacy Education*. Binghamton, NY: Haworth Press; 2003.

39. Berger BA, Butler SL, Duncan-Hewitt W, et al. Changing the culture: an institution-wide approach to instilling professional values. *Am J Pharm Educ.* 2004;68(1):article 22.

40. Brown, DL, Ferrill, MJ, Pankaskie MC. White coat ceremonies in US schools of pharmacy. *Ann Pharm.* 2003;37(10):1414–1419.

41. Eyler JS, Giles DE, Stenson CM, Gray CJ. *At a Glance: What We Know About the Effects of Service-Learning on College Students, Faculty, Institutions and Communities, 1993–2000*. 3rd ed. Boston, MA: Campus Compact. http://www.compact.org/wp-content/uploads/resources/downloads/aag.pdf. Accessed April 12, 2010.

42. Duke LJ, Francisco GE, Herist KN, McDuffie CH, White CA. Student professionalism: development and implementation of a curricular competency statement and professionalism policy at the University of Georgia College of Pharmacy. *J Pharm Teach.* 2005;12(2):5–24.

43. Hardigan PC, Lai LL, Arneson D, Robeson A. Significance of academic merit, test scores, interviews and the admissions process: a case study. *Am J Pharm Educ.* 2001;65(1):40–43.

44. Stolte SK, Scheer SB, Robinson ET. The reliability of non-cognitive admissions measures in predicting non-traditional doctor of pharmacy student performance outcomes. *Am J Pharm Educ.* 2003;67(1):article 18.

45. Latif D. Using the structured interview for a more reliable assessment of pharmacy student applicants. *Am J Pharm Educ.* 2004;68(1):article 21.

46. Hall FR, Regan-Smith M, Tivnan T. Relationship of medical students' admission interview scores to their dean's letter ratings. *Acad Med.* 1992;67(12): 842–845.

47. Sandow PL, Jones AC, Peek CW, Courts FJ, Watson RE. Correlation of admission criteria with dental school performance and attrition. *J Dent Educ.* 2002;66(3):385–392.

48. Eva KW, Rosenfeld J, Reiter HI, Norman GR. An admissions OSCE: the multiple mini-interview. *Med Educ.* 2004;38(3):314.

49. Reiter HI, Eva KW, Rosenfeld J, Norman GR. Multiple mini-interviews predict clerkship and licensing examination performance. *Med Educ.* 2007;41 (4):378–384.

50. Manasse HR, Stewart JE Jr, Hall RH. Inconsistent socialization in pharmacy—a pattern in need of change. *J Am Pharm Assoc.* November 1975; NS15: 616–621,658.

51. Boice B. Classroom incivilities. *Res Higher Educ.* 1996;37:453–486.

52. Hammer DP. So you only have one credit in your curriculum devoted to social–behavioral pharmacy issues? Strategies for a high-impact course. *Am J Pharm Educ.* 2002;66(suppl):85S.

53. Hammer DP, Paulsen SM. Strategies and processes to design an integrated, longitudinal professional skills development course sequence. *Am J Pharm Educ.* 2001;65,77–85.

54. Conrad WF, Doherty MB. Using pharmacy organizations to enhance student development. Poster presented at: American Association of Colleges of Pharmacy Annual Meeting; July 2003; Minneapolis, MN.

55. Charneski L, Congdon HB, Lebovitz L. Student engagement: participation of students at a distance education campus in student organizations. Poster presented at: American Association of Colleges of Pharmacy Annual Meeting; July 2008; Chicago, IL.

56. American Pharmacists Association, Academy of Student Pharmacists. Pharmacy professionalism toolkit for students and faculty, provided by the APhA-ASP/AACP Committee on Student Professionalism. http://www.pharmacist.com/AM/Template.cfm?Section=Professional_Committees. Accessed December 4, 2009.

57. Hammer DP. Improving student professionalism during experiential learning. *Am J Pharm Educ.* 2006;70(3):article 59.

58. American Association of Colleges of Pharmacy. Professional experience program (PEP) library of resources. http://www.peplibrary.vcu.edu/search.asp. Accessed December 4, 2009.

59. Kearney KR. Service learning. *Am J Pharm Educ.* 2004;68(1, theme issue): Articles 26–29,43–45,99.

60. Chretien KC, Greysen SR, Chretien JP, Kind T. Online posting of unprofessional content by medical students. *JAMA.* 2009;302(12):1309–1315.

61. Guseh JS II, Brendel RW, Brendel DH. Medical professionalism in the age of online social networking. *J Med Ethics.* 2009;35(9):584–586.

62. Cain J, Scott DR, Akers P. Pharmacy students' Facebook activity and opinions regarding accountability and e-professionalism. *Am J Pharm Educ.* 2009; 73(6):article 104.

63. Cain J, Fox BI. Web 2.0 and pharmacy education. *Am J Pharm Educ.* 2009; 73(7):article 120.

64. Cain J. Online social networking issues within academia and pharmacy education. *Am J Pharm Educ.* 2008;72(1):article 10.

65. Hall RH. Professionalization and bureaucratization. *Am Soc Rev.* 1968; 33(2):92–104.

66. Chisholm MA, Cobb H, Duke L, McDuffie C, Kennedy WK. Development of an instrument to measure professionalism. *Am J Pharm Educ.* 2006;70(4): article 85.

67. Hammer DP. Development of a general student survey to document professional socialization of pharmacy students and attitudes toward pharmacy curricula. *Am J Pharm Educ.* 2000;64(suppl):106S–107S.

68. Peeters MJ, Stone GE. An instrument to objectively measure pharmacist professionalism as an outcome: a pilot study. *Can J Hosp Pharm.* 2009;62(3): 209–216.

69. Rest J, Narvaez D. *Guide for DIT-2.* Minneapolis: University of Minnesota; 1998:1–43.

70. Phelan S, Obenshain SS, Galey WR. Evaluation of noncognitive professional traits of medical students. *Acad Med.* 1993;68(10):799–803.

71. Boyle CJ, Beardsley RS, Morgan JA, Rodriguez de Bittner M. Professionalism: a determining factor in experiential learning. *Am J Pharm Educ.* 2007;71(2): article 31.

72. Hammer DP, Jackson TR, Schreffler RS. Continued testing and validation of an instrument to assess behavioral professionalism of pharmacy students. Poster presented at: American Association of Colleges of Pharmacy Annual Meeting; July 2007, Orlando, FL.

73. Wood J, Collins J, Burnside ES, et al. Patient, faculty, and self-assessment of radiology resident performance: a 360-degree method of measuring professionalism and interpersonal/communication skills. *Acad Radiol.* 2004;11(8):931–939.

74. Joshi R, Ling FW, Jaeger J. Assessment of a 360-degree instrument to evaluate residents' competency in interpersonal and communication skills. *Acad Med.* 2004;79(5):458–463.

75. Hobson E, Hammer D, Lynch JC. Implementing teaching and learning strategies. Paper presented at: American College of Clinical Pharmacy Annual Meeting; April 21, 2007; Memphis, TN. Handout.

76. Anderson-Harper H. Dealing with boundary violations. In: Berger BA, ed. *Promoting Civility in Pharmacy Education.* Binghamton, NY: Pharmaceutical Products Press; 2003;9(3),105–117.

CHAPTER 11

What Matters in Advising and Mentoring Students?

Lisa A. Lawson, PharmD
Eric G. Boyce, PharmD

Introduction

Why does this chapter on student advising and mentoring matter? Because prospective, new, and existing pharmacy faculty members need a resource as they develop and provide academic advising and mentoring to students. Some institutions include advising and mentoring as an explicit faculty responsibility, but others do not have formal expectations. All faculty members will serve as academic advisors or mentors at some time during their career, and preparation to serve in this role will benefit both students and faculty.

The intent of this chapter is to provide answers to the following questions on student advising and mentoring:

- Why should I advise or mentor students?
- How does mentoring differ from advising?
- What are the major goals and outcomes associated with advising and mentoring?
- What pitfalls should I avoid as an advisor or mentor?
- What legal issues are associated with advising?

What Is the Difference Between Advising and Mentoring?

Advising and mentoring both involve a relationship between a more experienced and a less experienced person. Advising may be more targeted to specific outcomes associated with academic goals, whereas mentoring is more focused on long-term development. Student advising is also more likely to be

251

recognized as a documented role and responsibility of faculty, whereas student mentoring may be included within advising, inferred without specific mention, or not mentioned at all as a role or responsibility of faculty. For the purposes of this chapter, we will consider *student advising* to be a relationship between a student and a faculty member with the goal of developing a successful educational experience that allows the student to subsequently move toward achieving career and life goals. *Student mentoring* will be considered a relationship between a student and a faculty member with the goal of enhancing the student's long-term development and planning.

Student Advisement: General Philosophy and Goals

Before undertaking the role of advisor, it is important to appreciate the guiding principles of student advisement. With this understanding, you will be more likely to "meet" the student at his or her stage of learning and serve as an effective guide in the student's professional development.

Philosophy

Academic advising may be considered broader in nature than mentoring because faculty may advise on a variety of types of students (first-year undergraduate, professional, nontraditional, transfer, distance) in several areas. Advising can encompass goal setting, curricular and course selection issues, adjustment to independent living, career guidance, and learning skills. Some faculty advisors may work with students in majors outside their own discipline. Advising must be individualized to the student and is meant to assist the student in developing his or her own self-monitoring skills, life skills, and learning and study skills. Depending on the student's age or year of study, the developmental nature of advising may be the most important component of this activity. For example, first-year college students undergo a transition process as they learn to live and care for themselves on their own. They must learn to become independent problem solvers and thinkers rather than relying on advisors who provide reminders or direct them through independent living and learning. In contrast, an advanced professional-year student with a previously earned degree may require little or no personal development advising. The faculty advisor must meet the student at his or her stage of life and learning, and guide the student to independent problem solving and responsibility for learning and life.

An advisor also serves as a source of information about campus services and departments, academic regulations, and policies and procedures concerning student life and activities. Advisors should prepare by identifying sources or places that provide information on a variety of topics. A great starting place is to become familiar with your institution's policies or guidelines, which are typically found in the academic catalog and the student handbook either in print form or on the institutional Web site.

> To be an effective advisor, you must meet the student at his/her stage of life and learning.

Advising is considered to have such significance that the quality of advising is assessed in the National Survey of Student Engagement (http://nsse.iub.edu/index.cfm), a national survey of hundreds of colleges and universities that documents learning and personal development activities provided to students. A good advising relationship between a student and an advisor can contribute to the student becoming more engaged with his or her educational experience. The degree of student engagement is related to the quality of student learning and the overall educational experience.

Reflective Exercise

Using your institutional resources, where can you find the information listed in **Table 11–1**? The first column of the table lists common topics for discussion with students in your role as advisor. To be prepared for your role as advisor, list in the second column where information on each topic can be found at your institution (e.g., handbooks, online sources).

Table 11–1 Sources of Information for Advising Students

Topic	Source of Information
Curricular requirements	
Academic standards	
Registration information	
College or university calendar	
Student and faculty contact information	
Financial aid and billing	
Health and counseling	
Tutoring services	
Security	
Housing and meal plans	
Student conduct	
Learning disabilities and Americans with Disabilities Act (ADA)	
Substance abuse	
Student transcripts	
Attendance and leave policies	
Course requirements	
Career exploration	

Have you adequately prepared for your role as student advisor?

Goals

The overarching goal of advising is to assist the student in completing a successful academic experience. This may include guiding the student in developing educational plans, making course selections, and developing career and life goals. The advisor must be aware of the student's progress, aid the student in developing plans to handle academic problems, and work with the student to develop self-monitoring skills. An advisor also serves as a source of information about campus resources. The faculty member may be involved in all or some of these areas, depending on the nature of the institution and the program as well as the availability of other professional advisors.

What Are the Roles and Responsibilities of a Faculty Advisor?

The roles and responsibilities of a faculty advisor vary markedly among institutions. At some institutions, a faculty advisor may be the only advising resource available to students. Increasingly, many universities or colleges have departments or units composed of professional advisors whose primary job function is to provide a comprehensive advising support system for students. In those situations, a faculty advisor may only be involved with career planning, course selection, or how to approach difficult course work. Whatever the types of advising, faculty advisors should always be able to recognize a student in distress and be familiar with the institution's acute support services for such students.

Individual Faculty Member

As a faculty advisor, it is your responsibility to direct the advising relationship and provide consistent and appropriate feedback to the student. Initiation of the relationship usually involves time spent exchanging information so that you and the student can become better acquainted. Some institutions may provide initial assessment instruments that help students learn about their own strengths and areas that need improvement. The next step usually involves setting educational goals that may include an educational plan of courses, academic skills development (e.g., study skills), and career exploration. Shorter-term goals may include plans for the upcoming semester or quarter, such as course selection or course performance goals. A schedule of meetings, communications, and expectations should be mutually developed and agreed upon. As the year progresses, you should provide feedback and assessment appropriate to the level of the student. At the end of the year, both you and the student should assess the strengths and weaknesses of the year's activities and plan for the future.

You should develop a monitoring system to identify students at risk so that advising or another intervention may occur. For example, if a student fails to attend a scheduled meeting without any communication, you should consider methods to contact the student and work with him or her on improving this behavior. Identifying students in distress and referring them to appropriate campus resources is a responsibility of all faculty advisors.

A successful faculty advisor is committed to the development of students. Displaying a caring attitude, dedication, and strong communication skills are of great importance. You should be familiar with campus resources and support services. Keeping current on and learning about changes in academic policies and curricular requirements on a periodic basis is necessary.

Individual Student

The student should be an active participant in self-assessment and the setting of academic goals. The student should commit to communicating with the faculty advisor, meeting deadlines, attending appointments, and behaving in a professional manner.

What Types of Student Advising Might I Provide?

Advising programs vary tremendously depending on the available campus resources and support services. **Table 11–2** offers a description of the types of activities performed by advisors. Faculty advisors may be solely responsible for all advising activities (this is becoming less common) or participate in selected areas of advising. Student advising may be centralized on your campus in a department such as student affairs, or it may be decentralized to individual schools and colleges. Often the faculty member

Table 11–2 Advising Activities

Advising Activity	Description
Development of educational plan	Course selection, registration, academic policies and procedures
Students having academic difficulties	Identification of academic difficulty, development of improvement plan, monitoring progress of student
Intrusive advising	Collection of formative assessment information about the student to identify possible academic problems; advisor contacts the student as soon as problems are identified to work with the student to develop a prospective academic improvement plan
Distance advising	Advising relationship via technology, such as e-mail or videoconferencing
Special populations	May require additional or different advising techniques; includes groups such as athletes, nontraditional students, students with disabilities
Distressed students	Immediately secure the safety and health of the distressed student or others associated with the student; institutions should have a well-publicized plan in place
Graduate and professional students	Usually, a mentoring relationship develops to concentrate on long-term goals

works in partnership with a professional advisor. You should become familiar with the expectations of faculty advisors at your institution.

Academic Advising

Academic advising usually involves the development of an educational plan, course selection, registration, and other academic policies and procedures. Students need to understand the academic regulations governing their program of study, such as minimum course performance expectations, required cumulative grade point averages, and other academic regulations. Useful reference materials include the institution's student handbook and college catalog in print or electronic forms. A central advising department or individual academic programs often have additional information specific to certain courses of study. Information in these areas often changes, so advisors need to make sure to remain current.

Academic advising also includes assisting students with academic difficulties. The role of the faculty advisor is to guide the student in identifying problems, performing self-assessments to identify how the problems developed, and creating plans for improvement. Periodic follow-up (e.g., weekly or monthly) is helpful to ensure a successful outcome, and through follow-up students perceive that support is coming from a caring advisor. The following exercise can help you become familiar with the types of issues associated with academic advising.

Reflective Exercise

In the first column of **Table 11–3** on page 257, common factors contributing to academic difficulties are listed. Column 2 provides a sample question that an advisor could ask to better identify the issue. Column 3 provides a sample recommendation that an advisor may make to help a student with each of the areas. Complete the table by identifying additional questions in Column 2 and recommendations in Column 3 regarding each factor that contributes to academic difficulty.

Intrusive Advising

Advising models often assume that a student will seek help when needed. However, undergraduate students are still undergoing personal development and may not have developed independent coping skills or help-seeking skills. Some institutions have initiated intrusive advising systems where advisors reach out to students rather than waiting for students to self-identify problems. Formative assessment information (e.g., quiz grades, individual assignment grades) is collected, collated, and communicated to the advisors continuously throughout the semester or quarter. Advisors can monitor for trends of decreasing academic performance or poor attendance and contact the student as soon as a problem is identified.

Table 11–3 Advising Students with Academic Difficulties

Contributing Factor to Academic Issue	Questions to Identify Issues Associated with Each Contributing Factor	Recommendations to Improve Identified Issues
Academic study skills, course material, learning and teaching styles	Can you describe the process you use to take notes during class?	Consider utilizing the college or university's tutoring services.
Time-management skills	How much time do you spend studying each day or week?	Develop a weekly plan for studying ——— hours per week for the problem course(s).
Social	Do your friends understand or support the time you need to study?	Plan a meeting with your friends to ask for their support of your needed study time.
Financial	Has your work schedule increased?	Decide on the maximum number of hours that you can work each week and still maintain good grades.
Family	Is there a serious illness or problem at home that is affecting your studies?	Schedule a family meeting to discuss the issue.
Personal	Are there any other personal problems that are interfering with your studies?	Refer the student to the appropriate support service.
Relationship	Are there relationships with another student, friend, faculty, or family member that are interfering with your studies?	Meet with the dorm resident advisor to discuss approaches to solving roommate problems.
Physical and mental health	Are you experiencing any symptoms of illness?	See a healthcare provider for a checkup.

Source: Adapted from Thomas RA. Preceptor development: integrating students into your pharmacy practice. Paper presented at: 2006 Iowa Pharmacist Expo; January 28, 2006; Des Moines, IA.

Source: Adapted from Hobson E, Roth M, Harris I. Active learning to achieve abilities. *ACCP.* Presented at the American College of Clinical Pharmacy Annual Meeting, October 22, 2005; San Francisco, CA.

Intrusive advising systems allow for interventions with students on a periodic basis to avert academic problems.

Other information, such as residence hall problems or lack of use of a meal plan, can also signal a problem.

Students are asked to meet with their advisor, identify the problems, and develop plans for success as soon as possible. By intervening during the semester rather than waiting until final course grades are available, many academic problems can be averted or minimized in a more prospective manner. Vander Schee found that semester grade point averages of students who were on academic probation significantly improved after attending three to eight meetings in an intrusive academic advising approach compared to students who attended one or two meetings or no meetings.[1]

Distance Advising

Advising students at a different geographic location requires the use of technology that ranges from telephone calls to e-mail to videoconferencing. The advisor needs to determine the most effective means of communication with the student, such as oral or written, synchronous or asynchronous, or individual or group communication. Technology increases flexibility, but it does not deliver the same face-to-face interaction of a meeting. The advisor and student will need to develop guidelines for communication and expectations of advising. The advisor needs to be aware that underlying assumptions of communication may not be valid when the student and advisor do not have a face-to-face meeting. Nonverbal communication, such as body language, is not available. Advising programs for distance students should be designed with consideration for the available technology, the modes of communication and access, and the unique needs of this student population.[2]

Special Populations

Special student populations may require additional or different advising. Special populations may include athletes, students with disabilities, international students, nontraditional students, or transfer students. Many institutions have specific programs or advisors for these categories of students. Faculty advisors need to be aware of the special needs of these populations.

Distressed Students

Scenario: You are working in your office when one of your advisees, LT, appears at your doorway and asks if he can speak with you. You have known LT for two years and notice a marked change in his demeanor. He is listless and depressed and occasionally has to pause to prevent himself from crying. You calmly ask questions to determine the nature of the situation, which involves the terminal illness of his closest friend. LT states that he is so despondent that he "feels like just popping some pills and giving up." This expression of suicidal thoughts by LT causes you great concern. How should you respond?

Identifying and assisting distressed students is a responsibility of all faculty advisors. A distressed student is one whose health and safety or that of others are at risk. This may include urgent physical and mental health issues, personal issues such as the death of a loved one, or risky behavior (e.g., substance abuse). The immediate need is to secure the health and safety of the student or others associated with the student. The university or college should have plans and support systems developed and communicated frequently to all members of the student community.

In the case of LT, he needs to have immediate assistance to help him handle his personal situation. LT should immediately be personally escorted to the appropriate office or department (typically student health and counseling) to meet with a healthcare professional about his personal situation. If possible, escort the student yourself. The distressed student is typically comforted by your presence because you are someone who knows him or her and the nature of the situation. Stay with the student until the student sees the healthcare professional or is under observation by a trained staff member. Offer your assistance to the student for the near future to help him or her handle the problem. Sometimes the student may ask the advisor to be a part of the meeting with the healthcare professional, or the student may ask the advisor to speak with the healthcare professional at a later time or date. The student will have to give consent for the healthcare professional to speak with the advisor. Be sure to follow-up with the student as soon as feasible. Professional help should be sought at once to prevent any threats to the health or safety of the student and others.

Some institutions have special teams in place to handle these situations. For example, the institution of one of the authors of this chapter has a multidisciplinary team, SEIRT (Student Early Intervention Response Team), that meets weekly and monitors the progress of distressed students. The presence of the team and the referral process is widely publicized around campus. The team is chaired by the dean of students and includes representatives from student health and counseling, residence halls, academic programs, academic advising, and security. Faculty, staff, and students may contact any member of the team about students with potential problems. The team can be mobilized quickly to deal with the potential problem in a prospective, secure, and confidential manner. The affected student can be referred to appropriate medical care as needed for the acute or urgent problem. Another important component is the development of a long-term plan to assess and deal with the issue. The student is allowed to return to academic work only with the submission of documentation from the appropriate resources. For example, students with mental health problems must be evaluated by a licensed healthcare provider and deemed able to return to campus.

Graduate and Professional Students

The relationship between a faculty member and graduate or professional students is most commonly a mentoring relationship that concentrates on long-term development goals (see the mentoring section later in this chapter).

What Are the Legal Aspects of Advising?

Scenario: You are beginning your first year as a faculty member and have been assigned five students as advisees. At the beginning of the semester, you and each student met and spent some time getting to know each other and discussing each student's educational plan. One student, AJ, found high school to be very easy, studied less than five hours per week, and graduated with a cumulative grade point average of 3.89. At your meeting last week, you and AJ reviewed his exam grades for two of the four exams in his General Chemistry I class, which were 57 percent and 43 percent. You helped AJ develop an academic success plan that involved time management, meeting with the professor, and utilizing the on-campus tutoring services. You receive a telephone call from AJ's mother at 8:45 a.m. on the following Monday, and she is very worried about AJ. She relates that he was worried and stressed on his weekend visit, but he would only say that he was not doing well on his tests. She asks you to tell her what problems AJ is having. What is your response?

With first-year undergraduate students, a common situation that advisors encounter is communication with parents or families regarding the student's grades or academic progress. As an advisor, it is important to be aware that the communication procedures in higher education differ from those in secondary education. In higher education, the Family Educational Rights and Privacy Act (FERPA) governs confidentiality of student records. Each institution has a designated officer responsible for compliance with FERPA regulations, and all faculty advisors must be familiar with them. Under FERPA, most information concerning the student can only be communicated to families with the student's written permission. For example, the grades of a student cannot be discussed unless the student has given permission. Parents may not understand that although they are bearing the financial burden of their child's education, they are not entitled to information about grades without the student's permission.

Parents are often unfamiliar with the requirements of FERPA and may be frustrated that you cannot discuss the situation. As an advisor, you should explain that the specifics of a student's situation cannot be discussed with the parents without the student's written consent. You might want to discuss the situation in general terms. For example, you could share that the course has four exams, of which two have been administered.

You could discuss the definition of a passing grade. In general terms, you could also explain the type of advice you typically give a student in this type of situation, which might include meeting with the professor, using the tutoring service, and evaluating time spent on studying and other activities. Often the parents may persist with additional questions about their child's situation. If possible, arrange a meeting with the parents and the student. This is a very effective way to discuss the situation because when information is shared, all parties hear the same thing, and suggestions can be made to improve the situation. It is usually reassuring to the parents to speak directly with the advisor in the presence of the student so that they can get a reliable description of the problem.

> Are you familiar with the FERPA regulations?

Although the student's permission is needed to discuss information like academic performance with his or her parents, in acute cases FERPA regulations permit institutions to notify parents of situations involving drug and alcohol use without the student's consent.

What Are the Benefits of Advising?

Most faculty members are in the profession because of their commitment to helping others in a meaningful way. There is great satisfaction in assisting an advisee through the growing and learning process of higher education. In some cases, an advising relationship may be the beginning of a long-term professional relationship with a future colleague or collaborator. Depending on the institution, advising may also be a component of the expected workload in terms of teaching or service to the institution.

What Are the Pitfalls of Advising?

One of the goals of advising is to assist the student in progressing from a dependent individual to one who directs his or her own life and educational program. The role of the advisor is to facilitate this development, not to be prescriptive and directive. The advisor must be sure that the student is given and understands all the information and consequences of a particular issue or decision. The advisor should then allow the student to make the decision. Be sure to allow the student time and space to grow and learn. Encourage the student to be reflective about his or her activities and experiences. Help the student to connect new information and experiences with his or her personal and professional goals.

One responsibility of a faculty advisor is to stay current with changes in regulations, procedures, or curricula. Providing wrong or incomplete information can adversely affect a student's educational performance, length of the program, or even financial obligations. You should be familiar with the program's curricular requirements, academic standards, course requirements, student services, housing and meal plans, student organizations, and other

Faculty advisors are responsible for staying current with changes in regulations, procedures, and the curriculum.

areas that are specific to your institution. Preparing yourself with the correct information and storing the information in an easily accessible place will better enable you to have successful and efficient meetings with your advisees. Consider returning to Table 11–1 to ensure that you have thought through the advising process and have collected the necessary information. Most important, if you are not sure of the correct information to convey to the student, contact the student later with the answer.

The development of an inappropriate personal relationship between an advisor and a student must be avoided. You need to be mindful to keep the relationship on a professional level at all times. The advising relationship should be ended if this is not possible.

How Do I Assess and Document My Advising Activities?

Interactions with advisees should be documented in written or electronic form. Many institutions have required or suggested formats for documentation. Usually, the date, issues discussed, referrals, recommended actions, and follow-up are documented. Other material to include in an advisee's file are grade reports, transcripts, self-assessment information, conversations with other institutional faculty or staff regarding the student, and official communications (e.g., letter from the dean regarding academic probation). Many advisors e-mail the results of meetings to their advisees. Alternatively, the advisee can document the meeting and send it to the advisor for review, which can also serve as a learning opportunity. Documentation can prevent problems, serve as a memory aid, be used for monitoring the student's progress, and help develop the student's documentation skills.

The National Academic Advising Association (NACADA) considers the assessment of advising to be a required component of any advising program.[3] The institution may conduct a comprehensive review, or the faculty advisor can assess his or her advising responsibilities on an individual basis. Information such as demographics of advisees, types of problems or issues, outcomes of problem resolution plans, and academic performance could be collected. The faculty advisor will also need this information for his or her annual performance review, pre- and post-tenure reviews, and dossier for promotion or tenure.

What Resources Are Available to Learn More About Advising?

There are many resources available to develop academic advising skills. NACADA is a professional organization for academic advisors, faculty, and administrators who are involved in providing quality academic advising. Their Web site (http://www.nacada.ksu.edu/AboutNACADA/index.htm) provides a rich array of references, and the organization holds several meetings annually. The Council for the Advancement of Standards in Higher Education (www.cas.edu) has developed standards related to academic advising that have been endorsed by NACADA (http://www.naca-da.ksu. edu/Resources/Standards.htm#CAS). Several journals related to academic advising, including the *NACADA Journal*, provide review and research articles about advising. Finally, many institutions have an administrative unit that provides academic advising services. This unit may be a centralized department for the entire college or university that is often found in student affairs, or it may be decentralized to individual schools and colleges. Professional advisors whose primary job responsibility is advising are eager to provide training programs for faculty advisors and have in-depth knowledge about the theories of advising as well as extensive, practical knowledge of the institution's policies, procedures, programs, and services that are available to students.

> Remember to document your advising activities and your communications with students.

Student Mentoring: General Philosophy and Goals

Unlike student advisement, student mentoring focuses on long-term development, and the mentor–mentee relationship often extends beyond the student's completion of the curriculum. Before undertaking the role of mentor, it is important to recognize the philosophical approach and goals to mentoring.

Philosophy

A major role of faculty is to enhance the development of students. This generally occurs with the class as a whole during didactic courses; it can also occur with small groups of students in certain courses or with individual students in experiential education. However, mentoring a student is an opportunity to individualize the development of a student in very specific areas. Mentoring programs for students can be expected to enhance the student's long-term development, just as faculty mentoring programs have done for new or inexperienced faculty.[4] Therefore, faculty members should consider student mentoring as an important component of their responsibilities.

Goals

The goals of mentoring are generally to enhance the student's development— usually from a long-term perspective and in very select areas. Mentoring should target the development of the student as a professional in addition to specific abilities that will impact his or her academic or professional career. Additional goals may be to introduce students to a certain discipline or career path. Mentoring may also benefit the faculty mentor in numerous ways, such as satisfaction in assisting others, beginning the development of a long-term professional relationship, obtaining assistance with projects, and enhancing the culture of the institution. In general, mentoring

What are your roles
and responsibilities
in mentoring
students?

a student involves more direction from the faculty mentor than would be seen in mentorship of one faculty member by another more experienced faculty member.

What Are the Roles and Responsibilities of a Mentor?

Student mentoring may or may not be identified as a responsibility of faculty at your institution. However, some universities have developed formal student mentoring programs where faculty serve as mentors.[5] Each faculty member should consider mentoring students, as well as faculty and staff, a fundamental responsibility. We can extend our academic advising to include more mentoring for our advisees. We may also advise a student organization and should consider mentoring students for leadership roles within that organization.

Individual Faculty Member

As a mentor, it is your responsibility to work with the student and direct the development of the mentoring relationship and activities. First, discuss the goals of the mentorship and revise those goals as needed to meet both your and the student's needs. Next, determine the nature and schedule for activities, meetings, and communication. During the mentorship, be sure to provide fair and balanced feedback on a routine basis to assist students in their development (see Chapter 9 for a review of how to provide effective feedback). Be sure to reward successes as well as provide insights for how to improve. Also, ask the student for a self-assessment of his or her development as well as an assessment of the mentoring relationship and activities. Consider any changes that may be needed if you revise the overall mentoring activities or relationship.

Individual Student

The student mentees or protégés also have responsibilities. Their major responsibilities are to set goals, strive to meet those goals, and communicate openly and honestly with their faculty mentor. Students should provide reasonably accurate self-assessments and respond appropriately to accolades as well as critiques. It is also important that students recognize the need to meet deadlines, make appointments, and act in a professional manner.

> *Scenario*: JP is a doctor of pharmacy student about to start the third professional year, and she is interested in pediatrics, oncology, and ambulatory care. She is a good student with a grade point average of 3.2 and is vice president of the student chapter of the National Community Pharmacists Association (NCPA). The doctor of pharmacy curriculum includes a required course in oncology pharmacotherapy, but it offers pediatrics only as an elective course. JP asks (1) how to sort this

out, (2) whether or not she should do a residency, and (3) how best to prepare for a career in those areas.

Mentoring a student on career options, selection, and preparation is a multiple-stage process of discovery and discussion. There are numerous approaches, but consider the following. Initially, ask JP why she is interested in these specialty pharmacy areas and what she knows about each area. Does she know that she could be a pediatric oncology pharmacist in an ambulatory care setting, or does she prefer to look at these areas as separate career paths? Provide initial general information on each career path. During this initial discussion, assess her understanding, rationale, interest, and dedication in pursuing each of those career paths. Consider providing additional sources of information to more fully describe these career options, including referral to other faculty or practitioners in those areas, literature articles on those types of practice areas, and job or residency descriptions of those career paths.

Set up another meeting when JP has had time to look into each of the options. This second meeting could then focus on how to collect more information; for example, referral to a faculty member or practitioner who would allow JP to spend time in those practice environments. The second meeting may also be a time to discuss residencies (PGY1 and PGY2) and fellowships in terms of general descriptions, the application and selection processes, responsibilities and activities, and advantages and disadvantages. If JP continues to be interested in pediatrics, it would be very reasonable to recommend that she enroll in the elective pediatrics course.

Subsequent meetings should target continued discussions on training programs and career pathways in addition to options that may be available in the advanced pharmacy practice experiences (APPEs) so JP can gain experience in her areas of interest. A referral to the director of the experiential program for a continuation of this discussion would be very appropriate. JP should also be informed or reminded of the time line for applications to residencies (and fellowships) before she goes on to her APPEs.

The mentoring continues during the APPEs and after graduation either in person or through e-mail communications. You may be asked to write a letter of recommendation for JP, and you may even extend that offer before being asked. Continue to interact with JP by being supportive and asking general questions about her career path and decisions. Provide insights and advice, particularly when asked. It is important to allow JP to transition from being your student to becoming your colleague, but still be a mentor when needed. This mentor–mentee relationship may result in a career-long professional relationship with many benefits for both of you.

What Are the Attributes of a Successful Mentor?

A successful mentor displays attributes that promote and enable student development, such as dedication, enthusiasm, caring, and strong organization

Does your institution have a required mentoring program?

and communication skills. When dealing with topics outside your expertise, you should be able to provide general guidance, assist in finding additional information, and refer the student mentee to those with more expertise on those topics.

How Do I Get Started as a Mentor?

There are many types of student mentoring programs and mentor–mentee relationships for students and faculty.[6] Does your institution have a required mentoring program, structured mentoring program, guidelines for mentoring, or none of the above? Such information will help you in setting up a mentoring relationship. In general, consider student mentoring to be a one-on-one activity, although you may have multiple protégés or mentees at one time, and they may have more than one mentor at the same time.

How are mentors and mentees selected? This is a very important component to consider. Any faculty member can volunteer to be a mentor. How do you then select mentees? Are you willing to accept any student, or must the student demonstrate the needed interest, attitude, behaviors, or abilities? Such decisions are based on your general goals as a faculty mentor, the type of mentor–mentee relationship that you desire, the specific outcomes that you are expecting, and your prior experiences as a mentor. Initially, consider making this decision based on interest and attitude, keeping in mind that students are still in a developmental stage of their careers and may not have clear ideas of their long-term direction. Your mentor–mentee relationship is likely to provide the student with valuable insights into his or her academic and professional career path and help the student develop abilities in specific areas.

What Are the Essential Components of a Student Mentoring Program?

Essential components of a student mentoring program include goals, a mentoring plan, expectations of the student and faculty member, a schedule of activities and communications, and assessments of the student's development and needs. The mentoring relationship and program should also be assessed and revised as needed. Some mentoring programs are best served by a structured plan throughout, but others may benefit by starting with a structured plan and then allowing for more flexibility as the mentor–mentee relationship develops.

What Types of Mentoring Might I Provide?

As with advisement, mentoring takes many different forms ranging from individual student mentorship to group mentorship. Moreover, the focus of your mentorship will vary dependent on the setting and needs of your mentee(s).

Mentoring Students During Individualized Course Work or Projects

Working with students on research, scholarship, or other projects offers excellent opportunities for mentoring. Such projects have short-term and long-term implications. These projects may be centered on the faculty member's needs and direction, but they should be flexible enough to be individualized to enhance the student's development. These projects may or may not involve enrollment in independent study or research courses. If a course is involved, be sure to set the criteria for performance as well as the other needed elements previously described. Many projects will extend beyond the course semester or quarter.

Mentoring Students During Pharmacy Practice Experiences

An excellent opportunity for mentoring students is during introductory pharmacy practice experiences, and more so during advanced pharmacy practice experiences. Students are exposed to real-life situations and healthcare environments during these experiences. Therefore, these are excellent settings in which to provide mentoring on career planning, interaction with patients and other professionals, projects, and professionalism. A preceptor that provides mentoring and goes beyond the minimum expectations of directing and evaluating the experience can have a marked impact on a student's short-term and long-term development.

Mentoring Students in Professional Organizations

If you become an advisor for a student professional organization, you will be able to work closely with students in the administrative aspects and activities of that organization. This involvement also offers the opportunity for group mentoring as well as mentoring of individual student leaders. The goals of student mentoring in professional organizations include the development of specific abilities in different areas—such as leadership, administration, program development and delivery, communication, advocacy, career development, and professional organization involvement—beyond the confines of the college or school of pharmacy. Mentorship prior to, during, and after local, regional, national, and possibly international meetings of the organization can also be very useful for student development.

Mentoring Students in Career Planning

Mentoring for career planning is a major need for students. As previously noted, mentoring for career planning can occur during pharmacy practice experiences and student professional organization activities. However, mentoring students in career planning and development can also be part of an advising program or other select courses, or it can voluntarily be offered and provided to all students with interests that pertain to yours.

For example, consider assisting students who are interested in your areas of expertise or knowledge. During your teaching, make it known to students that you welcome questions about careers in your discipline—whether your field is pharmaceutical sciences, social and administrative sciences, or clinical practice. Students should be encouraged to come to you or your colleagues to discuss residencies, fellowships, and graduate education. Such efforts can have long-term benefits for the student, you, your institution, and even the profession and academy.

Informal Mentoring of Students

Whether or not we accept the role, each faculty member is a mentor for students on at least an informal level. Students will continuously look for direction and advice from faculty on course work, professional activities, careers, and other areas of need and interest. Therefore, faculty need to be cognizant of this role and treat students with respect, be consistent and reasonable, and look for clues to what types of mentoring are needed or requested.

What Are the Benefits of Mentoring?

The major benefit of mentoring is knowing that you have helped someone develop a better set of abilities or choose a career path. You may also benefit by getting assistance in the completion of projects or activities. Finally, you may develop a long-term professional relationship with a future colleague and collaborator.

What Are the Pitfalls of Mentoring?

The most significant pitfall is the development of an inappropriate relationship with your mentee. The relationship should stay firmly based at the professional relationship level. Be sure to make that clear, and make any needed adjustments if it appears that the relationship is becoming too intimate or too confrontational. If needed, you may need to end the mentorship. Another major pitfall is failing to consider the student's perspectives and ideas in developing or revising the goals, plans, and assessments. A mentor's major role is to facilitate the development of the student, not to create a clone or to mandate development in a certain manner. You can avoid these and other pitfalls by arriving at an appropriate and productive balance.

How Do I Assess and Document My Mentoring Activities?

It is becoming increasingly more important to fully document your activities, including your activities in mentoring students. Documentation is much easier if your institution values and describes student mentoring activities. However, you still need to document, assess, and plan your student mentoring activities for your annual review, pre- and post-tenure reviews, and dossier for promotion or tenure.

Summary

Student advising is often a required faculty responsibility, whereas mentoring may be more of an elective responsibility. Student mentoring activities may or may not be separate from advising, and they may serve as an extension of student advising. Advising activities vary and can range from serving as the student's sole advisor to working in partnership with a professional advisor. A successful advising relationship with a student involves setting goals, having regular meetings, monitoring the student's progress in terms of that individual student's place in the educational process, and completing assessments. In a similar manner, a successful mentoring relationship with a student involves setting goals, initial planning and organization, focusing on development in specific areas, following the plan and activities, and performing assessments and revisions in a formal or informal manner. Both you and the student can benefit from advising and mentoring relationships.

What can go wrong and how can you avoid common pitfalls?

References

1. Vander Schee BA. Adding insight to intrusive advising and its effectiveness with students on probation. *NACADA J.* 2007;27(2):50–59.

2. Dunn STM. A place of transition: directors' experiences of providing counseling and advising to distance students. *J Dist Educ.* 2005;20(2):40–57.

3. White ER. Using CAS standards for self-assessment and improvement. http://www.nacada.ksu.edu/Clearinghouse/AdvisingIssues/CAS.htm. Published 2006. Accessed July 24, 2009.

4. Zeind CS, Zdanowicz M, MacDonald K, Parkhurst C, King C, Wizwer P. Developing a sustainable faculty mentoring program. *Am J Pharm Educ.* 2005;69(5):article 100.

5. San Diego State University. Faculty–student mentoring program. http://dus.sdsu.edu/fsmp.html. Accessed July 8, 2009.

6. Haines ST. The mentor–protégé relationship. *Am J Pharm Educ.* 2003;67:1–7.

What Matters in Faculty Advancement?

CHAPTER 12

What Matters in Faculty Development?

Eric G. Boyce, PharmD

Introduction

Why does this chapter on faculty development matter? All faculty (prospective, new, and existing) benefit from the implementation of a career-long systematic plan for the development of needed abilities. Continual, progressive development of these abilities is fundamental to the role of a faculty member. Very few newly appointed faculty members enter an academic position with expertise in all areas of responsibility associated with the position. As such, you will greatly benefit from faculty development at the start of your career.[1,2] As your academic career progresses, you will need continual development to enhance your abilities. All faculty benefit from development in areas of advancement in teaching and learning, scholarship and research, service and administration, and in the roles and responsibilities of faculty members.[3]

The intent of this chapter is to provide answers to the following questions about faculty development:

- Why is it important for an institution and a faculty member to develop a philosophy and plan for faculty development?
- Who is responsible for faculty development?
- What can be learned during the initial employment orientation phase that will be useful in short- and long-term faculty development?
- Why should you consider finding one or more mentors?
- What types of faculty development opportunities exist to assist in the development of teaching and learning, research and scholarship, and service and administrative abilities?

- How should you document and manage your faculty development?
- How will your overall development be assessed and evaluated?

What Is Faculty Development?

Faculty development can be defined as a systematic process used to enhance faculty abilities in three major areas: teaching and learning, research and other scholarly activities, and service (to the university, college, school, department, profession, community, etc.). Faculty development can be considered a career-long journey to enhance our abilities and strive toward, but never reach, perfection.

Abilities can be defined as they relate, in combination, to the three domains of learning: knowledge or the cognitive domain, skills or the psychomotor domain, and behaviors and attitudes or the affective domain. For example, your abilities in the pharmacotherapy of osteoarthritis include the combination of what you *know* about osteoarthritis, its therapy, the drugs used, and the monitoring parameters; how you can *find* and *communicate* information about the patient, the disease, and the drugs used in the treatment of the disease; and how you *interact with* and *approach* patients with osteoarthritis or other healthcare providers who are also involved in the patient's care. An individualized faculty development plan should be directed at helping you enhance your knowledge, skills, and attitudes as they relate to teaching and learning, research and scholarship, and service.

What Is the General Philosophy and Approach to Faculty Development?

Throughout your academic career, you should strive to continue to develop your abilities in all areas in a continuous, prospective manner.[4] This philosophical approach to an academic career is very consistent with the philosophy of higher education in general. Higher education is directed toward enhancing the abilities of students, members of your discipline, other healthcare professionals, and the public. The goals of a faculty development program are, quite simply, to enhance our abilities as faculty. The ultimate goals are to enhance the success of faculty, students, and the institution.

The development of an institutional culture of faculty development is requisite for a successful faculty development program. A culture is defined by its shared values and beliefs, goals, attitudes, behaviors, and practices. Therefore, an institutional culture that supports faculty development will consistently demonstrate behaviors and practices that promote and support faculty development. Those behaviors and practices are built on values and the belief that the continual development of faculty is an important and necessary component of the institution. If the

What is your philosophy as an educator? Shouldn't this philosophy also apply to your own development and the development of your colleagues?

institutional culture is truly based on development, then these same elements should be in place to support student and staff development.

Who Is Responsible for Faculty Development?

Reflective Exercise

Why did you choose a career as an educator? What abilities do you have that will make you a good educator and faculty member?

_____

_____

_____

_____

Each of us, as an individual faculty member, is responsible for our own development. Therefore, you need to be honest, prospective, and insightful. You have the responsibility to honestly evaluate your own strengths and weaknesses and also to recognize that you need to continue to develop in your areas of both strengths and weaknesses. You need to develop a plan for your continued development and be prospective. Such a plan is likely to change over time as you become more knowledgeable and experienced. In the beginning of your career, you have the responsibility to listen to others and learn about how to be successful in an academic environment. It is also important to be able to react and alter your course when needed. Finally, you have the responsibility to be insightful in evaluating your progress and selecting your path.

Faculty as a Whole

Faculty as a whole sets the stage for faculty development in a number of ways. Is there a desire to continue to advance as individuals, as teams, and as an institution—or is there more desire to be highly competitive and aggressive without regard for others? The basis for a successful faculty development program lies in our colleagues. They not only provide support and guidance, but also serve as mentors and mentees.

Department Chair and Dean

Department chairs, deans, and other administrators set the stage and demonstrate the institution's commitment to faculty development.[5] The department chair is probably one of the most important individuals in faculty development in terms of his or her interactions with all department members, as well as his or her role in leading the department. Department chairs generally serve as a sort of mentor to each member of

What are your responsibilities in your own faculty development? Who has the ultimate responsibility for your development?

the department. They also are instrumental in setting up policies, procedures, and rewards, and allocating resources within the department. Deans are also important in faculty development because they set the general direction for the college or school in their interactions with each faculty member and in their actions to enable institution-wide programs.

Reflective Exercise

What do you perceive will be or is the most difficult thing about being an educator and faculty member? What is the most important aspect of your role as educator that you need to understand better?

_____

_____

_____

_____

What Are the Components of a Faculty Development Program?

Are there a set of essential components of a faculty development program? Probably, but those components may appear in different forms from one institution to the next. In general, the components include (1) developing an individualized development plan; (2) orientation upon starting the position; (3) mentoring; (4) opportunities for development in general areas; (5) documentation; and (6) reflection, assessment, and evaluation.

Creating an Individualized Faculty Development Plan

You should consider the creation of an individualized faculty development plan that provides prospective planning but is also flexible to allow for adjustments along the way. It may be best to attempt to formally document this plan, but many faculty mentally develop such a plan and document it only for an annual review or promotion or tenure dossier. A faculty development plan should include a set of long-term goals and a general plan to develop the abilities, experiences, and successes to meet those goals. General career goals will help direct the overall plan. Goals in teaching and learning, scholarship and research, and service and administration will help guide the specific aspects of the plan. Advice from mentors, the department chair, and other faculty are very useful in determining goals and a plan to attain those goals. It will also be important to evaluate promotion and tenure criteria. Teaching and course evaluations, grant and manuscript reviews, annual evaluations, prepromotion or pretenure reviews, and other feedback will also serve as useful sources of information in your development and adjustment of your development plan. As previously noted, it is also important to allow for flexibility based on changes in your goals, abilities, and opportunities.

To help you with the development of an individualized plan, please see **Table 12–1**. This table can be customized to your current situation as a prospective faculty member, new faculty member, or existing faculty member. As you progress through this chapter, consider revisiting this table to reflect on the various components and stages of faculty development.

> Why should I waste my time during orientation? I am ready to start my job and already have a lot to do to prepare for teaching and research.

Orientation Program

What can I expect from an orientation program? Why is orientation important? When you first start your position at a college or school of pharmacy, you should receive an orientation to your position and the institution to help you more completely understand your position and the institution, begin the process of becoming a part of the institution, and hopefully allow for a more efficient transition.[6] You should understand your roles and responsibilities, assignments and expectations, criteria for success, administrative structure and faculty governance, and be able to find your office and the bathroom, the exit, the library, support services, eating and recreational facilities, and the department chair and dean's offices. Initial developmental sessions on teaching and learning, scholarship and research, and select service responsibilities may also be desired and very useful.[4] Orientation is the time to begin to understand and to become a part of the institution's culture.

Formal Orientation Programs

Most institutions have developed formal orientation programs at the institution or specific academic unit level, but these programs vary considerably in length, design, and content. Common components in formal orientation programs include a general orientation to the institution or unit and its administrators, introduction to existing and new faculty, discussion and enrollment in the institution's salary and benefits programs, provision of an identification badge, and perhaps a tour of select physical facilities. A formal faculty orientation may also include initial descriptions of roles and responsibilities, faculty governance, administrative structure, and initial programming in faculty development in teaching and learning. Some of these formalized orientation activities may include online sessions or training, such as Family Educational Rights and Privacy Act (FERPA) training (to learn more about FERPA, see Chapter 11). These structured, formal sessions generally provide an overview of the fundamental aspects of the position and the institution. Formal orientation programs usually begin soon after the beginning of the academic year and may have a short, intensive phase of one to five days, possibly followed by a second phase of monthly sessions during the first year, for example.

Table 12–1 Individualizing Your Faculty Development Plan

	Teaching and Learning Abilities	Research and Other Scholarship Abilities	Service Abilities
Prior to hire • Define each of these areas. • List why each of these areas is important to you and your career.			
Orientation • List your strengths in each area. • List your weaknesses in each area. • List who can help you in each area.			
First and second years • List the criteria for promotion and tenure in each area. • List your goals in each area. • List your initial plans for development in each area. • List your accomplishments in each area.			
Third and fourth years or prepromotion and pretenure review • List your accomplishments in each area. • Assess your accomplishments in each area. • List what you need to do to meet the criteria for promotion and tenure.			
Later in your career • List your accomplishments in each area. • Assess your abilities in each area. • Make plans to continue to enhance your abilities in each area.			

Informal Orientation Activities

A less structured, informal series of activities are needed to complete the orientation process. The goals of these activities are to provide additional detail and structure to items covered in the formal orientation. These activities generally occur in one-on-one or small-group sessions and may more directly target the individualized needs of the new faculty member based on his or her needs, roles and responsibilities, and prior experience. These activities may also be individualized to the specific unit. If you are a new pharmacy practice faculty member, for example, then you will likely be oriented to your practice site as well as to experiential education. If you are a new basic pharmaceutical science faculty member without a background in pharmacy, then your orientation may include sessions on the pharmacy profession and education as well as an introduction to animal use and laboratory safety guidelines.

Mentoring

Reflective Exercise

Do you have a mentor or have you had a mentor in the past? If so, what did you gain from that relationship? If not, why?

_____

_____

_____

_____

A faculty mentoring program is designed to assist a less experienced faculty member in his or her development and may benefit both the mentee and mentor.[7–9] There are many types of mentoring programs and mentor–mentee relationships.[10–12] One category is the designation of a formal mentoring program where the selection, roles and responsibilities, and activities of the mentor and mentee are well defined. Formal mentoring programs may or may not require that all new faculty members have a mentor. Informal mentoring programs may or may not provide general guidelines for mentoring and do not require that all new faculty members have a mentor. Other types of mentorship include broad-based or focused mentoring. A broad-based mentor will provide insights into all the major aspects of a faculty member's roles and responsibilities. Focused mentoring is based on a specific aspect, such as scholarship and research or teaching and learning. Mentoring may be one-on-one or may involve a group of mentors. Finally, it is important to note that a mentee may have more than one mentor.

How can I benefit from a mentor? Can the institution force a mentorship onto me? Answers: A mentor can be very beneficial to provide insights into the roles of faculty and how to be successful as a faculty member. A mentor can also assist in socialization to the institution. Mentorship cannot be forced on a mentor or mentee (the one being mentored); instead, it must be a shared responsibility.

The fundamental design elements of mentoring support the concept that mentoring is for the development of the mentee but is not about the power of one person over another or about forced relationships. Mentor–mentee relationships are best set up and maintained only if both sides agree to develop and maintain the relationship. Effective communication is the key to a strong mentee–mentor relationship. As a mentee, you should listen to and carefully consider the advice or direction provided by your mentor but also be cognizant of the mentor's time and limitations. The mentor should provide the big picture and long-term implications as well as the smaller details and short-term implications to the mentee. Both parties need to realize that the mentee is responsible for his or her own actions. Hopefully, being a mentor is recognized and valued at the institutional, college, school, and department levels.

Later in your career, you may also consider seeking additional mentors based on your perceived needs, direction, strengths, weaknesses, and opportunities. Mentorship can be very beneficial in considering or making transitions into new responsibilities (such as leadership), new areas of research interest, or different phases in one's career. For example, after you are tenured, you might ask your mentor, where do I go from here?

Formal Versus Informal Mentoring Programs

As previously noted, the selection, roles, and responsibilities, as well as the activities of the mentor and mentee are well defined in a formal mentoring program. The selection of a mentor can be random, or preferably the mentor is selected following a meeting between the mentee and prospective mentors. A formal mentoring program should outline the roles and responsibilities of the mentee and the mentor, as well as examples of when to continue, modify, or stop the mentorship. A formal program may also provide guidelines for activities or examples of activities to consider during the mentorship. The duration of a formal mentoring program for new faculty may last from one to three years and then allow for some change in direction.

Should mentorship be required for all new faculty? It should definitely be *offered* to all new faculty, but it is not clear whether it should be *required*. A requirement for mentorship might create a forced mentoring relationship that could actually prove to be detrimental if any of the involved faculty thinks it is a waste of time, counterproductive, or invasive. Alternatively, most, if not all, new faculty members would likely benefit from a mentor during the first few years of their career in the academe.

A formal mentoring program generally provides policies and procedures on the structures and activities that guide the mentorship. A well-written, balanced, and flexible formal mentoring program can work very well. However, an overly directive or restrictive formal program may inhibit the success of mentoring and the mentoring program. Alternatively, an informal mentoring program may allow for a more natural process for mentor selection and mentoring activities. Guidelines are less structured, which may appeal to some, but it may not enable effective mentorship for some of those who need it most.

The most important consideration is to develop a culture that embraces mentorship as a component of faculty development. Each institution should develop a mentoring program that best fits the institution's culture and meets the needs of the faculty. For example, an institution that highly values and strongly promotes faculty development, mentoring, and collaboration may benefit more from an informal mentoring program than an institution that values and promotes mentoring activities at a lower level.

How does this apply to you as a new or prospective faculty member? In your search for a position, try to determine the type of mentoring program offered by the school of pharmacy and identify how that program fits with the culture of the institution.

What Opportunities Are Available for Development in Specific Areas?

Please refer back to the reflective exercises. In the series of exercises, you were asked to reflect on your current role as an educator and identify the specific aspects of your role that you feel least prepared to undertake. Which of the major responsibilities of your new position do you need to more fully develop? What are your strengths and weaknesses? Most likely, you come to your first academic position following success in your prior educational, training, and work experiences. If you were fortunate, your training or graduate program included some development in teaching and learning abilities.[13–15] Few of us are well prepared to meet all of the three major areas of responsibility (teaching and learning, scholarship and research, and service and administration) at a high level. Even within each category, we are likely to have a variety of levels of ability. Therefore, consider planning for the development of your abilities in each of the following three general areas of responsibility. The orientation program and your mentor, if you have one, are excellent resources for your development in each of these areas. This section provides additional methods by which to develop in each of these areas.

Reflective Exercise

Is the teaching philosophy statement that you created in Chapter 1 consistent with the teaching philosophy of your peers, the institution, and your own teaching practices to date?

Faculty Development in Teaching and Learning

What are your abilities as a teacher? Most faculty have little training in teaching when they begin their career in academia. Where can you learn more about teaching and learning? There are so many pathways to enhancing your abilities in teaching and learning. Start with some self-reflection. What do you know about teaching and learning? What is your teaching and learning philosophy? (Revisit your teaching philosophy statement that you drafted in Chapter 1.) Notice that this section is titled "Teaching and Learning." As was discussed in Chapters 1 and 2, you first need to understand learning before you can decide how best to teach. Another way to consider this is that you should learn how best to facilitate learning. Therefore, how best do you learn? (See Chapter 2 to revisit the learning style surveys.) Other items for reflection should include your prior experiences in teaching and your current responsibilities in teaching. Be honest as you determine your strengths and weaknesses in the following activities based on your future responsibilities:

- Lecturing
- Facilitating a discussion or laboratory session
- Writing examinations and quizzes
- Creating active learning exercises
- Grading papers
- Evaluating student presentations or experiential activities
- Creating a course syllabus
- Creating course exercises or activities
- Creating and using a grading rubric
- Managing a class and course
- Revising any of these activities

After each teaching experience, briefly assess your performance. At the end of a major block of teaching, at the end of your course, and in preparation for your annual review, provide an honest self-reflection of what went well, what could be improved, and any specific changes to make or training to undertake. You are now ready to look for some assistance and development opportunities.

There are a number of excellent resources to enhance your development in teaching and learning at your institution. Begin the discussion with your department chair and with other faculty who teach similar courses. Many institutions or academic units have experts, administrators, offices, or centers responsible for enhancing faculty abilities in teaching and learning. Take advantage of any workshops, discussions, or lectures on teaching and learning, particularly those that pertain to your own activities.[16] Well-developed, longitudinal faculty development programs in teaching and learning have demonstrated positive effects on teaching.[17] Experts or centers should also be contacted to see if they have individualized sessions or programs. Many provide direct classroom observation in conjunction with a review of your notes, slides, and other course materials. Peer and student evaluations of your teaching and your courses are excellent sources of information about how to become more effective in facilitating learning. If your college or school of pharmacy does not have a formal peer evaluation or teaching program, consider consulting references on this topic and request assistance from your peers to perform a peer assessment. Be sure to discuss your self-assessment and others' evaluations and assessments of your teaching with your department chair before or during your annual review, and also discuss them with your mentor.

External sources for faculty development in teaching and learning include online and hard copy publications and online and face-to-face meetings. There are numerous books on teaching and learning in various settings.[18] Based on your responsibilities, consider reading books on the philosophy of teaching and learning, active learning, teaching in large classrooms, using technology in teaching, and evaluating students. An excellent book on classroom assessment techniques will provide you with many methods to understand if and what students are learning. There are numerous online resources that provide information on these topics and others as static resources, interactive programs, or synchronous webinars. Pharmacy organizations such as the American Association of Colleges of Pharmacy (AACP), American College of Clinical Pharmacy (ACCP), American Society of Health-System Pharmacists (ASHP), and American Pharmacists Association (APhA) offer programming on teaching and learning at their national meetings. Pharmacy organizations have also developed programs to enhance faculty abilities in teaching and learning, including the Education Scholar program from AACP (http://www.aacp.org/career/educationscholar/Pages/default.aspx) and the Teaching and Learning Certificate Program from ACCP (http://www.accp.com/academy/teachingAndLearning.aspx).

How can you improve your abilities and performance in teaching and learning? How can you measure success? You can improve your abilities and most likely your performance in teaching and learning through experience alone. However, deliberate development in these areas will further enhance your performance. Student evaluations are not always the best measures of performance because they may be influenced by numerous factors not related to teaching and learning that include, but are not limited to, faculty popularity, faculty personality, perceived workload, perceived fairness of grades, course timing and scheduling, and certain student and faculty demographics. However, you should look for trends when making your assessment and considering what to change. Peer and expert assessments of your teaching can be very insightful

What are the requirements in scholarship and research for promotion and tenure? Answer: The research and other scholarly activity requirements are specific to each institution. Obtain and read the criteria for promotion and tenure, then talk to the department chair and senior faculty members to ascertain the reality and interpretation of those criteria.

and valuable. Success is also measured by winning a teaching award or recognition.

Reflective Exercise

Revisit Table 12–1. List your strengths and areas that need improvement in research and other scholarly activities.

Faculty Development in Scholarship and Research

In general, all pharmacy faculty are required to produce at least some level of scholarship or research. However, the level of prior development in scholarship and research abilities is highly variable, making self-assessment a very important component in creating a plan to develop these abilities. The initial consideration is to clearly identify what level of scholarship and research is needed for success annually and for promotion and tenure. Use these assessments to reveal gaps and identify areas in need of improvement.

How can you develop your abilities in scholarship and research? First, consider reading Boyer's book on scholarship redefined and other articles on scholarship to be able to more fully understand the broad spectrum of scholarship and research.[19–21] The next steps will be based on the expectations of your position as well as your identified needs. Consider each of the following as potential areas for development: determining what topics or projects to pursue, developing the research plan, pursuing funding, writing and revising grants, collecting and analyzing data, and writing and revising abstracts and papers. Each of these abilities may be developed in a number of ways.[17] A highly valuable method for development is to work with more experienced faculty, possibly starting out as a coinvestigator or coauthor and eventually working toward becoming the primary investigator or lead author. A careful review of instructions or guidelines for grants, papers, and abstracts, in addition to a review of similar grants to the same agency or articles in the same journal, will provide needed insights. Comments from presubmission reviews by colleagues and from a formal review of the grants or manuscripts will provide additional opportunities for development. This type of experience in scholarship and research is an excellent method of development.

Although there is no substitute for experience in scholarship and research as previously noted, there are other methods to enhance your abilities in scholarship and research. Professional organizations, granting agencies (such as the National Institutes of Health [NIH], National Science Foundation [NSF], etc.), universities, and other organizations provide workshops and training sessions on scholarship and research. For example,

ACCP offers the Research and Scholarship Certificate Program.[22] There are also a number of publications and online materials that are useful in developing scholarship and research.

Faculty Development in Service and Administration

> ### Reflective Exercise
> Are you an effective, contributing member of a committee?
> Could you effectively lead a committee or project?

An often-overlooked area for faculty development relates to the development in service, administrative, and leadership abilities. First, consider defining service broadly as service to students and colleagues, academic units and the institution, practice sites, the profession, and society. Student advising and mentoring may be the major service provided to students by faculty, although some institutions may classify advising as a component of teaching. Student advising abilities can be developed through workshops or training sessions offered by many universities, colleges, or schools; hard copy and online resources; and discussions with faculty or administrators involved in student advising. Some of those same general principles will apply to advising student professional organizations. Service to our colleagues may involve peer review or mentoring. Development in these areas is best performed through discussions with colleagues, a review of institutional documentation on those practices, and consulting hard copy and online resources. Service to your department, school or college, and university includes work on committees (or task forces) and participation in events. There are few resources to help you develop your abilities as an effective committee member, so the best method for development is to meet with other faculty, particularly the committee chair and your department chair. See Chapter 13 for a discussion of how to develop a service plan.

Professional pharmacy organizations offer numerous faculty development opportunities in practice, managerial, administrative, and related abilities. Leadership development programs include the Leadership and Management Certificate Program from ACCP, the Conference for Leaders in Health-System Pharmacy from ASHP, and the Academic Leadership Fellows Program from AACP.[23-25] Many pharmacy practice-based certificate, training, and development programs are available from professional organizations such as APhA, ACCP, and ASHP. The American Association of Pharmaceutical Scientists (AAPS) offers a professional development series during its annual meeting that focuses on the development of many administrative and managerial skills.

> Service activities only get in the way of performing my teaching and scholarship, so why should I care? Answer: Faculty responsibilities go beyond teaching and research and include advising, meeting institutional needs, and approving courses, curricula, admissions criteria, academic standards, promotion and tenure criteria, and other elements as defined in the policies and procedures of the institution. Therefore, each faculty member has responsibilities in service areas.

How Should I Document My Development?

It is becoming increasingly more important to fully document your development and developmental activities. Such documentation will be very useful in assessing your progress and future needs, such as preparing for your annual and pre- and posttenure reviews, preparing your dossier for promotion or tenure, and providing information to support future awards and potential changes in position. The basic methods of documentation include your curriculum vitae and required evaluation documents, including the aforementioned reviews and dossier. Portfolios are more supplementary or elective, but they can be used to more completely document your accomplishments, abilities, and development.

Curriculum Vitae

What is the main purpose of your curriculum vitae? It is an excellent vehicle to demonstrate your accomplishments, organizational skills, and individuality. Be sure to keep your curriculum vitae up to date, but also realize that it may change in form and organization over time. Consider having your colleagues review your curriculum vitae and provide ideas to improve its content, organization, and clarity.

Evaluation Documents

Annual faculty evaluation reports, pre- and posttenure reviews, and your promotion or tenure dossier must generally follow guidelines set by the institution and academic unit. However, these documents usually allow for some flexibility in style but not in content. These documents are used to evaluate your performance and are therefore opportunities to fully document your accomplishments and abilities. Most of these evaluation documents also provide you with an opportunity to reflect, self-assess, set goals, and develop plans to meet those goals. This is also an opportunity to promote yourself, but it is important to be honest. First, be sure to thoroughly review the institutional guidelines for creating these evaluation reports. Then work with your department chair and other faculty to obtain insights and recommendations on creating these reports.

Academic and Teaching Portfolios

Academic and teaching portfolios are methods to enhance the documentation of your accomplishments, abilities, activities, and plans. Portfolios are dynamic and should also include ongoing reflection and self-assessment. The use of portfolios is highly variable in colleges and schools of pharmacy, with extensive use in some institutions and essentially no use in others.

How do you know if you have been successful? Answer: To determine if you have been successful as a faculty member, list your goals and the criteria for performance in each area of responsibility (teaching, scholarship, and service). Perform an evidence-based self-assessment of your accomplishments. Next, discuss your self-assessment and accomplishments with your department chair, mentor, or other faculty (who are generally more senior than you) to determine a balanced assessment of your successes and shortcomings.

How Is Development Assessed and Evaluated?

What are the major measures of your accomplishments, progress, and development? Most of these measures were previously noted. Reflection and self-assessment are most important, should be performed on an ongoing basis, and are the best methods for revising goals and developing plans for future development. It is important to be honest and reasonable rather than overly positive or negative. Your annual evaluation by the department chair can be an excellent process by which to obtain additional information on your accomplishments, your progress in general, and your movement toward promotion or tenure. The annual review process can also help you in setting new goals and developing plans. The department chair should also provide you with assessments and general and specific methods by which to enhance your development and performance in a relatively continual manner.[26]

Pretenure reviews, promotion or tenure reviews and decisions, and posttenure reviews are more comprehensive evaluations of your accomplishments and performance. Pretenure reviews are extremely important in determining any deficiencies, concerns, or needs that you may have in your preparation for promotion and tenure. You can then work with the department chair, your mentor, and other faculty to determine how best to meet any deficiencies or concerns.

Awards and other honors are excellent ways in which your accomplishments, performance, and contributions can be recognized. Consider self-nomination or ask a colleague to nominate you if you have the qualifications, attributes, and accomplishments that fit the award or other recognition, but be honest in your assessment of the likelihood of becoming the recipient of the award or recognition. Your department chair and colleagues may assist in determining whether or not you should be considered for an award. Use this information to continue to plan for and develop your abilities.

Summary

Faculty development is important for all faculty members. A well-developed plan should include development in the major areas of responsibility: teaching and learning, scholarship and research, and service and administration. Reflection, documentation, and planning are fundamental components of faculty development plans. To help you develop a progressive plan for faculty development, **Table 12–2** provides key questions that you should ask at various stages of your development. By seeking answers to these questions and taking a proactive approach to your development, you will be more likely to progressively and successfully develop in all areas of faculty responsibility.

How can you put this all together? Plan, implement, and document your development plan.

Table 12–2 Questions to Ask at Various Stages of Your Development

Questions to ask during recruitment or the interview for the position	• What will be my responsibilities in teaching, scholarship, and service? • Does the college offer a formal faculty development program?
Questions to ask during orientation to the position	• What policies (institutional and departmental) do I need to be aware of? • Is there a formal mentoring program at the college? If so, how do I identify a mentor? • Does the university, college, or school offer support for my teaching responsibilities through a center for teaching and learning or with individuals who have expertise? • Does the university, college, or school offer support for my research and other scholarly activity responsibilities through a grant office or with individuals who have expertise?
Questions to ask during the first and second years in the position	• What is the basic departmental and institutional philosophy of education, scholarship, and service? • Who among the faculty are well-respected for each of the following: teaching, research and other scholarship, and service?
Questions to ask during the third and fourth years in the program or during prepromotion or pretenure reviews	• Am I meeting the expectations for promotion and tenure in the areas of teaching, research and other scholarship, and service? • What are my perceived strengths and areas in need of improvement? • How can I improve my abilities in teaching, research and other scholarship, and service?
Questions to ask throughout your career	• How can I improve my abilities in teaching, research and other scholarship, and service? • What major advances in teaching and learning do I need to know about? • What are the major advances or directions in my discipline and area of expertise? • What are my career options, what appeals to me the most, and how can I best plan to learn more? • How can I plan and work toward my career goals? • Should I go on sabbatical (an intensive period or 6 to 12 months to markedly enhance one's abilities)? If so, what could I do on sabbatical to make a difference in my career?

References

1. Raehl CL. Changes in pharmacy practice faculty 1995–2001: implications for junior faculty development. *Pharmacotherapy.* 2002;22(4):445–462.
2. MacKinnon GE. An investigation of pharmacy faculty attitudes toward faculty development. *Am J Pharm Educ.* 2003;67:49–71.
3. Dean Sorcinelli MR, Austin AE, Eddy PL, Beach AL. *Creating the Future of Faculty Development: Learning from the Past, Understanding the Present.* Boston, MA: Anker Publishing Company; 2006.
4. Draugalis JR, DiPiro JT, Zeolla MM, Schwinghammer TL. A career in academic pharmacy: opportunities, challenges, and rewards. *Am J Pharm Educ.* 2006;70(1):article 17.
5. MacKinnon GE. Administrator and dean perceptions toward faculty development in academic pharmacy. *Am J Pharm Educ.* 2003;67:1–14.
6. Glover ML, Armayor GM. Expectations and orientation activities of first-year pharmacy practice faculty. *Am J Pharm Educ.* 2004;68:1–6.
7. Zeind CS, Zdanowicz M, MacDonald K, Parkhurst C, King C, Wizwer P. Developing a sustainable faculty mentoring program. *Am J Pharm Educ.* 2005;69(5):article 100.
8. Chalmers RK. Faculty development: the nature and benefits of mentoring. *Am J Pharm Educ.* 1992;56:71–74.
9. Campbell WH. Mentoring of junior faculty. *Am J Pharm Educ.* 1992;56:75–79.
10. Morzinski JA, Simpson DE, Bower DJ, Diehr S. Faculty development through formal mentoring. *Acad Med.* 1994;69:267–269.
11. Morzinski JA, Diehr S, Bower DJ, Simpson DE. A descriptive, cross-sectional study of formal mentoring for faculty. *Fam Med.* 1996;28:434–438.
12. Haines ST. The mentor–protégé relationship. *Am J Pharm Educ.* 2003;67:1–7.
13. Romanelli F, Smith KM, Brandt BF. Teaching residents how to teach: a scholarship of teaching and learning certificate (STLC) program for pharmacy residents. *Am J Pharm Educ.* 2005;69:126–132.
14. Castellani V, Haber SL, Ellis SC. Evaluation of a teaching certificate program for pharmacy residents. *Am J Health-Syst Pharm.* 2003;60(10):1037–1041.
15. Unterwagner WL, Zeolla MM, Burns AL. Training experiences of current and former community pharmacy residents, 1986–2000. *J Am Pharm Assoc.* 2003:43(2):201–206.
16. Beza JB, Stritter FT, Caiola SM, McDermott JH, Thorn MD. The effects of a preceptor development program. *Am J Pharm Educ.* 1992;56:44–47.
17. Cole KA, Barker LR, Dolodner K, Williamson P, Wright SM, Kern DE. Faculty development in teaching skills: an intensive longitudinal model. *Acad Med.* 2004;79:469–480.
18. Cuéllar LM, Ginsburg DB, eds. *Preceptor's Handbook for Pharmacists.* Bethesda, MD: American Society of Health-Systems Pharmacists; 2005.
19. Boyer EJ. *Scholarship Reconsidered: Priorities of the Professoriate.* San Francisco, CA: Jossey-Bass; 1990.
20. Kennedy RH, Gubbins PO, Luer M, Reddy IK, Light KE. Developing and sustaining a culture of scholarship. *Am J Pharm Educ.* 2003;67(3):article 92.
21. Leslie SW, Corcoran GB III, MacKichan JJ, Undie AS, Vanderveen RP, Miller KW. Pharmacy scholarship reconsidered: the report of the 2003–2004 Research and Graduate Affairs Committee. *Am J Pharm Educ.* 2004; 68(3):article S6.

22. American College of Clinical Pharmacy. Research and scholarship certificate program. http://www.accp.com/academy/researchAndScholarship.aspx. Accessed July 7, 2009.

23. American College of Clinical Pharmacy. Leadership and management certificate program. http://www.accp.com/academy/leadershipAndManagement.aspx. Accessed July 7, 2009.

24. American Society of Health-System Pharmacists. Conference for leaders in health-system pharmacy. http://www.ashp.org/Import/MEETINGS/Leadership-Conference.aspx. Accessed July 7, 2009.

25. American Association of Colleges of Pharmacy. Academic leadership fellows program. http://www.aacp.org/career/leadership/Pages/default.aspx. Accessed July 7, 2009.

26. Latif DA. Using supportive communication to foster the department head/junior faculty relationship. *Am J Pharm Educ.* 2003;67(4):article 112.

CHAPTER 13

What Matters in Faculty Service?

John R. Reynolds, PharmD

Introduction

This chapter will delve into the world of service, one of the three primary elements of faculty contribution and evaluation. Unlike its counterparts, teaching and scholarship, service is not always consistently valued and rewarded, leaving one author to refer to service as the middle child of faculty roles.[1]

According to Palmer, service provides three distinct benefits to faculty: a sense of contributing to the greater good of the institution; opportunity for valuable interactions among individuals with varying levels of experience within disciplines; and engagement of the faculty member in the community of learners.[2] Additionally, through service, faculty members model good citizenship, which positively influences the professional development of students. When service is constructed as a component of professional development linked to one's teaching and research, it can take on greater value to the institution and may be seen as a form of scholarship.[3]

In this chapter, the following questions about service will be answered:

- What is service and how is it conducted?
- What kinds of service are available to me as an academic practitioner?
- What types of service will matter most in my faculty position?
- How should I develop my service plans and contributions to enable my success?
- What can I learn by providing service?
- How can I relate service to scholarship?

What Is Service?

So you have planned your lessons, thought through how you will deliver your educational sessions and engage students in learning, constructed your assessment instruments, and figured out how to include research and scholarship in your overall workload for the year. Now you have been asked to develop a plan for institutional, professional or scientific, and clinical service. What forms will your service take, and how will you fit service into an already ambitious teaching and scholarship plan? What you may not realize is that the bulk of your academic work, done alone or in combination with other activities and colleagues, may be a form of service to your institution or practice site. Such work may be considered service in that it addresses some type of *need* in your school or college. In the previously noted examples, a major focus of your efforts has been placed on achieving quality in student education. As you look beyond the boundaries of what is commonly understood about teaching and learning situations, you can begin to recognize how your educational initiatives contribute to the broader academic, clinical, and scientific communities, and the profession as a whole. By bringing your energy and ideas about learning strategies, assessment, and educational processes to the table with colleagues, you provide service. This service may manifest in the form of creating or revising a course or addressing a specific curriculum or course-related problem. In each of these ways, you have contributed service to your community of learners.

The definition of *service* in Webster's Online Dictionary includes several elements that are relevant to our discussion: an act of help or assistance and work done by one person or a group that benefits another.[4] In higher education, no uniform definition of service exists. Generally, academic service reflects the role of faculty in sharing their ideas and expertise, either alone or in organized groups, to move a school, college, or practice site forward or to address a short- or long-term institutional need. In higher education, service takes on many forms and is conducted in a variety of ways. Let us look at some examples.

Institutional service is a broad term that typically reflects formal work done by faculty and staff for and at the university, college, school, and department. Such service is often guided by an explicit set of responsibilities and instructions, referred to as a *charge* that may specify intended outcomes, work time lines, and reporting mechanisms. Institutional service often addresses matters of governance and is therefore guided by bylaws, operating policies and procedures, and administrative imperatives. Common names of governance and administrative groups that conduct this type of work include the faculty senate, faculty council, and executive committee. Examples of service groups that have specific functions concerning academic matters include the curriculum committee, assessment committee, academic affairs or standing committee, and admission committee. In all of these committees, specific subcharges may be assigned by a group or a person in a leadership or supervisory position. The subcharge is derived from the standing charge. It addresses a current need, problem, or opportunity that requires a resolution, recommendation, or policy within a defined period of time (e.g., in the course of the academic year, develop a new dual-degree option, create a new technology-based assessment system, or update the faculty development and mentoring program).

Clinical service is a term that signifies work provided either directly or indirectly to help patients and colleagues at, or in association with, a healthcare institution. It is common among individuals in the health professions to provide service that is aimed at improving health through the diagnosis, prevention, and treatment of diseases. Such service may take the form of direct patient care or the development of systems designed to ensure or improve the provision of quality patient care. For example, clinical service may include work in acute care and ambulatory care or participation on a pharmacy and therapeutics committee. Each of these functions involves some contribution to patient care. The term *clinical pharmacy* is useful as a point of reference when discussing specific forms of pharmacy service. As defined by the American College of Clinical Pharmacy, *clinical pharmacy service* addresses the discipline of clinical pharmacy and the associated personnel and roles.[5] Academic practice faculty, as practitioner educators, are often responsible for specific patient care functions and provide related services while teaching pharmacy students enrolled in introductory and advanced pharmacy practice experiences. In this regard, both clinical and educational services are being provided.

Association or *professional service* involves work provided by professionals to their representative local, regional, national, and international organizations and associations. One of the best ways to become involved in the advancement of the profession or your scientific discipline and to become recognized widely for service, research, and academic expertise is through participation in organizations. Such organizations represent specific interests and functions of the professional and academic communities and seek to advance agendas that improve the membership's standing and influence. Political advocacy, for example, is a major focus of many professional and scientific organizations that seek to enhance the involvement of pharmacists in the provision of health care or the expansion of funding for pharmaceutical and clinical sciences research. Achieving success in these areas requires the involvement and expertise of many members who work alone or in groups. Advocacy is offered as only one example of a common service area in pharmacy and scientific organizations. Other broad areas of opportunity include matters surrounding policy development, patient care, and research. One needs only to review the governance and committee structures of the

When should I
move my service
external to the
institution?

organizations to determine the extensive opportunities for association and professional service that are available to pharmacy faculty. Additional forms of professional service include serving as a manuscript peer reviewer or as an editorial board member for a professional journal.

Although service that is external to your institution will often require a major time commitment, it has numerous benefits. First, not only will you contribute to the activities of the professional or scientific organization, but frequently you will also interact with colleagues from other universities and gain new insights and approaches to areas of common interest. Second, if you are interested in attaining an elected or appointed office in an association, increased visibility through committee work will be an asset. And finally, when you contribute to the programs of the association and gain visibility, your institution will benefit from your involvement through the infusion of new ideas and wider recognition of the quality of the faculty.

> *Scenario*: After nine years as a full-time faculty member in a research-intensive university, you find yourself increasingly involved in professional association work and less so in research. You have served on multiple committees with one national association and, because of your strong contributions, you are now being nominated to serve as a member of its board of directors, a role that has great appeal to you. You have achieved tenure and promotion to the rank of associate professor, and it is your desire to pursue promotion to full professor within the next five years. To be successful in this endeavor, you will need to maintain excellence in teaching and funded research. Should you submit your name to be considered for an elected position with the national organization?

This scenario depicts a common occurrence for faculty in the middle to later stages of their careers. The call for service at higher levels in an organization comes with time and experience. Faculty typically build relationships with organizations starting at the membership level. With continued involvement as an active member, you may be recognized by the organization for your contributions and asked to provide a higher level of service. This may involve serving as an elected officer (e.g., president, vice president, secretary, treasurer, regional or national delegate), chair of a committee, or member of an advisory council or the board of directors. When presented with the opportunity for service as an elected officer, the following should be considered: total time commitment, term of office, travel requirements, existing commitments to your college or school during the term of office, and perceived value of the service to your institution and your professional development. In this scenario, because you have already earned promotions and tenure, this may be the appropriate time for you to take on such a significant outside service commitment. The most important steps to take before responding to this call for service are communication and planning. Talk to your department chair and dean to determine their level of support for this type of external service. In this scenario, where you are working for a research-intensive institution, you need to be sure that you are meeting the university's expectations for scholarship and funding. In this example, the department chair and dean may not support the external service commitment because of the demands for research and teaching. You may be more likely to gain their support if you construct a plan that ensures a balance between your existing responsibilities and this impending service commitment.

> The most important steps to take before responding to a call for external service are communication and planning.

Student advising and mentoring is another important service function provided by faculty. The successful educational and professional development of students requires the careful attention of faculty, yet it can occur in a less structured and more fluid way as students move through the program. Some examples of such service include advising students in their professional organizations and associations, career counseling and residency selection, and guiding leadership development activities. Each of these requires that faculty participate in some form of direct advising or informal facilitation. The benefits of such work are evident when you observe students' increased sophistication in their thoughts, behaviors, and actions as future practitioners and leaders. The time commitment for such work varies depending on the nature of the assignment, but usually it is less than that required for more formal committee work. This relates to the nature of the interactions, which tend to be mostly advisory and informal. (See Chapter 11 for more information on your role as a student advisor and mentor.)

Community service involves activities that typically go beyond the academic and practice settings and professional associations and organizations. Community service includes work, often done on a voluntary basis, conducted through local civic and religious organizations that may or may not relate directly to one's expertise as a faculty member. For example, service to a local library's board of directors, a school committee, a recreation council, high school science fairs, or a homeless shelter may or may not tie your expertise in higher education and health to a community need for service, but this type of service is nonetheless important to those being served and those providing the service.

Reflective Exercise

Before we proceed with our discussion of service, take a few moments to list and reflect on your *current* service commitments using **Table 13–1** as a guide. By completing this exercise, you will be better able to determine how service fits into your overall work profile and how to plan your service activities in the future.

Table 13–1 Developing an Individualized Service Plan

List Your Current Service Work (e.g., committees, projects, clinical work, associations)	Who Assigns the Service and Who Evaluates It?	What Percentage of Your Total Professional Workload Does This Represent? Is It the Right Amount?	How Important Do You Perceive This Work to Be for Your School, Practice Site, or Organization? (1 = least important; 5 = most important)	How Important Do You Perceive This Work to Be for Your Own Professional Development and Advancement? (1 = least important; 5 = most important)

How Are People Organized to Accomplish Service?

Service occurs in a variety of ways, from individual contributions to cooperative group endeavors. In the case of individual work, a person may be assigned a specific function by virtue of a job description or a unique strength. Group work, often done through committees, brings together individuals who provide strong and complementary contributions in addressing a given charge. The following are some of the common group forums used to organize and advance service work within institutions.

A *standing committee* functions on an ongoing basis, with regularly scheduled meetings, and usually has a primary function or charge (e.g., curriculum development, assessment, research) with elected and appointed members, sometimes with representative membership guided by bylaws. Standing committees are typically comprised of more experienced faculty. Greater degrees of formality (e.g., use of Robert's Rules of Order,[6] voting on written resolutions, development of policies, compilation of minutes that require committee approval) are noted in the proceedings of standing committees. Such committees deal with matters that often require lengthy discussions and deliberations, particularly when the agenda items have ramifications for the professional and intellectual lives of students, faculty, and staff.

An *ad hoc committee* or *task force* addresses a specific problem, need, or issue, usually on a short-term basis. As a point of comparison, *ad hoc* committees tend to be less formal than standing committees. Members usually volunteer for service based on their interests or position on the applicable matter. To that extent, it is important to have balance on the *ad hoc* committee or task force so that multiple viewpoints and positions are considered. For example, your curriculum committee (a standing committee) may be considering a university proposal to include a new biomedical ethics course in its health science programs. It appoints a task force and charges it to compile a list of credit hours dedicated to pharmacy ethics in schools of pharmacy nationwide. The findings and recommendations of the task force are directed to the standing committee, an administration group, and then to the entire faculty for consideration.

A *focus group* provides ideas, reactions, and perspectives as a form of qualitative study that is often used to formulate a plan about a concept or product. Focus groups are typically comprised of 6 to 10 individuals from outside or inside the institution or a combination of both. The work of the group is typically short-lived and often time-consuming. The group will be given a task or charge to consider and will work in an inductive way to explore the matter, considering questions of feasibility and rationale of a given concept. For example, a focus group comprised of prominent alumni who have succeeded in positions of hospital pharmacy leadership may consider the best ways to prepare future hospital pharmacy managers and directors. They may seek to determine the best practices in graduate didactic learning and experiential learning in preparing future pharmacy directors. The group would conduct interviews with prospective and current leaders using open-ended questions to gather information and opinions about the desirable approaches. Part of the success of focus groups relates to the effective interaction of its members and the generation of new ideas. Other examples of work conducted via focus groups include assessment of the need for and utility of a student-developed honor code or the degree of alumni engagement in continuing professional development.

What Are the Motivations to Serve?

Individuals have a variety of motivations and reasons for providing service. While some are motivated by altruism and an associated regard for the welfare of others (i.e., intrinsic motivation), others do so based on a sense of duty and obligation imposed on them by their supervisors or in association with expectations in their positions (i.e., extrinsic motivation). In many cases, it is probably a combination of both intrinsic and extrinsic factors that motivate faculty to provide service.

Most pharmacy faculty, as teachers and often as pharmacists, possess characteristics of healthcare professionals, such as a genuine desire to help others and an accompanying sense of compassion and commitment. These characteristics may represent long-standing personal values or perhaps grow out of academic and professional experiences. With this in mind, it is

> Motivation and experience play important roles in choosing service assignments.

What does it mean to be a good citizen in an academic setting?

not surprising to see the high levels of service that pharmacy faculty typically provide in academic and clinical settings. It is not uncommon for a new faculty member to eagerly offer his or her service on a committee or task force or initiate a new activity that will help students, patients, or colleagues. As you gain experience in a faculty position, it is important to think about the best ways of applying time and energy to service and how to make the most worthy contributions to those being served.

Relationships can be made between professional and practice service and citizenship service.[1,7] The term *citizenship* refers to the core nature of belonging and contributing to a group or community. In the context of professional service, a good citizen commits time to the workings of the group, takes responsibility for membership in the group, and is accountable. One can easily see how notions of citizenship play out in academic environments. When you agree to serve or are assigned to serve on a professional committee, your contributions are twofold: as a citizen and as an expert in your field of study. Your contributions as an expert in your field are usually apparent to you; however, the goals of good citizenship are not typically stated and are often unclear, especially to new faculty. To make the distinction between professional service and citizenship service, consider the elements described in **Table 13–2**.

The nuances of good citizenship become clearer as you gain more experience. The challenge for a new faculty member is to find the best balance between trying to be a team player (i.e., willingness to help out and be a good citizen) and providing expertise from the aspect of your clinical or science background. As you progress in your career, you may achieve a

Table 13–2 Sample Activities Constituting Professional Service and Citizenship Service

Criteria	Professional Service	Citizenship Service
General description of service	Contribute expertise and knowledge to the committee as a clinical practitioner or scientist	Volunteer to record committee minutes, distribute the agenda, and schedule the meeting room
Outcomes of service	Modify the professional curriculum	Ensure the successful completion of the committee's charge(s)
Measures of excellence	Evidence of improved student learning	Requests to serve again or to be on another committee with greater responsibility; reappointment as committee member or chair
Judgments about service	Evaluations from colleagues; publications	Evaluations of citizenship behavior by other members of the committee

Source: Adapted from Brazeau GA. Revisiting faculty service role—is "faculty service" a victim of the middle child syndrome? *Amer J Pharm Ed*. 2003:67(3):article 85.

Source: Adapted from Braskamp LA, Ory JC. *Assessing Faculty Work Enhancing Individual and Institutional Performance*. San Francisco, CA: Jossey-Bass; 1995:33–113.

closer alignment between your professional service contributions and your role as a citizen, resulting in a greater degree of motivation to serve.

How Should You Respond to a Call for Service?

Scenario: You have recently joined the clinical faculty at a relatively new school of pharmacy in an educationally progressive university. At the first department meeting of the year, the department chair asks for volunteers to serve on a new *ad hoc* committee that will be comprised of full-time faculty, adjunct faculty preceptors, and students. The committee will develop an instrument to measure student performance during advanced pharmacy practice experiences (APPEs). Although you had some experience as a preceptor in your just-completed post-graduate year 1 residency, it was under the direct supervision of your residency director; otherwise, you have no experience in designing APPEs and assessing students in the experiential setting. Just the same, you are interested in participating in this committee because you can contribute the perspective of someone who recently completed pharmacy school and a residency, and you think it will be a good learning experience. You eagerly volunteer to serve, and you notice that only one other person, the assistant dean for academic affairs, offers her name. Your department chair seems disappointed with the response and successfully presses two midcareer faculty members to serve. During the first committee meeting, you again note hesitancy on the part of your fellow committee members when the department chair asks for volunteers to serve as chair and secretary of the committee.

This scenario raises two important questions specific to responding to a call for service. First, as a new faculty member, should you volunteer as chair or secretary of this committee? It is not uncommon for a department chair or dean to get unenthusiastic reactions when a committee is being constituted and a call is made for volunteers to serve. Moreover, members are more hesitant to accept the responsibilities associated with serving as chair (i.e., the person who advances the agenda) and secretary or scribe (i.e., the person who prepares the minutes and maintains other forms of written information) due to the time commitments associated with these positions. As a new faculty member, you may feel obligated to take one of these roles as a way of showing collegiality and goodwill. But be aware of the time commitment and expected level of knowledge and expertise needed to be successful with the work, particularly when taking on the role of chair. As a new faculty member serving on a committee, all that is generally expected of you is to be well prepared for meetings, engage in discussions, and produce timely results. Moving into the role of secretary and then chair of a committee will usually occur as a natural order of progression, particularly if you do good work and are recognized as being a good citizen and contributor. Assuming these responsibilities before you are ready may overwhelm you, thereby compromising your credibility and potentially limiting your opportunities for advancement.

This scenario also raises a second question. Should you have talked privately to your department chair after the meeting rather than offering your service when it was first mentioned? Driven by your interests in experiential education, your strong desire to develop something better than what you may have experienced in your own APPEs, and your desire to be a good citizen, you offered to serve on this committee. But is this a good fit for your talents? How often will this committee meet, and do you know and understand the charge? As a new faculty member, it would be advisable to discuss service opportunities directly with your department chair before volunteering to serve on any committee. The department chair is in the best position to determine whether your service on a committee is appropriate and desirable. By noting the motivating factors to serve and asking about other responsibilities that will compete for your time, a joint determination can be made about whether it is best to proceed with the assignment. In this scenario, a discussion with the chair may have revealed whether his response signified disappointment with the lack of faculty interest in the committee or if there was concern about your lack of experience in the area of experiential education delivery and assessment. Asking key questions will help you determine the kinds of service that will be required and the time commitment. In a discussion with your supervisor or mentor, consider posing the questions listed in **Table 13–3** regarding a potential or actual service commitment.

Table 13–3 Questions to Ask Regarding Service

Primary Question	Secondary Question	Answers and Considerations
What is the charge?	Is it clear and specific, and can the results of the work be measured?	
What is the time commitment and time line?	How much time is required, and is it reasonable?	
Who is sharing in the service work?	Are committee members qualified and committed to the work?	
Who will oversee the group's work?	Is it a supervisor or a peer?	
Who has served in this group in the past?	What was their experience?	
Does the work relate to my expertise?	Will the work help me with regard to professional advancement?	
What motivates me to do this work?	Is it internal or external motivation?	
Is the work balanced with my overall workload?	If not, how should I address the challenge, and with whom should I consult to discuss it?	

How Can You Balance Service Commitments with Other Commitments?

Responding to the multiple and sometimes competing service demands of the school or college, research laboratory, and practice site is one of the greatest challenges for practice faculty. A substantial amount of planning and time is needed to successfully contribute to service at the school or college and practice site. The following scenario illustrates the challenges of serving both institutions.

> *Scenario*: You are in the second year of an appointment as a cofunded (50/50) clinical track faculty member and have teaching responsibilities at a large acute care hospital and the university, but you are still not sure how much service is expected at each institution. Being a practitioner, you understand that most of your service work will be in the area of patient care. For most of your first year, you spent upward of 90 percent of your time at the practice site. The dean is now asking you, along with two more senior members of the practice faculty and a computer science faculty member, to serve on a task force regarding the development of an electronic clinical intervention documentation system. This will involve weekly campus-based meetings for most of one semester and then monthly meetings afterward to assess the program's success. When you discuss this with the pharmacy director at the practice site, she says she understands the value of the initiative but is concerned about any reduction in your clinical service time at the site.

This scenario describes a typical situation for a practice faculty member whose primary service responsibility is in the area of patient care. In this case, the association between clinical work and potential scholarship is evident. By collaborating to develop an electronic clinical intervention documentation system, you as the faculty member have established a link between service to the college and scholarship at the practice site. In this scenario, such a link needs to be explained to the director of pharmacy. In addition, the director of pharmacy needs to be assured that the project will be short-lived (because it is a task force) and that it will benefit you as a practitioner and educator at the practice site. If the concerns prevail, it would be beneficial to discuss the matter with the department chair to determine the best way to proceed. In some cases, a joint meeting with the director of pharmacy and the department chair may be warranted to talk through the details of the project and the time expectations, as well as the potential benefit of the project to both institutions. To build credibility with the director and alleviate her concerns, you should provide periodic updates on the project and note the positive impact that the project will have on the department's operations when it is implemented. Such dialog builds credibility and should facilitate buy in.

General Recommendations and Guidelines on How to Approach Service

As a new faculty member, you can ask lots of questions while you get acclimated. Asking good questions (and getting good answers) is a worthwhile undertaking in that it gets you on the right track early in your academic career. The following recommendations are offered to help you choose and assess your service responsibilities.

Conduct an Inventory of Your Service Work

From time to time, and especially as you begin an academic year, it is worthwhile to list your service activities and determine if they represent part of a reasonable and balanced workload. Faculty sometimes find themselves overextended and overwhelmed with committee and project work. When this happens, they may be unable to fully attend to other aspects of their work, and frustration is likely to set in. Some faculty actively seek out service work because they find it more satisfying than other aspects of their work, and this can potentially be detrimental to their standing and progression. In effect, they get caught in a type of service trap where their teaching and scholarship may suffer, thereby limiting their success in areas such as promotion and professional advancement. As a new faculty member, it is useful to have discussions about such matters with more seasoned colleagues, the chair, or your mentor.

Identify the Expectations and Time Line of Service Commitments

Service is typically done voluntarily or as part of an assignment by an administrator. Department chairs routinely offer opportunities, assign workloads, and specify expectations in areas such as patient care, clinical teaching, and research. Service that is solicited or assigned by other members of the academic or practice communities should be discussed with the chair first. Although all members of the academic community are expected to participate in some form of service, practice faculty often have a higher degree of service by virtue of their work as clinicians. The chair and other persons who assign workloads should specify the amount of time required, in hours or as a percentage of the total workload, before service work begins. The assigner of workload is often the person who evaluates service contributions at the end of the year. As such, it is important to know the specific nature of the work, the expectations in terms of outcomes, the time commitment, and the time line to address the functions or charge, if applicable.

Assess the Value and Importance of the Work and Reflect on Your Motivations for Doing It

Returning to Table 13–1, consider the responses that you provided in the last two columns of the table. The results give you a good sense of the alignment of your own interests within the larger academic or practice community and may help you better understand your motivations for doing the work. It is a useful and often enlightening exercise to see how your interests and expertise relate to institutional needs. In the ideal situation, there is strong alignment between the two and, therefore, the motivation to serve is high. In other cases, a faculty member may do the work because it is seen as something that will help with promotion and advancement, though it may not necessarily be appealing.

Consider the Link Between Service and Scholarship

Service can contribute to your professional advancement in an academic practice position and may constitute a legitimate form of scholarly activity. Brazeau noted that "as an academy, we need to develop processes, complete with institutional standards and expectations, that can guide junior and senior faculty members to effectively document service activities as a form of scholarship for annual evaluations, tenure and promotion and post-tenure review" and that "teaching, research and service are not mutually exclusive activities."[1] *Scholarship*, in its broadest definition, is work that is conducted in a systematic and rigorous way that is held up for critical review by peers through publications and presentations. Boyer notes that service-based scholarship must relate to the faculty member's special field of knowledge and flow out of associated professional activity.[3] Service that reflects good citizenship but is associated with effort outside of one's professional domain, though meritorious, will not generally be recognized and rewarded as a form of scholarship.

Consider an example of how service and scholarship can be related in the area of clinical practice. Let us suppose that you learn about the need for improved medication adherence in a diabetes clinic in the community health center where you practice. As a first step, you identify a team of individuals (e.g., physicians, pharmacists, nurses, dieticians) who share interest in addressing the problem with medication adherence. You design a program that compares patient care outcomes (e.g., HbA1c results) between patients who have been receiving the usual care and those who receive enhanced pharmacist-directed care. By developing a scientifically based method to compare these patient outcomes, you are providing service to patients and may be able to share your findings with the professional community in the form of presentations and publications; it also may provide the foundation for a follow-up study supported by a grant. The opportunities for such practice models as a form of service and scholarship abound in the health care area. Service provided directly to the school or college of pharmacy may also result in scholarship. For example, national surveys conducted by

> How do you integrate service with your scholarship?

curriculum or assessment committees that compare credit in disciplinary areas, as well as benchmarking of assessment systems and innovative teaching strategies, may meet the definition of scholarship of integration and application and lead to publication in pharmacy education journals.

Learn When and How to Say No

Most faculty will experience the challenge of selecting—or being selected for—service. In some situations involving service assignments, you may have the choice to serve or not serve. Saying no to service requests and assignments is not easy, and successfully doing so takes time, effort, and experience. One needs to do so thoughtfully and tactfully, but most importantly with a clear and compelling rationale. Remember that you will be asked to do things in your job that you may not enjoy, but at the same time recognize that your contributions will likely benefit others, such as colleagues and students, the institution, and the profession. The expectation to be a team player prevails in most schools of pharmacy, and academic culture places importance on processes that include both individual and joint efforts. You do not want to be in a situation where you are seen as resisting this mindset. But when the time comes, how do you say no?

Begin by carefully reviewing your workload profile for the semester or the year. Make your own assessment of how balanced it is and how effectively you can attend to each element. Do you think you will be able to achieve your workload goals within the given time period? If not, another responsibility, of course, is going to make it even more difficult. Next ask yourself how excited you are about the requested service work. In some cases, it may be something you genuinely want to do, but you do not think you will be able to give it your full effort. If that is the case and you are not able to work with your chair to modify your workload, you should explain your hesitation, respectfully decline, and ask to be considered for future assignments in this area. If you are not interested in the project, and that is the reason for your hesitation, you should express that to your chair. It is important to signify that you do not think you can give it your full attention because it is not your interest or passion. Realize that when you attempt to decline an assignment, you may get it anyway. Keep in mind that even in cases where you are required to do something you do not wish to do, it could be an excellent learning experience. Finally, an attempt to trade off other assignments in this situation may be a worthwhile approach to ensure balance. A good department chair will consider your abilities, interests, and motivations in light of institutional needs when making an informed decision about your workload assignment. The key is to make

> You can respectfully decline service and still be seen as a good citizen.

cogent and persuasive statements when discussing such matters with your chair and to keep an open mind.

Summary

Now that you have learned more about service, take a few moments to revisit Table 13–1. Is your service plan balanced in consideration of your responsibilities in the areas of teaching and scholarship? What service do you value the most, and is this service commitment in alignment with the mission and goals of your department and school or college? In what areas do you need growth? As you reexamine your plan, consideration should be given to the following general strategies for optimizing service:

- Determine what value your institution assigns to specific forms of service, and participate in those types of service as often as possible.
- Ask for descriptions of service and related expectations.
- Seek advice and mentoring when choosing and evaluating service.
- Talk with seasoned faculty to determine what service roles were beneficial to them professionally and how service can contribute to success in the areas of promotion and tenure.
- Reflect regularly, in writing, on your service and service-related contributions, and note the reflections in your performance evaluations and promotion documents.

Schools and colleges of pharmacy, as institutions of higher education, are complex organizations that require multiple forms of expertise and commitment to be successful in meeting their missions and goals. Schools and colleges benefit from, and often require, faculty members' participation in institutional and clinical service to ensure that goals are achieved. The ideal situation for you, as a member of the academic community, is to find an alignment of your interests and passions with institutional needs in meeting goals. As we have discovered in this chapter, achieving a balance of service with your overall workload is often challenging. By applying a deliberative and thoughtful approach to service, you can gain valuable experience that fosters your professional success while serving your institution.

References

1. Brazeau GA. Revisiting faculty service role—is "faculty service" a victim of the middle child syndrome? *Amer J Pharm Ed*. 2003:67(3):article 85.
2. Palmer PJ. *The Courage to Teach: Exploring the Inner Landscape of a Teacher's Life*. San Francisco, CA: John Wiley and Sons; 1998.
3. Boyer EL. *Scholarship Reconsidered: Priorities of the Professoriate*. Lawrenceville, NJ: Princeton University Press; 1990:21–25.
4. Webster's Online Dictionary. Definition: service. http://www.websters-online-dictionary.org/definition/service. Accessed December 6, 2009.

5. American College of Clinical Pharmacy. The definition of clinical pharmacy. http://www.accp.com/docs/positions/commentaries/Clinpharmdefnfinal.pdf. Accessed December 7, 2009.

6. Rules Online.com. Welcome to Robert's Rules of Order. http://www.rulesonline.com/. Accessed December 6, 2009.

7. Braskamp LA, Ory JC. *Assessing Faculty Work Enhancing Individual and Institutional Performance*. San Francisco, CA: Jossey-Bass; 1995:33–113.

CHAPTER 14

What Matters in the Scholarship of Teaching and Learning?

Donna M. Qualters, PhD
Judith T. Barr, ScD, MEd

Introduction

Our book opened with the phrase "You have chosen the path of a teacher," and as you have been reading, that phrase encompasses knowing much more than just your subject matter. Over the course of this book you have read about student-centered learning; active learning; assessment, teaching, and learning in large classrooms, small discussion groups, and laboratory-based courses; technology; clinical precepting; and the myriad of duties associated with being a teacher. In this chapter we take you to a new place—a place that will bring all of these elements together in a way that will enrich your teaching, your students, your colleagues, and hopefully your institution and profession.

This chapter will help you answer the following questions:

- What is the scholarship of teaching and learning? What is the difference between scholarly teaching and the scholarship of teaching and learning (SoTL)?
- Why is SoTL important today?
- How do you conceptualize an SoTL project?
  - How do you frame a good SoTL question?
  - How do you choose methods?
  - What components are important in analysis?

> The scholarship of teaching and learning . . . means viewing the work of the classroom as a site for inquiry.[7]
>
> M. Huber,
> P. Hutchings

- How do you disseminate SoTL?
- What ethical considerations are there in SoTL?

What Is the Scholarship of Teaching and Learning (SoTL)?

The scholarship of teaching and learning has its origins in the work of Ernest Boyer. His seminal text, *Scholarship Reconsidered*,[1] challenged higher education to think differently about what constituted scholarship. Beyond the traditional scholarship of discovery, Boyer added three other dimensions of faculty work that, in his experience, are examples of faculty scholarship: "The work of the professoriate might be thought of as having four separate, yet overlapping functions. These are: the scholarship of discovery, the scholarship of integration, the scholarship of application, and the scholarship of teaching."[1]

Boyer made the case that teaching, done in a scholarly manner, qualifies as a form of scholarship. There are many definitions of SoTL, but there are common elements that define the essence of SoTL.[2–6] Huber and Hutchings, in their book *The Advancement of Learning: Building the Teaching Commons*, state it most succinctly: "Though employed in different ways and to different degrees, the scholarship of teaching and learning entails basic but important principles. . . . It means *viewing the work of the classroom as a site for inquiry, asking and answering questions about students' learning in ways that can improve one's own classroom and also advance the larger profession of teaching*"[7] (emphasis added).

In general when considering SoTL, we are talking about study, application, and communication of results; deep reflection; and a public sharing of findings about teaching and learning. Although much has been written about SoTL, one point less often made that we would like to emphasize is the *learning* piece of SoTL. It is more about what improves student learning than a prescription for how to teach. Teaching is contextual; what works in one environment may not work in another. The composition of the course, the physical setting, the student demographics, and the teacher's style all contribute to what makes a successful learning environment. Through SoTL, you can examine, question, and study if the input and process elements inherent in a course and the environment produce the desired learning. SoTL asks us to be open to trying change in our teaching and learning system, to be willing to critically evaluate the effectiveness of this change, to engage with others about teaching and learning, and to publicly share our findings.

What Is the Difference Between Scholarly Teaching and SoTL?

Many teachers take a scholarly approach to their teaching. They talk to colleagues, they read articles about new methodologies, they reflect on their classes and make adjustments as needed, they attend workshops, and they ask peers to give them feedback. These are all elements of good teaching, and as Richlin tells us, scholarly approaches to teaching and learning are important if we are to understand learning, enhance curriculum, and assess our student learning in a thoughtful manner.[4] These activities of reflection and revision are the hallmark of scholarly teachers. However, SoTL takes the scholarly approach to a more rigorous level. According to Shulman, "an act of intelligence or of artistic creation becomes scholarship when it possesses at least three attributes: it becomes public; it become an object of critical review and evaluation by members of one's community; and members of one's community begin to use, build upon, and develop those acts of mind and creation."[8]

> Research is formalized curiosity. It is poking and prying with a purpose.
> Zora Neale Hurston

There are a number of challenges inherent in this definition. First, to do SoTL you must be willing to challenge your assumptions about teaching and learning by publicly scrutinizing your own work. Next, defining one's community can be complex. Traditionally, your discipline colleagues constitute your academic community. SoTL asks you to broaden that community to include those from other disciplines who might gain in wisdom and knowledge through your work, as you will from theirs. Last, you must find the appropriate venues to disseminate your work if others are to use and build upon your findings. A good example of this is the work done on cold calling.[9] This was an interdisciplinary effort between communication studies and business faculty to study a teaching method that is now used universally in every discipline.

To be considered SoTL, then, the project must contain carefully crafted research questions, have appropriate methodologies to study the question, and have thoughtful analysis that leads to useful information about learning that can be employed across disciplines.

Reflective Exercise

Reflect on your last year and identify the scholarly elements of your teaching. For example, when did you talk to a colleague about teaching or invite a colleague to observe your class? When did you attend a session on a new idea or technique and then tried it in your course? When did you read anything about teaching or learning? Or when did you join colleagues to explore teaching and learning more deeply? Now reflect on your motivation to engage in scholarly teaching practices—what were the reasons that led you to seek information about your teaching?

_____

_____

_____

_____

> If a child can't learn the way we teach, maybe we should teach the way they learn.
>
> Ignacio Estrada

Why Is SoTL Important Today?

Much has been written about the Millennial student, Generation Y, and the Net generation.[10,11] This literature was prompted when faculty noticed that students of various generations had different approaches to learning in and out of the classroom. Although the differences in the Millennial generation have led to a lot of complaining about classroom behaviors, the reality is that teaching and learning are evolving as technology and cognitive science advance. As teachers, we can entrench ourselves in our current practices and tough it out, or we can try to adapt our teaching to this generation of learners. Faculty must find ways to facilitate the achievement of the learning goals of their students while engaging today's students in a way that is relevant to them; in other words, teaching and learning are changing, and bridge building is necessary if we are to be successful.[12]

Another reason to engage in SoTL involves our professional responsibilities. As faculty we choose our own textbooks, design our own curricula, choose our own methodologies, and decide what content we are going to teach and what methods we will use to assess our students' learning. Because many of us have never studied the extensive educational research on these topics, we often make decisions and choices based on our experiences either as a learner or teacher. In many ways, although we are hired for our content expertise, our work is to teach and to bring the most evidence-based practices to this activity. We therefore have ethical obligations to be sure that what we choose to do results in student learning.[13] One of the best ways to meet our professional and ethical responsibilities is to engage in SoTL.

Reflective Exercise

Reflect on the students you have taught this past year—did you notice anything different about their approaches to the classroom, their learning, or the subject? Were there particular classroom issues that you were concerned about or any challenges you have not faced before?

_____

_____

_____

_____

How Can I Do SoTL?

Because there is no one right way to teach, there is no one right way to examine learning. Faculty who are not trained as educational researchers often feel that they do not have the tools to do educational research. But as you will see, SoTL projects reflect the discipline in which they are conducted, and many of the elements of the skill set you bring to your discipline can be applied to the scholarship of teaching and learning. In the following sections, we will take you through a set of exercises and guide you in identifying an SoTL project in your area of expertise. These are based on the three-phase continuum of growth toward SoTL identified by Weston and McAlpine.[14]

Phase 1: Intention to Grow and Develop Knowledge About Your Own Teaching

Step 1: Identify a Possible Project

In the last two reflective exercises, you identified areas that you have either begun to explore or challenges that you are having with your classes. Now expand on these observations by reviewing your teaching evaluations and write down any patterns you see in the responses over the last three years. Then ask yourself which of these areas you are most interested in examining. Although you may want to answer the big questions in your discipline research, in your SoTL research you want to answer the questions that you think impede your students' learning. For new faculty, consult with a mentor during your first teaching experiences to identify questions that you could examine the next time you have a teaching assignment.

Step 2: Have Conversations

Because meaningful SoTL research has broad applicability and opens up the classroom, begin discussing this topic with colleagues from your discipline, from other disciplines, and from the teaching and learning center. These conversations will allow you to understand the importance of your inquiry, the resources that are available to help you, possible interdisciplinary connections to your idea, and colleagues in your discipline who may want to collaborate with you because they also have the same interests or challenges.

Phase 2: Transition from Thinking About to Discussing and Conceptualizing a Study

Step 1: Choose Your Research Topic

Because any rigorous discipline research begins with choosing topics that are important to the field, so too does SoTL research. Thompson and colleagues outlined two approaches to formulating good SoTL research.[15] The first is the goal approach. Using this approach, you define a goal for your research, list the questions you wish to explore to answer that goal, and create a one- or two-sentence summary of the goal. The second approach is the issue approach. In this approach, you set criteria to study by asking questions, such as, Is the topic investigatable? or What is the

> Somewhere, something incredible is waiting to be known.
> Carl Sagan

significance of the topic? You then consider the length of time needed, the complexity of the procedures, the availability of subjects, and the availability of support. In reality, these approaches are intertwined, and both are necessary to define a project in which you are interested, that is important, and for which you have the resources to accomplish the work.

Reflective Exercise

Look back at your previous reflective writing in this chapter. Based on these writings, choose a topic that you think meets the criteria of both the goal approach and the issue approach. In other words, choose something you have identified that interests you and that you have the time and resources to investigate.

_____

_____

_____

_____

Step 2: Formulate Clear Questions

This may take some time, but the more focused your question, the easier it will be to determine how to study it and what resources you will need. There are many different kinds of questions to consider. Hubball and Clarke list four types of questions[16]:

1. *Context questions.* These questions focus on the critical structures that shape the educational experience, such as course admissions requirements, course prerequisites, or the conceptual framework for a course.
2. *Process questions.* These questions focus on periodic assessments of issues of importance, such as investigating the sequence of course activities or the use of technology.
3. *Impact questions.* These questions focus on results, such as the impact of an educational innovation.
4. *Follow-up questions.* These questions focus on issues resulting from longer-term initiatives.

Hutchings offers four types of questions as well but frames them in more direct language[5]:

1. *What works questions.* These questions seek to identify or validate approaches to learning.
2. *What is questions.* These questions are less about proving and more about describing what something looks like, such as documenting students' approaches to applying abstract concepts to concrete examples and situations.

3. *Vision of the possible questions.* These questions seek to answer the what if scenarios. What if I try to get students to understand the ethical responsibilities in the field, or what if I teach in a way that makes students more empathetic with patients?

4. *Vision of the future questions.* These questions help to formulate new conceptual frameworks for shaping thoughts about teaching and learning practices.

> I never teach my pupils; I only attempt to provide the conditions in which they can learn.
>
> Albert Einstein

What both approaches have in common is the desire to answer an important question about student learning that has significance for a wider audience: What are the conditions that can improve learning?

For example, perhaps in your earlier reflective exercises you identified that students seem to be having trouble with problem solving and critically analyzing clinical cases when patients have several comorbidities. From this, you ask yourself, What can I do to improve my students' analytic and problem-solving abilities? Although this is a good starting point, this question is not investigatible. So now you need to ask yourself, Will incorporating student response systems with embedded small-group discussions in my class improve the students' analytic and problem-solving abilities? From here you need to determine how you will know if better learning has occurred, so now the question becomes, Will incorporating student response systems with embedded small-group discussions in my class improve the students' analytic and problem-solving abilities as measured by their scores on the clinical case section of the examination?

Step 3: Determine the Context

As any good researcher knows, to answer a question you must know what has already been done in the field. The same holds true for SoTL. You need to see if there are any studies or relevant literature that will help you design your SoTL study. In the previous example, you may want to explore the literature on student response systems (clickers) to see if there are any useful studies that can help you plan your study. You might also want to look at literature on the development of critical thinking and problem-solving skills. Another avenue might be to explore the educational literature of other healthcare disciplines to see what strategies they have used to develop these skills. Because you are not an expert in these areas, now is the time to look for help. Find colleagues who may be experts in that field or who may be experts in education, cognitive science, teaching, and learning. Consult and collaborate with the staff in your teaching and learning center. By grounding your study in the literature and research, you will save yourself time and energy as you move down the road toward being an expert teacher.

Reflective Exercise

From the previous exercises, refine your question until you have something you think you can study. Write that question (or those questions) down, and then find a colleague and discuss the question with him or her. Encourage your colleague to ask you questions about your study, the resources you might need, or any concerns he or she may have before you start reading the literature in the field.

_____

_____

_____

_____

Phase 3: Intention to Share Expertise and Develop Scholarly Knowledge About Teaching That Has a Significant Impact on the Institution and the Field

Although initially you may start your SoTL activity as a small internal project, the underlying goal behind the word *scholarship* in the phrase *the scholarship of teaching and learning* is that your findings will be shared. They may benefit colleagues in your institution as well as other members of the pharmacy and general educational communities. Therefore, your SoTL studies should be well designed so that they will meet publication guidelines, such as those set forth in 2009 by the *American Journal of Pharmaceutical Education* (*AJPE*).[17] You should consult these guidelines as you begin to plan, and pay particular attention to incorporating an assessment component into any study that attempts to improve student learning. As stated in the *AJPE* publication guidelines, "For scholarship to be truly revered as such, the outcomes of such efforts must be peer-reviewed and publically disseminated with the intention that the scholarly efforts could be reproduced by others."[17]

Step 1: Design the Study

Now you are ready to begin designing your SoTL study. Your first task is to conceptualize how you will study your topic. You need to think about what kind of data you can gather to answer your question. Our suggestion is that you start with your own disciplinary models of research. Most SoTL research uses a mixed methodology of quantitative and qualitative data, so whatever mode you feel most comfortable with should be your starting point. As you will see, some designs are more difficult to implement than others, but initially, thinking in your discipline will get you started.

Qualitative information will allow you to understand the why behind your study question; it is a more flexible design and allows you to generate a hypothesis. Quantitative data gathering will allow you to make comparisons, to conduct statistical evaluations, and to test your hypothesis. Thompson and colleagues express it this way,[15] as summarized in **Table 14–1**.

As you can see from Table 14–1, most of the work you want to investigate will need both types of data if you are to have a study that captures the complexity of the teaching–learning environment. For example, to study how students use the podcasts of your lectures that you meticulously upload after every class, you would need quantitative data about the number of times the podcasts were listened to and how much of the podcasts the students listened to. You could then correlate these numbers with the test scores students received on the podcast topic. Does listening to the podcast and the amount of time listened relate to the students' test scores? However, to understand how students use the podcasts or why they do not listen, you would need to interview a student and perhaps observe a student listening to one of the podcasts.

Meaningful SoTL involves many methodological approaches from action research models, to case studies, to quasi-experimental design, to phenomenological studies, to an occasional control study. The point here is not to determine the superior design but to choose the design that will help you best answer your research question. However, be aware that research designs with evaluative components are preferred by journals such as *AJPE*.

Step 2: Practical Considerations

Now that you have some idea of the what and the how of the study, you need to be practical. How much time will the study take? What resources will you need to carry out the work? What resources are available on campus to assist you? What will you need to submit to your institutional review board (IRB) before you can start the study?

Here is an example. With the help of your institution's teaching and learning center, you are able to acquire student response systems (clickers). In class, you present a complex clinical case, and then using a series of clicker questions with increasing complexity (each one followed

Table 14–1 Comparison of Characteristics of Qualitative and Quantitative Research Approaches

	Qualitative	Quantitative
Sample	Small, purposeful	Large, representative
Measures	Interviews, observations	Scales, tests, surveys
Findings	Rich, deep	Precise, reliable

Source: Adapted from Thompson S, Nelson C, Naremore R. Toward coherence from alpha to omega in the scholarship of teaching and learning. Paper presented at: Professional Organization and Development Network in Higher Education (POD); October 2000; Vancouver, British Columbia.

by small-group discussion), you lead the class through the deconstruction of the case into its important elements and finally guide them to identify therapeutic recommendations.

This practical approach only required the time to learn the clicker and discussion strategy and was relatively easy to add to your class. But did the students' learning improve? Did they gain the increased analytic and problem-solving skills that you intended? Isn't that the goal of your efforts—to improve the students' learning and analytic skills? What is missing? You do not have an assessment component. Without that component, you cannot determine if the clicker and discussion approach improved the students' learning. You have a descriptive study, but a more rigorous study design should be considered.

Step 3: Collaborate and Share

You identified your question, chose a research design, and did a pilot descriptive study. But now you realize that your study lacked an assessment component. Wouldn't it have been better if you had sought input for your design from the staff at the teaching and learning center or others who, based on their expertise, could collaborate with you to strengthen the study? Be sure to take advantage of the resources on campus or within your institution and collaborate with others in sister academic institutions who have similar interests.

Because it is difficult to conduct randomized controlled studies in the educational world, your collaborators suggest that you consider two quasi-experimental designs that both contain an assessment component. First, you could do a group comparison of the class performance with and without your clicker–discussion intervention. For example, within the same course and with the same group of students, what about using the traditional case analysis in one clinical area (e.g., hypertension) and then trying the new clicker–discussion method for the next clinical area (e.g., diabetes)? Did the students' problem-solving abilities increase with the use of the clicker–discussion approach? How was improvement in clinical problem solving measured or assessed? This design adds some rigor to your study; now you have a self-controlled pre- and postdesign. But it also leaves room for internal validity issues that could lead to other explanations, such as whether the students gained some problem-solving skills from the hypertension cases so that they were more prepared for, and hence performed better on, the diabetes cases (maturation effect). Be careful of assuming that the changes you observed relate only to your new teaching–learning methods.

If you had two sections of the class, you might be able to answer that question by doing a concurrent pre- and postcontrol study. But more likely, you have one large class, so that approach is not possible. Your collaborators

> Experience does not ever err; it is only your judgment that errs in promising itself results which are not caused by your experiments.
> Leonardo da Vinci

suggest that if you taught this course last year, and if the cases and testing methods you used then were of similar complexity to this year's, and if you think the students' abilities are similar, you could consider a historical-controlled design. Notice that this design has a lot of ifs, each having an effect on the comparability of results between the two years as well as the internal validity of your conclusions. But if you are comfortable that the ifs hold true and that the two classes are similar, then your collaborators suggest that you could compare the test scores from last year's class to this year's class in both clinical areas.

Reflective Exercise

What other study designs could you use to answer the SoTL question in this example? Could you incorporate a qualitative component to answer your question?

_____

_____

Reflective Exercise

For your research question, outline the SoTL study process. Indicate the specific questions, study design and methodology, time line in the semester, resources needed, and colleagues with whom you will seek input or collaboration.

_____

_____

_____

_____

_____

_____

Step 4: Obtain Institutional-Specific IRB Guidelines, Write the Study Proposal, Submit It to Your IRB, and Wait for IRB Approval

Just as teaching is contextual, so too are the ethical considerations of SoTL. Conducting SoTL research raises many questions about the privacy of student data, the ability to share information, and the possibility of identification of courses, faculty, or students. But even more to the point, there is a question about the ethics of SoTL data collection. Think of the previous example where you measure the learning effect of a new method that you sincerely believe will produce better learning for your students. As you conceptualize the project, you begin to wonder if you should use a control group. Is it right to introduce one group of students to something that might make their learning more efficient or effective? Conversely, it is right to try something with a group of students that might not produce the desired results? These are not easy questions. Students are not subjects; they are our professional responsibility, and determining what constitutes that responsibility is a deep and serious discussion.

Pharmacy faculty are familiar with the need to receive IRB approval for clinical trial protocols prior to the initiation of a clinical study, but you may not have a similar level of awareness that many SoTL studies require IRB submission and approval. The same U.S. Department of Health and Human Services (HHS) general regulations (45CFR46) apply to the protection of human subjects in research, independent of location and type.[18] Although we do not want to consider students as subjects, for purposes of scholarly investigation of teaching and learning strategies, we must. If the study involves human subjects, defined as "living individuals about whom an investigator obtains data through intervention or interaction or obtains identifiable private information,"[18] and if the study is classified as research, defined as "a systematic investigation, including research development, testing and evaluation designed to develop or contribute to generalizable knowledge,"[18] then an IRB review will likely be needed. It does seem ironic that SoTL activities, intended for internal university purposes only, generally do not require IRB review, but as soon as you want to "contribute to generalizable knowledge"[18] through a presentation of your findings at a meeting or a publication in the literature, you must have IRB approval for the initial study.

IRB approval is not retroactive. You cannot perform a course intervention to improve student learning, find that the intervention was successful, present it to your department head, who encourages you to publish the results, and then submit the protocol to the IRB for approval so that you can submit the study for publication. Although IRB approval is generally not needed for internal curricular improvement and evaluation purposes, when you generalize your results to share them with an external audience, IRB approval is needed. Therefore, the message is clear: if you are going to conduct a well-designed SoTL study, submit your protocol to the IRB for approval so that you can share your findings at the completion of the study.

If you plan to share your SoTL findings beyond your institution, obtain IRB approval before you begin the study.

Several suggestions may help you to become acquainted with these requirements. First, take the National Institutes of Health online course called Protecting Human Research Participants, which you can access at http://phrp.nihtraining.com/users.login.php. Second, learn the distinctions[18,19] among exempt, expedited,[20] and full IRB review and what study design elements would trigger the more rigorous full reviews. Knowing these distinctions is a valuable input as you design your study so that your IRB submission may be handled as efficiently as possible. Third, learn the purpose, content, and alternate methods of obtaining informed consent from students. And fourth, introduce yourself to the staff at your institution's office of human subjects and IRB and become familiar with institution-specific policies, regulations, IRB submission materials, and other documents, as well as the board's meeting dates. Remember that if you plan to present or publish your findings, no SoTL activity should start until you have an approval letter from your IRB.

Even if you believe your study is exempt, wait until you receive the IRB letter stating that the study is exempt before you start. If you proceed without IRB approval, you do so at your own peril. Scholars at one institution collected student data, believing that their data collection efforts were exempt from human subjects regulations as part of a national geriatrics curriculum evaluation. Although the investigators had sent a letter to the IRB requesting exempt status, the letter was not answered at the time of their study. Students complained to the IRB about some aspects of the data being collected. The IRB issued formal allegations of research misconduct against the involved faculty and stopped further data collection.[21] The faculty's self-determination of an exemption status without the independent judgment of the IRB precipitated this unfortunate experience.[21]

Each institution is responsible for ensuring that the submitted educational protocol receives the appropriate level of review. But unfortunately, several studies indicate that institution-specific IRB decisions can be quite idiosyncratic, and the same protocol can lead to different decisions at different institutions. Three brief examples follow: two are in health services research and one is in medical education research. All involve multicenter studies with the same common study protocol, and all IRB submissions were made by the local principal investigator to the IRBs at the participating sites.

In the first instance, a multicenter study of the IRBs at 15 participating sites, 9 approved a common telephone survey protocol through an expedited process, but 6 sites required full IRB review. Several requested changes to the protocol (thus negating a common protocol across all 15 sites).[22] The elapsed time between submission and the issuance of the IRB letter ranged from 5 to 172 days. In the second case, investigators designed a multicenter study to qualify for expedited review status by the IRBs associated with the 43 Veterans Administration primary clinics that were participating in the study. However, only 10 IRBs expedited the common protocol, 31 required full reviews, one rejected it, and one exempted it. Here the review process took between 52 and 798 days, with 23 IRBs requiring that the consent form be modified.[23] And in the third example, faculty at six medical schools proposed to invite medical students to participate in a Web-based

> No longer can the educator or the institutional leadership make the determination that medical education data are exempt from the human subjects review process.[21]
> J.M. Tomkowiak, A.J. Gunderson

survey of the effect of medical school on the students' quality of life. Four IRBs expedited the review of the common protocol, and two gave it a full review; five IRBs asked for a median of 13 changes to the protocol, with 33 percent of these requests being made by only one institution.[24]

The overall message is that if you are going to invest the time and effort to conduct an important and well-designed study involving your students that will likely be of value to the greater educational community, you owe it to yourself, your students, and your colleagues to submit the protocol to your IRB and gain its approval. However, given the variability within the IRB decision process, you would benefit from consulting with the IRB staff at your university prior to submission of your protocol so that institution-specific IRB issues are addressed in your study.[25]

Reflective Exercise

Consult with the staff at your institution's office of human subjects protection and the IRB. Obtain the requirements for the format of your study protocol submission. Do you think your proposal meets the definition of exempt, expedited, or full review status? Determine if and how you will deal with obtaining informed consent from the students. Convert your study outline into a full proposal for IRB consideration.

_____

_____

_____

_____

Step 5: Conduct the Study and Analyze the Results

You have received IRB approval for your research design, and you have located the test results of the students in last year's class on the analytic questions in the hypertension and diabetes sections. Although informed consent was not required by the IRB, you have told students not only what you are doing, but *why* you are doing this type of work and the important role they play in this work. You start the study by presenting the hypertension content in the traditional way and then introduce the clicker–discussion approach with the diabetes unit. You administer the tests, compare this year's to last year's results, and summarize your findings in **Table 14–2**.

Last year's traditional class averaged a two-point improvement from hypertension to diabetes, and this year's clicker–discussion diabetes class had an eight-point improvement over the traditional hypertension teaching approach. Next, based on the sample size and standard deviations, you can determine whether the six-point difference between these teaching methods is statistically significant. With your new methodology, you have improved the design of your study and evaluated the effectiveness of your new teaching strategy.

Table 14–2 Average Class Scores for Analytic Questions in Hypertension and Diabetes Clinical Cases with Traditional and Clicker–Discussion Teaching Strategies Across Two Years

	Hypertension Analytic Questions	Diabetes Analytic Questions	Change in Test Score	
Last year	Traditional approach Mean score = 80%	Traditional approach Mean score = 82%	2-point improvement	6-point improvement in the difference between differences
This year	Traditional approach Mean score = 81%	Clicker–discussion approach Mean score = 89%	8-point improvement	

You also have IRB approval to run a focus group of randomly selected students, and in coding the data you determined that the use of clickers created a more active learning environment. Triangulating your data from the quantitative and qualitative methods, you realized that introducing clickers improved both the actual learning and the learning environment of the course.

Step 6: Write Up the Study

This is the step that often differentiates SoTL from traditional scholarship. You have already been exposed to reflection as a key element of good teaching. Reflective practice is also a hallmark of SoTL work. Hutchings advises faculty to use a format that contextualizes the findings.[5] SoTL is an ongoing process of reflection and improving practice; studies are seen as part of a continuum in which the results from one study often lead to a cycle of continuous course improvement, especially when conducted on a single class or a single segment of the curriculum. Hutchings also encourages faculty to think about the broader context or significance of the results.[5] How does your study inform the larger world of higher education? In the spirit of collaboration that is a critical element of SoTL work, faculty are also encouraged to write about the benefits of their work and how it promotes student learning, then share the lessons learned with their colleagues. Remember, this is a newer form of scholarship, and we are all learning how to do this together.

Step 7: Get the Word Out

Getting SoTL work published can be challenging, but it is getting much easier. There are a number of journals devoted entirely to SoTL, such as the *International Journal for the Scholarship of Teaching and Learning*, *Excellence in Teaching Journal*, and the *Journal of Scholarship of Teaching and Learning*. However, as this form of scholarship has grown, so have the types of publications that will publish SoTL work. Within pharmacy education, the *American Journal of Pharmaceutical Education*, *Pharmacy Education: An International Journal for Pharmaceutical Education*, *Currents in Pharmacy Teaching and Learning*, and discipline-specific journals provide opportunities for publication. Check with your professional organization,

> Follow effective action with quiet reflection. From the quiet reflection will come even more effective action.
>
> Peter Druker

departmental colleagues, and teaching center personnel to find the appropriate journal. A particularly helpful Web site designed by Kathleen McKinney is located at http://www.sotl.ilstu.edu/resLinks/sotlMats/getPub. shtml. This Web site lists 22 excellent tips on getting your article published.

There are many other methods of disseminating your findings to improve teaching and learning. There are newsletters, such as the *Teaching Professor* or the *National Teaching and Learning Forum*. There are also educational conferences with workshops and poster sessions, such as the American Association of Colleges of Pharmacy annual meeting, the Teaching Professor national conference, the International Society for the Scholarship of Teaching and Learning, Lilly Conferences, and the London Scholarship of Teaching and Learning (SoTL) International Conference. In the spirit of SoTL, presenting your work to your home department, college, or campus is extremely valuable in promoting the concept of improving student learning as scholarship. As colleagues learn how this work will enrich their students' learning, a culture can be created that promotes and values SoTL and encourages further SoTL activities.

What Are Other Ethical Considerations in SoTL?

In addition to the IRB issues, what are other ethical considerations in SoTL? When you disseminate your information, you must be aware of your audience and tailor your work. For example, if you are presenting data from your course, be sure that you protect the identity of your students; especially in smaller settings, it is often too easy to identify outliers in your data. We recommend that you do not use SoTL to identify ineffective practice, but always think of your research in the positive light of identifying and improving practice. This approach will avoid the ethical dilemma of doing something you think will not work just to prove that point. For a more complex and complete description of the ethical issues in SoTL, we recommend that you read Hutchings's work, *Ethics and Aspiration in the Scholarship of Teaching and Learning*, from the Carnegie Foundation for the Advancement of Teaching.[26]

Reflective Exercise

Take a moment to consider your SoTL project. What ethical issues can you identify in your project? Who will help you solve these issues?

_____

_____

_____

_____

Summary

Teaching is difficult, fascinating, frustrating, rewarding, challenging, joyful, and mysterious. Yet as professionals we need to approach our teaching and our goal of improving student learning as we approach all of our professional responsibilities—as scholars. The scholarship of teaching and learning is one way to meet our professional responsibilities, grow and develop as teachers, and contribute to the larger higher education context.

References

1. Boyer E. *Scholarship Reconsidered: Priorities for the Professoriate.* San Francisco, CA: Jossey-Bass; 1990.
2. Cambridge B. What is the scholarship of teaching and learning? *AAHE Bull.* 1999;52(4):7–10.
3. Kreber C, Cranton PA. Exploring the scholarship of teaching. *J Higher Educ.* 2000;71(4):476–495.
4. Richlin L. Scholarly teaching and the scholarship of teaching. In: Kreber C, ed. *Scholarship Revisited: Perspectives on the Scholarship of Teaching and Learning.* San Francisco, CA: Jossey-Bass; 2001:57–68
5. Hutchings P. Approaching the scholarship of teaching and learning. In Hutchings P, ed. *Opening Lines: Approaches to the Scholarship of Teaching and Learning.* Menlo Park, CA: Carnegie Foundation for the Advancement of Teaching; 2000:1–10.
6. Martin E, Benjamin J, Prosser M, Trigwell K. Scholarship of teaching: a study of the approaches of academic staff. In Rust C, ed. *Improving Student Learning: Improving Student Learning Outcomes.* Oxford, England: Oxford Centre for Staff Learning and Development, Oxford Brookes University; 1999: 326–331.
7. Huber M, Hutchings P. *The Advancement of Learning: Building the Teaching Commons.* San Francisco, CA: Jossey-Bass; 2005.
8. Shulman L. Taking learning seriously. *Change.* 1999;31:10–17.
9. Dallimore E, Hertenstein J, Platt M. Classroom participation and discussion effectiveness: student-generated strategies. *Commun Educ.* 2004;53:1–11.
10. Twenge J. *Generation Me.* New York, NY: Free Press; 2006.
11. Oblinger DG, Oblinger JL, eds. *Educating the Net Generation.* Washington, DC. EDUCAUSE; 2005. http://www.educause.edu/books/educatingthenetgen/5989. Accessed June 12, 2009.
12. Qualters, D. Building bridges to learning. Keynote address to the Learning Assistance Association of New England (LAANE); October 2007; Wellesley, MA.
13. Pecorino P, Kincaid S. Why should I care about SoTL? The professional responsibilities of post-secondary educators. *Int J Scholarsh Teach Learn.* 2007: 1(2). http://www.georgiasouthern.edu/ijsotl/current.htm. Accessed June 15, 2009.
14. Weston C, McAlpine L. Making explicit the development toward the scholarship of teaching. *N Dir Teach Learn.* 2001;86:89.
15. Thompson S, Nelson C, Naremore R. Toward coherence from alpha to omega in the scholarship of teaching and learning. Paper presented at: Professional Organization and Development Network in Higher Education (POD); October 2000; Vancouver, British Columbia.

16. Hubball H, Clarke T. Diverse methodological approaches and considerations for SoTL in higher education. http://www.cte.hawaii.edu/handouts/ CJSoTL_Paper.pdf. Accessed November 16, 2009.

17. Poirier T, Crouch M, MacKinnon G, Mehvar M, Monk-Tutor M. Updated guidelines for manuscripts describing instructional design and assessment: the IDEAS format. *Am J Pharm Educ.* 2009;73(3):article 55.

18. US Department of Health and Human Services, Office for Human Research Protections. Title 45 part 46. Basic HHS policy for protection of human subjects. www.hhs.gov/ohrp/humansubjects/guidance/45cfr46.htm. Accessed January 15, 2010.

19. US Department of Health and Human Services. Office for Human Research Protection (OHRP). Human subjects regulations decision charts. www.hhs.gov/ohrp/humansubjects/guidance/decisioncharts.htm. Accessed January 15, 2010.

20. US Department of Health and Human Services, Office for Human Research Protections. Categories of research that may be reviewed by the institutional review board (IRB) through an expedited review. www.hhs.gov/ohrp/humansubjects/guidance/expedited98.htm. Accessed January 15, 2010.

21. Tomkowiak JM, Gunderson AJ. To IRB or not to IRB? *Acad Med.* 2004; 79:628–632.

22. Dziak K, Anderson R, Sevick MA et al. Variations among institutional review board reviews in a multisite health services research study. *Health Serv Res.* 2005;40:279–290.

23. Green LA, Lowery JC, Kowalski CP, Wyszewlanski L. Impact of institutional review board practice variation on observational health services research. *Health Serv Res.* 2006;41;214–230.

24. Dyrbye LN, Thomas MR, Mechaber AJ et al. Medical education research and IRB review: an analysis and comparison of the IRB review process at six institutions. *Acad Med.* 2007;82:654–660.

25. Henry RC, Wright DE. When do medical students become human subjects of research? The case of program evaluation. *Acad Med.* 2001;76:871–875.

26. Hutchings PA. Ethics and aspiration in the scholarship of teaching and learning. http://www.carnegiefoundation.org/elibrary/docs/ethics_of_inq-intro.pdf. Accessed April 6, 2010.

Additional Resources

1. A PowerPoint tutorial on SoTL with audio description supplements and faculty project examples is provided online by the International Society for the Scholarship of Teaching and Learning at http://www.issotl.org/tutorial/sotltutorial/intro/intr01.html.

2. Murray R, ed. *The Scholarship of Teaching and Learning in Higher Education.* Berkshire, England: Open University Press, McGraw-Hill Education; 2008.

3. US Department of Health and Human Services, Office of Inspector General. Institutional review boards: a time for reform. http://oig.hhs.gov/oei/reports/oei-01-97-00193.pdf. Accessed January 15, 2010.

4. Byerly WG. Working with the institutional review board. *Am J Health Syst Pharm.* 2009;66:176–184.

Index

A

AACP. *See* American Association of Colleges of Pharmacy

abilities, 274

abilities-based outcomes (ABOs)
definition of, 89
as input for systems approach to developing topic-specific longitudinal curricular content, 75

ABIM. *See* American Board of Internal Medicine

ABOs. *See* abilities-based outcomes

abstract conceptualization, in experiential learning, 200–201

academic advising, 255–257

Academic Leadership Fellows Program, 285

academic portfolios, 286

accountability, assessment for, 85, 87

ACCP. *See* American College of Clinical Pharmacy

ACCP Academy Teaching and Learning Certificate Program, for preceptors, 205–206

ACCP Professional Experience Program Library of Resources, for preceptors, 206

Accreditation Council for Pharmacy Education (ACPE)
experiential education goals set by, 203
pharmacy education program standards set by, 77–78, 100, 176
professionalism and, 232

Accreditation Standards and Guidelines for the Professional Program in Pharmacy Leading to the Doctor of Pharmacy Degree (ACPE), 77–78

ACPE. *See* Accreditation Council for Pharmacy Education

active experimentation, in experiential learning, 200–201

active learning
in experiential education, 210
high-threshold strategies for, 125–126
for laboratory learning and teaching, 179–182, 186
in laboratory settings, 176
in large classroom teaching, 106–111, 116–126
in lectures, 108–111
low-threshold strategies for, 119–123
medium-threshold strategies for, 123–125
strategies for, 128
student push back against, 127–128
in systems approach to teaching a class, 67–68
in teaching and learning relationship, 7

active–reflective dimension, of Felder's Dimensions of Learning Style, 39–40

activities, within large classes, 121

actors, for laboratory learning and teaching, 187–188

ad hoc committee, 296–297

A.D.A.M. computer simulations, 189

adjourning, of groups, 162

administration, faculty development in, 285

administrators, faculty development and, 275–276

admission process, professionalism and, 235

advanced pharmacy practice experiences (APPEs), 197–222, 265
assessment for entry into, 208–209
assessment tools and instruments for, 217–219
characteristics of, 204
curriculum allocation to, 197
feedback in, 220–221
goals of, 203

advanced pharmacy practice experiences
(APPEs) (*Continued*)
    outcome statements for, 206–207
    practice environment for, 203–206
    setting realistic expectations for, 207–209
adverse drug reporting, professionalism
        development and, 240
advising, student; *See also* faculty advisor
    academic, 255–257
    benefits of, 261
    distance, 258
    of distressed students, 258–259
    goals of, 254
    of graduate and professional students, 260
    introduction to, 251
    intrusive, 256, 258
    legal aspects of, 260–261
    mentoring *v.*, 251–252
    philosophy of, 252–253
    pitfalls of, 261–262
    resources for, 262–263
    roles and responsibilities in, 254–255,
        261–262
    as service, 285, 295
    sources of information for, 253
    summary for, 269
    types to provide, 255–260
affective learning domain, 28–31
    personal inventory of, 47
    in student-centered teaching, 32
aim
    of a class, 63–64
    of a course, 71
    of curriculum review, 76
    in systems approach, 59
    of topic-specific longitudinal curricular
        content, 73
American Association of Colleges of Pharmacy
        (AACP)
    2009 Curricular Change Summit white
        papers of, 78
    CAPE Educational Outcomes of, 76, 190
    faculty development resources from, 283
    leadership development with, 285
American Board of Internal Medicine (ABIM),
        professionalism according to, 229
American College of Clinical Pharmacy
        (ACCP)
    experiential education goals set by, 203
    faculty development resources from, 283

    leadership development with, 285
    professionalism according to, 230
    scholarship and research and, 284–285
American Pharmacists Association (APhA),
        faculty development resources from, 283
American Society of Health-System
        Pharmacists (ASHP)
    faculty development resources from, 283
    leadership development with, 285
analyzing stage, of cognitive learning domain,
        29
annual review process, of faculty development,
        287
APhA. *See* American Pharmacists Association
APPEs. *See* advanced pharmacy practice expe-
        riences
application, in laboratory learning and teaching,
        177
application-based learning, 155
applying stage, of cognitive learning domain,
        29
ASHP. *See* American Society of Health-System
        Pharmacists
assembly effects, 156–157
assessment, 85–100
    for APPEs, 217–219
    of course, 88, 96–100
    of curriculum, 98–100
    definition of, 87–91
    for entry into IPPEs and APPEs, 208–209
    in experiential education, 217–220
    of faculty, 283–284, 287
    of faculty mentor, 268
    of instruction, 96–100
    introduction to, 85–86
    for IPPEs, 217–219
    in laboratory learning and teaching,
        183–186, 188, 192–193
    levels of, 87–88
    models of, 89–91
    of patients, 180–181
    of preceptor, 220
    professionalism and, 231–233, 242–244
    purpose of, 85, 87
    in small-group teaching and learning,
        166–167
    of student mentoring, 268
    in systems approach to teaching a class, 69
    of teacher, 96–100
    techniques and tools of, 91–98

technology for, 148–150
terms and concepts associated with, 87–97
timing of, 219
use of technology in, 133
association service, 293–295
Astin's inputs, environment, outcomes model, 89
attention span, of today's students, 110–111
attitudes, in learning, 30–31
attitudinal attributes, of professionalism, 230
attributes, of faculty mentor, 265–266
audience response systems, 242
    for classroom assessment, 97, 148–149
    evidence for use of, 124
    for large classes, 123–125
Austin's Pharmacists' Inventory of Learning Styles (PILS), 41–44, 54–56
    in integrated theory and educational model, 47–50
    in student-centered teaching, 43–44
awards, for faculty assessment, 287

B
Baby Boomers, teaching of, 45
Becoming a Critically Reflective Teacher (Brookfield), critical reflection defined by, 18
behavioral attributes, of professionalism, 230–231
beliefs, in learning, 30–31
benchmark, 89
bidirectional relationship, of teaching and learning, 8
blended learning, 147
    for active learning in large classes, 125
Bloom's Taxonomy, 28–33, 47–50
    cognitive learning domain in, 28–30, 32
    in experiential education, 208
    in integrated theory and educational model, 47–50
    for professionalism development, 232
    psychomotor learning domain in, 28–30, 32
    in student-centered teaching, 32–33
    in systems approach to teaching a class, 67–68
bookending of lectures, for large classes, 120–121
Boyer, Ernest, 308
brain, learning effects on, 115

broad-based mentoring, 279
business orientation, of pharmacists, 228–229
buzz group strategy, 165

C
CAPE. *See* Center for the Advancement of Pharmaceutical Education
capstone projects, for active learning in large classes, 125–126
career
    individualized faculty development program for, 276–278
    mentoring for, 264–265, 267–268
case-based learning, 155
CATs. *See* classroom assessment techniques
Center for the Advancement of Pharmaceutical Education (CAPE), 2004 Educational Outcomes of, 76, 190
checklist, for assessment in experiential education, 218
Chickering and Gamson seven principles for good practice in undergraduate education, 10
    for large classes, 112
    for Millennials, 46
Chickering and Reisser's Seven Vectors, 52
Chronicle of Higher Education, as resource for technology implementation, 138
circular questioning, 165
citizenship service, 298–299
civility
    in classroom, 237–238
    professionalism *v.*, 231
class
    aim of, 63–64
    components of, 64–70
    input elements of, 65–67
    output elements of, 65, 68–70
    process elements of, 65, 67–68
    systems approach to teaching of, 62–70
class size, professionalism and, 236–238
classroom; *See also* large classroom teaching
    civility in, 237–238
    as input for systems approach to teaching a class, 66
    as input for systems approach to teaching a course, 71
    management of, 236–238
    wired, 138

classroom assessment techniques (CATs), 96–97

classroom response systems. *See* audience response systems

clickers. *See* audience response systems

clinical pharmacy, 293

clinical service, 293

close-ended discussions, 168

coaching, in experiential education, 211, 214

Code of Ethics for Pharmacists, 230

cognitive development
    in experiential education, 208
    intellectual ability *v.*, 26
    professionalism and, 232
    progression of, 33–35

cognitive learning domain, 28–30
    personal inventory of, 47
    in student-centered teaching, 32

cognitive maps, for laboratory learning and teaching, 177

cognitive psychology, teaching insights from, 114–115

cognitive theories of learning, 33–38
    in integrated theory and educational model, 47–50
    Kitchner and King's Reflective Judgment Model, 36–38, 47–50
    Perry's Schemes of Intellectual and Ethical Development, 33–36, 47–50

cohesiveness, in groups, 157–158

collaboration, in SoTL, 316–317

collaborative learning activities, for active learning in large classes, 125–126

college mission, professionalism development and, 234

commitment in relativism, in Perry's Schemes of Intellectual and Ethical Development, 34–35

committees, 296–297

communication, in groups, 157–158

community education, professionalism development and, 240

community service, 295

competency, 89

components, of classes, 64–70

compounding, professionalism development and, 240

compounding laboratories, 189–191

computer simulations, in laboratory learning and teaching, 189–190

concrete experience, in experiential learning, 200–201

Conference for Leaders in Health-System Pharmacy, 285

conflict, in small-group teaching and learning, 161, 169–171

connectedness, in effective teaching, 13

constructivism theory
    in experiential education, 200
    learning process explained by, 27–28
    teaching based on, 7

content
    as input for systems approach to developing topic-specific longitudinal curricular content, 73–75
    as input for systems approach to teaching a class, 66–67
    as input for systems approach to teaching a course, 72–73
    as process for systems approach to teaching a class, 67

context determination, for SoTL, 313

context questions, 312

continual refinement stage, of psychomotor learning domain, 30

continuity, in experiential education, 199–200

contracts, for group work and learning, 163

conversations, for SoTL, 311

cooperative learning, for active learning in large classes, 125–126

coordinating stage, of psychomotor learning domain, 30

corroborating evidence, for assessment, 96

The Courage to Teach (Palmer)
    good teaching defined by, 15
    questions for developing a teaching philosophy, 19

course
    aim of, 71
    assessment of, 88, 96–100
    definition of, 70
    input elements of, 71–73
    as input for systems approach to teaching a class, 66
    systems approach to teaching of, 70–73

course coordinator, for laboratory learning and teaching, 187

course mapping, for laboratory learning and teaching, 179, 186

course work, student mentoring for, 267

creating stage, of cognitive learning domain, 29

creators, in Austin's PILS, 56

critical reflection, as effective teacher trait, 18

critiquing stage, of cognitive learning domain, 29

cross-disciplinary curriculum projects, systems approach to, 79

crossover strategy, 165

curriculum mapping, 73, 100

curriculum review, 98–100
    aim of, 76
    input elements of, 76–80
    systems approach to, 75–80

curriculum vitae, 286

cycle of teaching and learning, 6–8

D

dean, faculty development and, 275–276

democratic discussion, in small-group teaching and learning, 158

department chair, faculty development and, 275–276

development
    faculty advisor and, 255
    of professionalism, 227–246

development level, intellectual ability *v.*, 26

developmental psychology, teaching insights from, 114–115

Dewey's theory of experiential education, 199–200

didactic course work, professionalism and, 235–236

digital capture, of class delivery, 147–148

direct assessment, 88
    techniques and tools of, 91–95

directors, in Austin's PILS, 55

discussion
    in experiential education, 210
    in large classes, 119–122
    open-ended *v.* closed-ended, 168
    patient, 240
    in small-group teaching and learning, 158

dispensing, professionalism development and, 240

distance advising, 258

distance learning, 142–143
    professional socialization and, 242
    professionalism and, 241–242

distressed students, faculty advisor and, 258–259

doing–reflecting dimension, of Austin's PILS, 41–42, 44

domains of learning. *See* learning domains

dualism, in Perry's Schemes of Intellectual and Ethical Development, 34–35

E

ECAs. *See* extracurricular activities

Education Scholar, for preceptor training, 205

educator-centered teaching. *See* teacher-centered teaching

Educause, as resource for technology implementation, 138

effective teaching and learning, 3–21
    common ideas on what constitutes effectiveness, 12–13
    evidence on what constitutes effectiveness, 10–12
    introduction to, 3–4
    teacher characteristics needed for, 9–18
    teaching *v.* learning, 4–8
    tools for drafting a teaching philosophy statement, 19–21

e-folios, 149–150

empathy assignment, professionalism development and, 240

enactors, in Austin's PILS, 55

end-of-lecture summaries, for large classes, 120

engagement; *See also* interactive engagement
    for effective teaching, 14–15
    in large classes, 118–126
    student push back against, 127–128

environment; *See also* external environment
    for experiential education, 203–206
    as input for systems approach to teaching a class, 66
    for laboratory learning and teaching, 177
    in laboratory teaching and learning, 185–186
    learning, 135–137
    in small-group teaching and learning, 156, 171–172

e-professionalism, 241–242

equipment, for laboratory learning and teaching, 186–187

ethical development, progression of, 33–35

evaluating stage, of cognitive learning domain, 29

evaluation. *See* assessment
evaluation documents, 286
examination
    for direct assessment, 91–92
    in laboratory learning and teaching, 183
    online, 149–150
    in systems approach to teaching a class, 69
experiential education, 197–222
    assessment for entry into IPPEs and
        APPEs, 208–209
    assessment in, 217–220
    definition of, 198–199
    design of, 203–209
    feedback in, 220–221
    goals of, 203
    mapping of, 198–199
    One-Minute Preceptor technique in,
        213–217
    outcomes-focused, 206–207
    practice environment for, 203–206
    preceptor role in, 198, 200–201, 209–212
    principles of, 199–202
    setting realistic expectations within,
        207–209
    Socratic method of teaching in, 212–214
    strategies for promoting learning in,
        212–217
    summary of, 222
experiential learning cycle, 202
experiential programs, professionalism and,
    239–241
experimentation, in laboratory learning and
    teaching, 177
expert assessments, for faculty assessment,
    283–284
external environment
    as input for systems approach to curricu-
        lum review, 76–79
    as input for systems approach to developing
        topic-specific longitudinal curricular
        content, 74
    of system, 62, 64
external review, teacher openness to, 18
extracurricular activities (ECAs), professional-
    ism and, 238–239

F
facilitation, in experiential education, 211–212
facilitator, in small-group teaching and
    learning, 155–158, 163–166

faculty
    as input for systems approach to teaching a
        course, 72
    in professionalism development, 241
    technology use by, 138–140
faculty advisor
    development and, 255
    distressed students and, 258–259
    family issues and, 257
    financial issues and, 257
    graduate students and, 260
    mental health and, 257–259
    personal issues and, 257
    physical health and, 257
    professional advisor training of, 263
    professional students and, 260
    relationship issues and, 257
    roles and responsibilities of, 254–255,
        261–262
    self-assessment and, 256
    social skills and, 257
    study skills and, 257
    time-management skills and, 257
faculty development
    assessment and evaluation of, 287
    definition of, 274
    introduction to, 273–274
    maintaining documentation of, 286
    philosophy and approach to, 274–275
    program components for, 276–281
    questions for stages of, 288
    responsibilities for, 275–276
    in scholarship and research, 284–285
    in service and administration, 285
    specific area opportunities, 281–285
    summary for, 287–288
    in teaching and learning, 282–284
faculty development program, 276–281
    individualized, 276–278
    mentoring, 279–280
    orientation program, 277–279
faculty mentor
    assessment and documentation for,
        268
    attributes of, 265–266
    benefits for, 268
    benefits to, 263–264
    mentoring types for, 266–268
    pitfalls for, 268
    program components for, 267

roles and responsibilities in, 264–265
starting as, 266
faculty mentoring program, 279–280
formal *v.* informal, 280–281
faculty service. *See* service
Family Educational Rights and Privacy Act
(FERPA)
student records and, 260
training for, 277
family issues, faculty advisor and, 257
feedback
in experiential education, 220–221
in laboratory learning and teaching, 177,
191–192
in systems approach to teaching a class, 69
on teaching, courses, and curriculum,
96–99
via One-Minute Preceptor technique,
216–217
feedback sandwich, 221
Felder's Dimensions of Learning Style, 39–41
active–reflective dimension in, 39–40
inductive–deductive dimension in, 39–40
sensory–intuitive dimension in, 39–40
visual–verbal dimension in, 39–40
FERPA. *See* Family Educational Rights and
Privacy Act
financial issues, faculty advisor and, 257
fishbowl strategy, 165
fixed standards, for assessment in laboratory
learning and teaching, 184
focus group, 297
focused mentoring, 279
follow-up questions, 312
forced choice examination, 91–92
formal mentoring, 279–281
formative assessment, 87
in experiential education, 219
in small-group teaching and learning,
166–167
forming, of groups, 160
free response examination, 91–92

G
games, for learning assessment, 149
General Systems Theory (von Bertalanffy), systems approach defined by, 58–59
generation, learning influenced by, 44–46
Generation X, teaching of, 45
Generation Y. *See* Millennials

goal(s); *See also* aim
definition of, 88
of experiential education, 203
for small-group teaching and learning session, 168
in systems approach, 59
graduate students, faculty advisor and, 260
group(s)
configuration of, in small-group teaching
and learning, 156–157
conflict in, 161, 169–171
developing contracts for work in, 163
discussion, in large classes, 119–120
getting learning started in, 158–159
process roles within, 157
size of, in small-group teaching and learning, 156
stages of formation of, 160–162
structure of, in small-group teaching and
learning, 157
group capstone projects, for active learning in
large classes, 125–126
group round strategy, 164–165
group work
contracts, 163
for service, 296–297
group-based assessment, 167

H
handouts, for lectures, 110
hardware, for use in education, 139–140
Health and Human Services (HHS), SoTL
and, 318
honors, for faculty assessment, 287
horseshoe strategy, 166
humanism, as effective teacher trait, 17
humor, in teaching, 159, 171–172
hybrid learning. *See* blended learning

I
IE. *See* interactive engagement
imitating stage, of psychomotor learning
domain, 30
impact questions, 312
implementing stage, of cognitive learning
domain, 29
improvement
assessment for, 85, 87
in experiential education, 220
in laboratory learning and teaching, 191–192

in-class discussion, in large classes, 119–122

independent learning, in experiential learning, 201

indirect assessment, 88
  techniques and tools of, 95–96

individualized faculty development program, 276–278

inductive–deductive dimension, of Felder's Dimensions of Learning Style, 39–40

informal mentoring, 279–281

inputs
  in systems approach to curriculum review, 76–80
  in systems approach to developing topic-specific longitudinal curricular content, 73–75
  in systems approach to teaching a class, 65–67
  in systems approach to teaching a course, 71–73

institution, assessment of, 88

institutional culture, of faculty development, 274–275

institutional good practices, 112–116

institutional review board (IRB)
  SoTL considerations for, 315–316
  SoTL submission to, 317–320

institutional service, 292–293

instruction. *See* teaching

instructor. *See* teacher

integrated practice skills laboratory. *See* laboratory learning and teaching

integrated theory and educational model, of student-centered teaching, 46–50

intellectual ability, cognitive development *v.*, 26

intellectual development, progression of, 33–35

intellectual skill acquisition. *See* cognitive learning domain

interaction, in experiential education, 199–200

interactive engagement (IE), 125–126

internal environment, of system, 62, 64

internalizing stage, of affective learning domain, 30

interpreting stage, of cognitive learning domain, 29

interprofessional curriculum projects, systems approach to, 79

interrater reliability, of laboratory assessments, 188

interview process, professionalism and, 235

introductory pharmacy practice experiences (IPPEs), 197–222
  assessment for entry into, 208–209
  assessment tools and instruments for, 217–219
  characteristics of, 204
  curriculum allocation to, 197
  feedback in, 220–221
  goals of, 203
  outcome statements for, 206–207
  practice environment for, 203–206
  setting realistic expectations for, 207–209

intrusive advising, 256, 258

IPPEs. *See* introductory pharmacy practice experiences

IRB. *See* institutional review board

J

JCPP. *See* Joint Commission of Pharmacy Practitioners

Joint Commission of Pharmacy Practitioners (JCPP), future vision of pharmacy practice developed by, 77

journal club, professionalism development and, 240

journaling, in experiential education, 219

just-in-time learning, 155

K

Kitchner and King's Reflective Judgment Model, 36–38, 47–50
  in integrated theory and educational model, 47–50
  prereflective stage in, 36, 38
  quasi-reflective stage in, 36–38
  reflective stage in, 36–38
  in student-centered teaching, 37–38

knowledge acquisition. *See* cognitive learning domain

Kolb Learning Style Inventory, 52
  for identifying student learning style, 39

Kolb's experiential learning model, 200–201

Krathwohl's Taxonomy of the Affective Domain, for professionalism development, 232

L

laboratory
    coordinating multiples evaluators and sections in, 188
    operation of, 185–189
    people involved in running of, 187–188
    safety in, 188–189
    supply and equipment maintenance in, 186–187
    use of space in, 185–186
laboratory learning and teaching, 175–193
    activity planning for, 179–182, 186
    advantages of, 175
    applications to, 189–191
    assessment in, 183–186, 188, 192–193
    compounded laboratories, 189–191
    course mapping in, 179, 186
    feedback in, 177, 191–192
    foundational principles of, 178–185
    future of, 192–193
    introduction to, 175–176
    objectives for, 179, 182, 186
    pharmacy skills and topics covered in, 180–181
    planning and design of, 178–185
    purposes of, 176–177
    quality improvements in, 191–192
    recommended resources on, 193
    research evidence on, 175–176, 178
    simulation laboratories, 189–190
    summary of, 192–193
large classroom teaching, 105–129
    active learning in, 106–111, 116–126
    increasing active learning experiences in, 116–118
    insights on teaching from physics education reform efforts, 126–127
    introduction to, 105–106
    moving to active learning in, 106–111
    student engagement in, 118–126
    student push back in, 127–128
    traditional passive lecture for, 106–111
    transformation from teaching to learning in, 111–116
leadership, faculty development in, 285
Leadership and Management Certificate Program, 285
learner. *See* student
learner-centered teaching. *See* student-centered teaching

learning; *See also* effective teaching and learning; experiential education; laboratory learning and teaching; scholarship of teaching and learning; small-group teaching and learning; systems approach to learning and teaching
    application-based, 155
    case-based, 155
    cognitive theories of, 33–38
    definition of, 4–5
    faculty development in, 282–284
    generation influence on, 44–46
    just-in-time, 155
    location of, 142–143
    organizing experiences using technology for, 146–148
    as outcome, 4–5
    problem-based, 154
    as process, 4–5, 27–28
    professionalism and, 231–233
    responsibility for, 5
    role of technology in, 135–137
    selecting experiences using technology for, 145–146
    skills-based, 155
    teaching relationship to, 6–8
    teaching *v.*, 4–8
    transformation from teaching to, 111–116
    use of technology in, 133
learning contracts, 163
learning domains, 27–33
    affective domain, 28–32, 47
    in Bloom's Taxonomy, 28–33, 47–50
    cognitive domain, 28–30, 32, 47
    in experiential education, 208
    in integrated theory and educational model, 47–50
    personal inventory of, 47
    psychomotor domain, 28–30, 32, 47
    in student-centered teaching, 32–33
learning objectives. *See* objectives
learning outcomes
    assessment of, 85–86, 99–100
    writing of, 86
learning strategies
    as input for systems approach to teaching a class, 66
    as process for systems approach to teaching a class, 67–68

learning styles
Austin's PILS, 41–44, 54–56
definition of, 5, 38–39
educational strategies aligned with, 43–44
Felder's Dimensions of Learning Style, 39–41
identification of, 39
in integrated theory and educational model, 47–50
intellectual ability v., 26
in student-centered teaching, 38–44
learning taxonomy. *See* Bloom's Taxonomy
Learning-Centered Teaching (Weimer), on selecting new teaching strategies, 116
lecture
appropriate uses of, 107
audience response systems in, 123–124
bookending of, 120–121
in large classroom teaching, 106–111
objectives for, 108
online capabilities blended with, 125
pacing of, 110–111
postclass assignments for, 122–123
progression of content within, 109
providing active learning in, 108–111
rewriting notes of, 122–123
teacher-centered strategies for improvement in, 109
written summaries of, 120
lifelong learning, technology for development of, 143–144
linear relationship, between teaching and learning, 6–7
listening stage, of affective learning domain, 30
longitudinal curricular content development
aim of, 73
input elements of, 73–75
systems approach to, 73–75

M
Maki's Assessment Loop, 90–91
managerial skills, faculty development in, 285
manipulating stage, of psychomotor learning domain, 30
mapping
for experiential education, 198–199
for laboratory learning and teaching, 179, 186

medication therapy management (MTM), 77
mental health, faculty advisor and, 257–259
mentoring, faculty, 279–280
formal v. informal, 280–281
mentoring, student; *See also* faculty mentor
advising v., 251–252
assessment and documentation of, 268
benefits of, 268
in career planning, 267–268
goals of, 263–264
during individualized course work or projects, 267
informal, 268
introduction to, 251
during pharmacy practice experiences, 267
philosophy of, 263
pitfalls of, 268
in professional organizations, 267
professionalism and, 232–233
program components for, 267
roles and responsibilities in, 264–265
as service, 285, 295
summary for, 269
types of, 266–268
Millennials
in integrated theory and educational model, 47–50
student-centered teaching for, 44–46
technology for, 135–136, 140–141
minute paper, for classroom assessment, 96
mobile learning, 142–143
modeling, in experiential education, 210–211
modeling stage, of psychomotor learning domain, 30
moral development, professionalism and, 232
motor skill learning. *See* psychomotor learning domain
MTM. *See* medication therapy management
muddiest point
for classroom assessment, 96, 111
for large classes, 120
multiple-choice examination, guidelines for writing of, 92–93
multiplism, in Perry's Schemes of Intellectual and Ethical Development, 34–36
Myers-Briggs Type Indicator, for identifying student learning style, 39

N

NACADA. *See* National Academic Advising
Association
NAPLEX. *See* North American Pharmacist
Licensure Examination
National Academic Advising Association
(NACADA), 262–263
National Survey of Student Engagement
(NSSE), 15, 113
neuroscience, teaching insights from,
114–115
nonconscious learning climate, in large
classrooms, 129
nonverbal skills, for effective teaching, 169
norming, of groups, 161–162
North American Pharmacist Licensure
Examination (NAPLEX), Blueprint and
Competency Statements of, 78, 190
NSSE. *See* National Survey of Student
Engagement

O

Oath of a Pharmacist, 230
objective structured clinical exam (OSCE), 92
for entry into IPPEs and APPEs, 208
in laboratory learning and teaching,
183–184
professionalism and, 235
objectives
definition of, 88
for laboratory learning and teaching, 179,
182, 186
for lectures, 108
writing of, 86
objectivism theory, teaching based on, 7
observation, in experiential education, 199
occupation, profession *v.*, 229
One-Minute Preceptor technique, 213–217
online examination, 149–150
online learning
for large classes, 125
location of, 142–143
open-ended discussions, 168
operation issues, of laboratory, 185–189
organization, for effective teaching, 171
organizing stage
of affective learning domain, 30
of cognitive learning domain, 29
orientation program, for faculty development
program, 277–279

OSCE. *See* objective structured clinical exam
OTC formulary, professionalism development
and, 240
outcomes
assessment of, 85–86, 99–100
definition of, 88–89
for IPPEs and APPEs, 206–207
learning as, 4–5
writing of, 86
outputs
in systems approach, 59
in systems approach to teaching a class, 65,
68–70

P

parents, FERPA and, 260–261
participating stage, of affective learning
domain, 30
partnership, in effective teaching, 13
passion, as effective teacher trait, 16–17
A Passion for Teaching (Day), passion defined
in, 16–17
The Passionate Teacher (Fried), passion defined
in, 16–17
patient assessment skills, for pharmacists,
180–181
patient care laboratory. *See* laboratory learning
and teaching
patient contact, in experiential learning environments, 204–205
patient counseling, professionalism development and, 240
patient discussions, professionalism development and, 240
patients
simulated, 187–189
standardized, 188
virtual, 189
PCAT. *See* Pharmacy College Admission Test
peer evaluation
for active learning in large classes, 124
for faculty assessment, 283–284
in laboratory learning and teaching, 191
of teaching, 97
Pendleton Four-Step Model, for providing
feedback, 221
PEP. *See* Professional Experience Program
performance assessment, 92
in laboratory learning and teaching, 183
performing, of groups, 162

Perry's Schemes of Intellectual and Ethical
Development, 33–36, 47–50
commitment in relativism in, 34–35
dualism in, 34–35
in integrated theory and educational
model, 47–50
multiplism in, 34–36
relativism in, 34
in student-centered teaching, 35–36
personal issues, faculty advisor and, 257
personality, as effective teacher trait, 15–16
pharmaceutical-care laboratory. *See* laboratory
learning and teaching
pharmacy, profession of, 228
pharmacy association, student chapters of, 239
Pharmacy College Admission Test (PCAT),
professionalism and, 235
pharmacy education, systems approach to,
61–80
pharmacy management, professionalism development and, 240
pharmacy practice experiences, student mentoring during, 267
PharmD degree, professionalism and,
231–232
philosophy statement, of teacher, 19–21
physical environment. *See* environment
physical health, faculty advisor and, 257
physics education, insights on teaching from,
126–127
PILS. *See* Austin's Pharmacists' Inventory of
Learning Styles
podcasts, of lectures, 125
portfolios
for assessment, 92–95
in experiential education, 218–219
postclass assignments, for large classes,
122–123
posttenure review, 287
PowerPoint presentations, for lectures, 110
practical examination, in laboratory learning
and teaching, 183
practice, in laboratory learning and teaching,
177
practicing stage, of psychomotor learning
domain, 30
preceptor(s)
assessment of, 220
in experiential education environment,
205–206

in professionalism development, 241
realistic expectations set by, 207–209
resources for development of, 205–206
role of, 198, 200–201, 209–212
in team-based approach to precepting, 205
precision stage, of psychomotor learning
domain, 30
preclass assignments, for large classes, 120
prereflective stage, in Kitchner and King's
Reflective Judgment Model, 36, 38
pretenure review, 287
problem-based learning, 154
process
learning as, 4–5, 27–28
in systems approach to teaching a class, 65,
67–68
process questions, 312
producers, in Austin's PILS, 55
profession
characteristics of, 228
occupation *v.*, 229
pharmacy as, 228
professional advisors, faculty advisor training,
263
professional competence, 203
Professional Experience Program (PEP), 241
professional organizations
faculty development with, 285
student mentoring in, 267
professional service, 293–295, 298
professional students, faculty advisor and, 260
professionalism
assessment and, 231–233, 242–244
attributes of, 229–230
civility *v.*, 231
definition of, 229–231
development of, 233–242
as effective teacher trait, 17
importance of, 228–229
improvement of, 229
introduction to, 227–228
learning and, 231–233
reasons for discussion of, 227
summary of, 246
teaching, learning, and assessment relation
to, 231–233
teaching and, 232–233
unprofessional behavior, 244–246
proficiency, 89
program, assessment of, 88

program outcome, professionalism development and, 234

projects, student mentoring for, 267

promotion review, 287

psychology, teaching insights from, 114–115

psychomotor learning domain, 28–31
personal inventory of, 47
in student-centered teaching, 32

Q

qualitative assessment, in experiential education, 217–218

qualitative research, quantitative *v.*, 315

quality improvement
in experiential education, 220
in laboratory learning and teaching, 191–192

quantitative assessment, in experiential education, 217–218

quantitative research, qualitative *v.*, 315

quasi-reflective stage, in Kitchner and King's Reflective Judgment Model, 36–38

question formulation, for SoTL, 312–313

question-and-answer sessions, in large lectures, 111, 119–121

questioning stage, of affective learning domain, 30

questions
redirection of, 170–171
reflection and deflection of, 169–170
as teaching strategy in experiential education, 212–214

R

recalling stage, of cognitive learning domain, 29

receiving stage, of affective learning domain, 30

recruitment strategies, professionalism and, 234–235

reflection
as effective teacher trait, 18, 116, 168–169
in experiential learning, 201
in laboratory learning and teaching, 191

reflective observation, in experiential learning, 200–201

reflective stage, in Kitchner and King's Reflective Judgment Model, 36–38

reflective writing, in experiential education, 219

relationship issues, faculty advisor and, 257

relative standards, for assessment in laboratory learning and teaching, 184

relativism, in Perry's Schemes of Intellectual and Ethical Development, 34

remembering stage, of cognitive learning domain, 29, 32

research
conduct, and analyze results of, 320–321
faculty development in, 284–285
formulate clear questions for, 312
IRB submission for, 317–320
practical considerations for, 315–316
publish, 321–322
qualitative *v.* quantitative, 315
study design for, 314–315
topic selection for, 311–312
write up of, 321

Research and Scholarship Certificate Program, 284–285

residency training, goals of, 203

resources, for using technology in education, 137–138

responding stage, of affective learning domain, 30

role models, professionalism and, 232–233

rubrics
for assessment, 92, 94–95
in experiential education, 218
in laboratory learning and teaching, 183–185

S

safety, in laboratory, 188–189

scheduling, as input for systems approach to teaching a course, 71

scholarly teaching, scholarship of teaching and learning *v.*, 308–309

scholarship
definition of, 303
faculty development in, 284–285
service link to, 303–304

scholarship of teaching and learning (SoTL)
collaboration and sharing, 316–317
conduct study and analyze results for, 320–321
conversations for, 311
definition of, 308
determine context for, 313

scholarship of teaching and learning
(*Continued*)
discussing and conceptualizing study for,
311–314
ethical considerations in, 322
grow and develop knowledge about teaching,
311
importance of, 310
introduction to, 307–308
IRB submission, 317–320
performance of, 310–322
practical considerations for, 315–316
project identification for, 311
publish, 321–322
question formulation for, 312–313
research topic selection for, 311–312
scholarly teaching *v.*, 308–309
study design, 314–315
summary for, 323
write up study, 321
school mission, professionalism development
and, 234
scientific teaching, 113–114
SEIRT. *See* Student Early Intervention
Response Team
self-appraisal. *See* self-reflection
self-assessment
in experiential education, 219–220
faculty advisor and, 256
self-knowledge, as effective teacher trait,
15–16
self-monitoring skills, development of, 254
self-reflection
as effective teacher trait, 18, 116,
168–169
in laboratory learning and teaching, 191
sensory–intuitive dimension, of Felder's
Dimensions of Learning Style, 39–40
sequential–global dimension, of Felder's
Dimensions of Learning Style, 39–40
service
assessing value and importance of, 302–303
association, 293–295
balancing commitments of, 301
citizenship, 298–299
clinical, 293
community, 295
conduct inventory of, 302
definition of, 292–295
faculty development in, 285

general recommendations and guidelines
for, 302–305
identifying expectations of, 302
individualized plan for, 295–296
institutional, 292–293
introduction to, 291
motivations for, 297–299
organizing people for, 296–297
professional, 293–295, 298
questions to ask regarding, 300
refusing, 304–305
responding to call for, 299–300
scholarship link to, 303–304
summary for, 305
service learning opportunities, professionalism
and, 239–241
Seven Principles Faculty Inventory, for evaluating effective teaching, 10
Seven Principles Institutional Inventory, for
evaluating effective teaching, 10
sharing, in SoTL, 316–317
shushers, professionalism and, 236–237
simulated patients, for laboratory learning and
teaching, 187–189
simulation laboratories, 189–190
skills laboratory. *See* laboratory learning
and teaching
skills-based learning, 155
small-group discussion, in large classes,
120–122
small-group teaching and learning, 153–173
assessment of, 166–167
conflict in, 161, 169–171
definition of, 154
facilitators and students working together
in, 163–166
how to get groups started, 158–159
introduction to, 153–154
role of facilitator in, 155–158
role of students in, 159–163
summary of, 172–173
tips for use of, 167–172
snowball group strategy, 165
social skills, faculty advisor and, 257
socialization, professional, 242
Socratic method of teaching, 212–214
software, for use in education, 139–140
Solomon and Felder's Index of Learning Styles
Questionnaire, 41
SoTL. *See* scholarship of teaching and learning

staff role, in professionalism development, 241
standardized patients, for laboratory learning
      and teaching, 188
standards
      for assessment in laboratory learning and
            teaching, 184
      definition of, 89
standing committee, 296
storming, of groups, 161
structural attributes, of professionalism, 230
student
      advising responsibilities of, 255
      assessment of, 88
      attention span of, 110–111
      balance of power between teacher and,
            14–15
      as input for systems approach to teaching a
            class, 66
      as input for systems approach to teaching a
            course, 72
      mentoring responsibilities of, 264–265
      redirection of, 170–171
      setting realistic expectations for, 207–209
      in small-group teaching and learning,
            159–166
      teacher knowledge of, 13
      technology use by, 140–142
      uncomfortableness among, 169
      willingness to learn in, 5
student advising. See advising, student
student chapters, of pharmacy association,
      239
Student Early Intervention Response Team
      (SEIRT), 259
student engagement
      for effective teaching, 14–15
      in large classes, 118–126
      student push back against, 127–128
student evaluations, for faculty assessment,
      283
student feedback
      in laboratory learning and teaching, 191
      on teaching, courses, and curriculum,
            97–99
student mentoring. See mentoring, student
student records, FERPA and, 260
student response system. See audience response
      system
student-centered discussion, in large classes,
      119–122

student-centered teaching, 7–8, 25–56
      closing thoughts on, 50
      cognitive theories of learning and, 33–38
      coordinating class schedules and content in,
            71
      definition of, 25
      generational influence and, 44–46
      integrated model of, 46–50
      introduction to, 25–27
      learning domains and, 27–33
      learning styles and, 38–44
      in lecturing, 109
      progression from teacher-centered teaching
            to, 116–118
      resources for, 51–52
      scenarios of, 50–51
      student push back against, 127–128
      teacher-centered teaching *v.*, 7, 25
      using Austin's PILS in, 43–44
      using Bloom's Taxonomy in, 32–33
      using Kitchner and King's Reflective
            Judgment Model in, 37–38
      using learning styles in, 43–44
      using Perry's Schemes of Intellectual and
            Ethical Development in, 35–36
study skills, faculty advisor and, 257
summative assessment, 87
      in experiential education, 219
      in small-group teaching and learning, 167
supplies, for laboratory learning and teaching,
      186–187
support, of student contributions, 170
survey, for assessment, 95
syllabus, as input for systems approach to
      teaching a course, 71–72
system
      boundaries of, 61–62, 64
      definition of, 58–60
systems approach to learning and teaching,
      57–80
      for a class, 62–70
      for a course, 70–73
      for cross-disciplinary curriculum projects,
            79
      for curriculum review, 75–80
      definition of, 58–60
      evidence supporting use of, 60–61
      for interprofessional curriculum projects,
            79
      introduction to, 57–58

systems approach to learning and teaching
(*Continued*)
   in pharmacy education, 61–80
   purpose of, 60–61
   summary of, 80
   for topic-specific longitudinal curricular
     content, 73–75
systems thinking, 58–60

T

TAs. *See* teaching assistants
task force, 296–297
taxonomy, learning. *See* Bloom's Taxonomy
teacher
   assessment of, 96–100
   balance of power between student and,
     14–15
   characteristics influencing effectiveness
     of, 9–18
   common ideas on what constitutes effec-
     tiveness of, 12–13
   evidence on what constitutes effectiveness
     of, 10–12
   focus of, 13–14
   knowledge of students by, 13
   of laboratory, 187
   nonverbal skills of, 169
   openness to external review of, 18
   organization of, 171
   outstanding, 10–11
   passion of, 16–17
   personality of, 15–16
   philosophy statement of, 19–21
   reflectiveness of, 18, 116, 168–169
   self-knowledge of, 15–16
   student engagement by, 14–15
teacher-centered discussion, in large classes,
    119–120
teacher-centered teaching
   in lecturing, 109
   progression to student-centered teaching
     from, 116–118
   student-centered teaching *v.*, 7, 25
teaching; *See also* effective teaching and learn-
    ing; experiential education; laboratory
    learning and teaching; scholarship of
    teaching and learning; small-group
    teaching and learning; student-centered
    teaching; systems approach to learning
    and teaching; teacher-centered teaching

   assessment of, 96–100
   discipline-specific for the sciences, 113–114
   in experiential education, 210
   faculty development in, 282–284
   grow and develop knowledge about, 311
   humor in, 159, 171–172
   implementation of technology in, 137–141
   learning relationship to, 6–8
   learning *v.*, 4–8
   professionalism and, 231–233
   reasons for using technology in, 141–150
   role of technology in, 135–137
   teacher-centered *v.* student-centered, 7, 25
   transformation to learning from,
     111–116
   use of technology in, 133
teaching assistants (TAs), for laboratory learn-
    ing and teaching, 187
teaching portfolios, 286
teaching strategies
   as input for systems approach to teaching a
     class, 66
   as process for systems approach to teaching
     a class, 67–68
technology
   application of, 146–148
   for assessment, 148–150
   educational purposes attained by use of,
     144–145
   implementation of, 137–141
   as input for systems approach to teaching a
     class, 66
   as input for systems approach to teaching a
     course, 71
   introduction to, 133–135
   for large classes, 123–125
   in learning environment, 136–167
   online resources for educational use of,
     136–137
   organizing learning experiences using,
     146–148
   as process for systems approach to teaching
     a class, 67
   in professionalism development,
     241–242
   reasons for using, 141–150
   role of, 135–137
   selecting learning experiences using,
     145–146
   summary of, 150

tenure review, 287
test. *See* examination
textbook, as input for systems approach to teaching a course, 72
think–pair–share, in large classes, 120–121
360-degree assessment, of professionalism, 243
time-management skills, faculty advisor and, 257
toxicology sleuthing, professionalism development and, 240
Traditionalists, teaching of, 45
triangulation, for assessment, 96
true–false examination, 92

U

unconsciously using stage, of psychomotor learning domain, 30
understanding stage, of cognitive learning domain, 29, 32
UNESCO. *See* United Nations Education, Scientific and Cultural Organization
United Nations Education, Scientific and Cultural Organization (UNESCO), on systems approach in education, 59
unprofessional behavior, dealing with, 244–246
unstructured–structured dimension, of Austin's PILS, 41–43

V

values, in learning, 30–31
valuing, of student contributions, 170
valuing stage, of affective learning domain, 30
virtual patients, 189
vision of the future questions, 313
vision of the possible questions, 313
visual–verbal dimension, of Felder's Dimensions of Learning Style, 39–40

W

Walvoord's Three Steps of Assessment, 90
Web-based assignment, for active learning in large classes, 125
what is questions, 312
What the Best College Teachers Do (Bain)
    definition of outstanding teachers in, 10–11
    on personality in successful teaching, 15–16
what works questions, 312
white coat ceremony, for professionalism, 234, 236
wholes, in systems approach, 59
willingness to learn, 5
wired classrooms, 138
workshop method, 166

CPSIA information can be obtained at www.ICGtesting.com
Printed in the USA
BVOW06s0014161213

339123BV00003B/26/P